• How do you make a wise decision about taking a particular medication? On pages 18–19, check the list of questions to ask your doctor *before* you begin drug therapy.

• If there are ten widely available drugs that treat depression, how do you know which one may be right for you? See "A Practical Guide to Antidepressants" on pages 33–37 to learn how your doctor makes such choices.

• What if a drug doesn't work? Does this mean there is no remedy for your problem? Not at all. Pages 19–21 explain why this is a fairly common response to mind/mood drugs, and why an alternative drug—or combination of drugs— often proves effective.

• If you have a medical disorder that makes a specific drug hazardous for you, does this leave you without a remedy for your mind/mood condition? It does not. Because there is often a range of drug therapies that can treat such conditions, your doctor can usually find a medication that is safe for you to take.

• What if you are pregnant or planning to become pregnant? Does this mean it is unsafe for you to take a drug for your mind/mood problem? Every drug profile specifies whether the drug is suitable for use during pregnancy and nursing; see also the discussion in Chapter 10.

• How should you assess the claims made for "natural" herbal remedies? Are they pure? Safe? Effective? Review Chapter 9 for answers about these often hyped substances.

DISCOVER THE LATEST INFORMATION ON
ALL THE MOST POPULAR MIND/MOOD DRUGS
IN A FORMAT THAT IS EASY TO USE FROM
AUTHORITIES YOU CAN TRUST.

Also by Robert E. Hales, M.D., and Dianne Hales

Caring for the Mind:
The Comprehensive Guide to Mental Health

THE
Mind/Mood Pill Book

ROBERT E. HALES, M.D.
AND DIANNE HALES

BANTAM BOOKS
New York Toronto London Sydney Auckland

This edition contains the complete text of the original trade edition.
NOT ONE WORD HAS BEEN OMITTED.

THE MIND/MOOD PILL BOOK

A Bantam Book

PUBLISHING HISTORY

Bantam trade edition / October 2000
Bantam mass market edition / October 2001

Selected general information about medical disorders and terminology has been adapted from *Caring for the Mind: The Comprehensive Guide to Mental Health,* by Dianne Hales and Robert E. Hales, M.D., copyright © 1995.

All rights reserved.
Copyright © 2000 by Robert E. Hales, M.D., and Dianne Hales.
Book design by Jessica Shatan.
Icon illustrations by Jackie Aher.

ISBN 0-553-58035-3

Published simultaneously in the United States and Canada

Bantam Books are published by Bantam Books, a division of Random House, Inc. Its trademark, consisting of the words "Bantam Books" and the portrayal of a rooster, is Registered in U.S. Patent and Trademark Office and in other countries. Marca Registrada. Bantam Books, 1540 Broadway, New York, New York 10036.

PRINTED IN THE UNITED STATES OF AMERICA

OPM   10   9   8   7   6   5   4   3   2   1

CONTENTS

ACKNOWLEDGMENTS

A NUMBER OF PEOPLE MADE THIS BOOK POSSIBLE. TINA Marshall typed the entire manuscript, developed the icons and format used for the drug profiles, and conscientiously compared information within drug classes to ensure conformity in both style and content. Her meticulous attention to detail and her unflappable response to numerous changes and drafts were remarkable. The book could not have been accomplished in such a fine and timely fashion without her considerable efforts.

Our editor, Ann Harris, edited the entire manuscript in her usual scholarly and insightful fashion. Her editorial suggestions greatly improved the overall quality of the book. We have had an outstanding twenty-year collaboration with Ann, and we continue to enjoy our working relationship with her. We are grateful to our agent, Joy Harris, for enabling us to work again with Bantam Books. Joy is simply the best.

Every effort was made to ensure accuracy of the information contained in this book. Each chapter was reviewed by both a pharmacist and a physician who possesses special expertise with the class of medications that was summarized in the chapter. In addition, the material contained for all of the drugs was compared with other references. When discrepancies were found, we sought other references to ensure the accuracy of the data.

We would like to thank the members of our Editorial Board—Drs. Lloyd Benjamin, Donald Hilty, Ladson Hinton, Martin Leamon, Richard Maddock, Thomas Neylan, Charles Scott, Mark Servis, Michael Wise, and pharmacist Robert Chew—for their invaluable help and guidance. We are grateful for their time, effort, and expertise.

EDITORIAL BOARD

THE

Mind/Mood
Pill Book

INTRODUCTION

How to Use This Book

NEARLY 1 IN EVERY 2 AMERICANS WILL DEVELOP A mental disorder in the course of their lifetimes. Approximately 25 percent of these men, women, and children will take medication as part of their treatment. This book provides concise and easily accessible information about the major mind/mood medications used in the United States.

To get the most benefit from this book, begin with Chapter 1, which provides essential information about the drugs described in Chapters 2 through 9. Chapter 1 also discusses the concepts and terms used both in the book and by physicians who prescribe mind/mood medications.

Chapters 2 through 9 cover the major categories of psychiatric medications in use today: antidepressants (Chapter 2); medications to treat anxiety (Chapter 3); mood stabilizers, called anti-manic agents (Chapter 4); medications to treat sleep disorders (Chapter 5); antipsychotic medications (Chapter 6); medications for attention deficit disorders (Chapter 7); cognitive-enhancing agents (Chapter 8); and herbal medications with mind/mood effects (Chapter 9). Each chapter begins with a brief introduction about the mental disorders that the medications are designed to treat and provides a general overview of the drugs discussed in the chapter.

After reading Chapter 1, turn to the chapter that focuses on the particular category of medication of interest to you. We encourage you to read the chapter introduction first, since this will give you an overview of all medications in the same category. About half of all patients have difficulty tolerating the initial medication prescribed for their problem; about a third find that the medication does not work for them. An overview of the range of medications available may be helpful in evaluating alternatives if they should be needed. Each medication is presented in a uniform format, with an icon that identifies each category of information:

 Generic name: The chemical or pharmaceutical name of the medication.*

 Available in generic form: Whether or not the medication is available in a generic form.

 Brand name: The trade name the manufacturer has given the medication for marketing to the consumer.

Source: In Chapter 9, the origin of an herbal medication or "natural" mind/mood pill. These substances are usually sold in health-food stores and are not regulated by the FDA.

Drug class: The classification of the drug (for example, tricyclic antidepressant), applicable to a group of drugs similar in chemical formulation, mode of action, and uses.

*The generic names of the drugs profiled in this book are accurate for both the United States and Canada. However, some of these drugs may be marketed under different brand names in Canada, so readers there should check with their physicians for the names of Canadian equivalents.

Rx Prescribed for: Indications—reasons to take the medication—approved by the Food and Drug Administration (FDA), as well as other accepted "off-label" uses by physicians.

General information: An overview of the medication, including how it works, why it was developed, and its general advantages and disadvantages.

Dosing information: Concise information concerning how the medication is prescribed, including dosage forms and strengths, when it should be taken, and how the dose should be increased. Many mind/mood drugs are initially given in low doses and then gradually increased.

Common side effects: The most common side effects noted during clinical trials and in clinical practice. These listings do *not* include every side effect listed in the *Physicians' Desk Reference (PDR)*, a comprehensive summary of the manufacturers' package inserts of most prescription medications approved by the FDA. It is also possible that you may experience additional side effects; if so, you should report these to your physician.

Precautions: Cautionary advice concerning the medication you are taking and other drugs you should avoid while taking this medication. The information in this section does not necessarily imply that you should not take the medication; its purpose is to make you aware of these risks when taking a particular drug or class of drug.

Warnings: Medical conditions for which the drug is contraindicated—should not be taken—or other medications that should not be taken with this drug.

Alcohol: Whether or not you can drink alcohol while taking the medication, and interactions with the medication if you do drink.

Food and beverages: Whether or not you should take this medication with food and beverages and whether doing so may either lessen some of the side effects or decrease or increase the amount of medication absorbed into your blood. This section also lists any foods or beverages that should not be taken with a specific medication.

Possible drug interactions: Mind/mood medications can interact with other drugs you are taking, increasing or decreasing their effectiveness or possibly causing dangerous reactions. This section alerts you to other drugs that may be of concern or that should be avoided altogether when taking a medication.

Use in pregnancy and breast-feeding: Whether or not the medication should be taken if you are contemplating pregnancy or are pregnant, and whether you should take it while breast-feeding. As an indication of pregnancy-related risks, the FDA has categorized medications on a scale from A to D, and X. Mind/mood medications are almost never systematically studied in pregnant women. Potential effects on humans are usually drawn from research conducted in mice or other animals. Category A means that controlled studies show no risk to humans. Most mind/mood pills have been classified by the FDA as Category B—"No evidence of risk in humans but adequate human studies have not been performed"—or Category C—"Risk cannot be ruled out." Category D is used when there has been proven risk to humans but the risk of potential harm to the fetus may be outweighed by the potential benefit to the mother. Category X signifies that the medication should not be used during pregnancy.

See Chapter 10, page 406 and Table 10-1, for more information.

Use in children: Whether or not the medication should be used in children and, if so, the conditions for which it is prescribed and the customary doses, if known.

Use in seniors: Whether the medication needs to be taken in lower doses by adults over the age of sixty-five. This entry also notes whether some side effects of certain medications may be more bothersome or potentially harmful to seniors, or whether the drug should be avoided altogether. Because the capacity to metabolize and excrete medications declines with age, certain medications may need to be taken in lower doses. See Chapter 10, page 428, for more information.

Overdosage: General information concerning the signs and symptoms of overdose, and what to do if someone you know takes too much of a prescribed medication.

Special considerations: A concise review of the medication discussed and a summary of some of its unique advantages and disadvantages.

Because of widespread interest in alternative preparations to treat mood/mind symptoms, Chapter 9 reviews the more common herbal agents used in the United States today. Chapter 10 discusses special considerations for women, children, and seniors.

The book also includes color photographs of the twenty-five most commonly prescribed mind/mood medications. The majority are antidepressants, anti-anxiety agents, or medications for sleep. At the back of the book are an index of all the medications discussed in the book, a concise glossary of terms and phrases used in the text, and a resource directory with addresses and phone numbers of organizations you may turn to for more information concerning a particular mental disorder or to obtain more information about mental illness and mental-health professionals.

CHAPTER 1

Mind, Mood, and Medications

WHY DO I FEEL THIS WAY? WHY AM I SO MOODY? Is there anything I can do to feel better? Can anyone help?

At some point in life, almost everyone asks these questions. We all experience sadness, worry, rage, self-doubt, even despair. Often these feelings are short-lived, but sometimes they continue for days or weeks, coloring the way we view ourselves and the world. A life crisis—an accident or illness, a huge financial setback, the loss of someone dear—may be responsible. In other cases, gloom or anxiety may descend for no apparent reason.

Like physical problems, persistent emotional aches and pains can affect every aspect of life. More than 1 in every 4 Americans suffer from a mind/mood problem so severe that it interferes with their ability to keep up with their daily routines, do their jobs, care for their families, or relate to others as they once did. No one, regardless of age, gender, education, or income, is immune.

According to the National Institute of Mental Health's (NIMH) landmark Epidemiologic Catchment Area (ECA) Survey, about 27 million adults and 7.5 million children in the United States have a diagnosable mental disorder; this is more than the combined total of individuals with cancer, heart disease, and lung disorders. In another major study, the National Comorbidity Survey (see Table 1-1), almost half of those queried reported having at least one mental disorder over the course of their lifetimes; almost 30 percent had been troubled by a disorder in the previous twelve months. Adults are not the only ones affected. According to some reports, the number of troubled children has increased to as many as 11 to 14 million youngsters.

Table 1-1: How Common Are Mind/Mood Disorders?

DISORDER	IN A GIVEN YEAR (% affected)	AT SOME POINT IN LIFE (% affected)
Anxiety disorders (panic disorder, agoraphobia, social anxiety disorder, specific phobia, generalized anxiety disorder)	17.2	24.9
Depressive disorders (major depression, manic depression, dysthymia)	11.3	19.3
Alcohol dependence or abuse	9.7	23.5
Drug dependence or abuse	3.6	11.9
Any mental disorder	29.5	48.0

Source: Kessler, R., et al. "Lifetime and 12-Month Prevalence of DSM-III-R Psychiatric Disorders in the United States." *Archives of General Psychiatry,* vol. 51, January 1994.

The most surprising—and disheartening—fact is not that so many people are troubled but that so few get help. According to NIMH statistics, 7 in every 10 Americans with a mental disorder do not receive any treatment. These individuals may never realize why they cannot function the way they once did or why their lives have become difficult and joyless. They may try to tell themselves that they are simply overworked or stressed out. Even when they suspect that something more serious is wrong, many hate to admit, even to themselves, that they have a problem. They blame themselves, as if becoming anxious or depressed or feeling out of control is somehow their fault in a way that a medical condition such as diabetes or arthritis could never be. Often they fear that no matter where they might turn, no one will be able to help them. And nothing could be farther from the truth.

During the last two decades the mental-health field has undergone a quiet but profound revolution that has produced new forms of help and new reasons for hope. We now have a much better understanding of how the mind and the brain work and of what can go wrong and why. We know more about the complexity and variety of problems that can develop. We have identified patterns of vulnerability and the biological components of many mental illnesses. And we have an impressive collection of highly specific, carefully tested, and scientifically proven medications that can help most of those who seek treatment.

Diagnostic Developments

In 1840, in the first official attempt to gather information about mental illness in the United States, the Census Bureau recorded the frequency of a single category: idiocy/insanity. By the beginning of the twentieth century, early psychiatrists had identified more than a dozen mental illnesses. For decades, however, American psychiatry viewed all mental illnesses, as psychiatrist Karl Menninger put it, "as being essentially the same in quality, although differing quantitatively and in external appearance." This view has since given way to a search for greater specificity and precision in both diagnosis and treatment.

One of the major advances in the quest came in 1980, not in the form of theory, technique, drug, or doctrine, but in a book: the third edition of the American Psychiatric Association's *Diagnostic and Statistical Manual of Mental Disorders,* or *DSM,* as it is commonly called. A revised version of this edition, published in 1987, and a completely overhauled fourth edition, *DSM-IV,* published in 1994, spell out explicit characteristics, or diagnostic criteria, for almost 300 disorders. Rather than focusing on the whys of mental illness, *DSM* emphasizes the whats—the specific signs and symptoms that characterize various psychiatric disorders. As a result, even when mental-health professionals disagree about or do not know the possible causes of a disorder, they can agree on how it manifests itself, and this common base enables them to assess treatments most likely to bring about recovery. *DSM* has given mental-health professions a shared language. Because its criteria are widely accepted, physicians; psychology, psychiatry, and social work trainees; and medical and nursing students use *DSM* as a textbook. Insurance companies base reimbursements on it. Research agencies and foundations fund investigations according to the *DSM* criteria.

New Treatments

Mental illness, as well as attempts to cure it, dates back to the oldest societies. The ancient Greeks pushed depressed individuals from the tops of cliffs into the sea to shock them out of their despair. In the Middle Ages, priests used exorcism to cast out the "demons" of madness. With the dawn of modern psychiatry, treatments were developed that were more humane but not necessarily more helpful. Only in recent years have mental-health professionals been able to offer a wide range of therapies—more numerous, more varied, and more precisely targeted than ever before— that have proved effective against common and often crippling disorders. These include new psychiatric medications that correct chemical imbalances in the brain and new psychotherapies that use cognitive, interpersonal, behavioral, and other techniques to produce lasting benefits within weeks or months. The combination of drug and psychological treatments—an approach that, not very long ago, many doubted would ever work—has proved even more helpful for many individuals than either psychotherapy or medication alone.

Although most people do not realize it, treatments for severe mental illnesses, such as major depression, bipolar (manic-depressive) illness, panic disorder, and schizophrenia, are as effective as or more effective than those available in other branches of medicine, including surgery. Therapies tailored to an individual's particular condition and needs can help 70 to 80 percent of those who suffer from depression, bipolar disorder, or panic disorder. More than 60 percent of those with schizophrenia can be relieved of acute symptoms with proper therapy, and advances in medication are pushing this percentage even higher.

The revolution that has brought so much excitement and hope to the mental-health field is far from over. The coming years will undoubtedly yield new insights, advances, medications, and therapies to treat common disorders and prevent recurrences. In the past, those with manic-depressive illness typically spent half of their adult lives disabled, often in psychiatric hospitals. Thanks to medications that prevent debilitating mood swings, 75 to 80 percent now live essentially normal lives—a change that has saved the United States economy more than $40 billion since 1970. Similar progress has been made in major depression. As recent studies have shown, as many as 80 percent of those who become depressed experience a recurrence within ten years and face increased risk of job loss, marital breakups, and suicide. Maintenance treatment with antidepressants can prevent these terrible problems and keep individuals well.

The Mind/Mood Center: The Brain

To understand how medications work requires some basic information about the brain. The last and greatest biological frontier, more complex and more challenging than anything else in the entire universe, the brain represents the sum of human knowledge, emotion, memory, experience, and creativity. It enables us to think and talk, to remember and anticipate, to work and play, to express our needs and control our desires. Some describe the spongy mass of gray and white matter within the skull as an enlightened machine that combines the analytic ability of a computer, the organizational skills of a filing system, and the communications network of a telephone switchboard. Yet no machine or invention, however sophisticated, can crack a joke, dream of daffodils, write a poem, believe in a hereafter, or fall in love.

The brain has intrigued scientists for centuries, but only recently have its explorers made dramatic progress in unraveling its mysteries. Leaders in neuropsychiatry, the field that brings together the study of the brain and the mind, note that 95 percent of what is known about brain anatomy, chemistry, and physiology has been learned during the last decade. These discoveries have reshaped our understanding of the organ that is central to our identity and well-being, and they have fostered great hope for more effective therapies for the more than 1,000 disorders, psychiatric and neurological, that affect the brain and the nervous system.

There is so much scientific excitement centering on the exploration of the brain that some mental-health professionals worry that the powers and potential of the mind will be neglected. In fact, the study of the brain is not only changing our understanding of mental illness, but it is also challenging the conventional view that the mind and brain are distinct from each other. We are learning that these two aspects of consciousness work as one, and that mental experiences affect brain processes, and vice versa. The more we discover about the molecular mysteries of the brain, about the energy that causes tiny clumps of cells to make an idea blossom or a feeling form, the more we understand about how we think, learn, create, communicate—in essence, how the mind does all the things that make human beings unique.

Inside the Brain

Each human brain contains hundreds of billions of nerve cells, or neurons, and support and scavenger cells, called glia. Most are present at birth, when the brain weighs less than a pound. The brain grows rapidly to its full weight of about three pounds over the first six years of life—the period during which we acquire more knowledge more rapidly than ever again. Thereafter, over the course of time, brain weight decreases gradually (about 10 percent in a normal lifetime) as neurons die.

The neurons are the basic working units of the brain. Like snowflakes, no two are exactly the same. Each consists of a cell body containing the nucleus; a long fiber called the axon, which can range from less than an inch to several feet in length; an axon terminal, or ending; and multiple branching fibers called dendrites. The glia assist in the growth of neurons, speed up the transmission of nerve impulses, and engulf and digest damaged neurons.

The brain is the master control center for the body, constantly receiving information and relaying messages to various parts of the body. Some of these messages travel through the spinal cord, which extends from the neck down about two-thirds of the length of the spine. The brain and spinal cord comprise the central nervous system.

Historically, scientists have focused on the anatomy and structures of the brain in their attempts to understand how it functions and why it sometimes malfunctions. That emphasis has now changed, and modern neuropsychiatrists have shifted much of their attention to biochemical processes within the brain, particularly those involved in communication between neurons.

Communication within the Brain

Neurons "talk" with each other by means of electrical and chemical processes. An electric charge or impulse travels along an axon to the terminal, where packets of chemicals called neurotransmitters are stored in tiny sacs called vesicles. When released, these "messenger molecules" flow out of the axon terminal and cross the synapse, a tiny space where the axon terminal of one neuron comes extremely close to a dendrite projecting from another neuron. On the surface of the dendrite are receptors, protein molecules designed to bind with specific neurotransmitters. It takes only about one ten-thousandth of a second for a neurotransmitter and a receptor to come together. Neurotransmitters that do not bind to receptors may remain in the synapse until they are broken down by enzymes or reabsorbed by the neuron that produced them—a process called reuptake.

Receptors relay a message—which can elicit a wide variety of responses, from a physical signal to a thought, feeling, sensation, or behavior—from a neurotransmitter (the "first" messenger) to the rest of the neuron via chemical intermediaries known as G-proteins and effectors. A "second" messenger then triggers a cascade of chemical reactions to process the information.

A malfunction in the release of a neurotransmitter, in its reuptake or elimination, or in the receptors or second messengers, may lead to abnormalities in thinking, feeling, or behavior. Some of the most promising research in neuropsychiatry is focusing on correcting such malfunctions. For example, the neurotransmitter serotonin and its receptors have been shown to affect mood, sleep, behavior, appetite, memory, learning, sexuality, and aggression, and to play a role in several mental disorders. The discovery of a possible link between low levels of serotonin and some cases of major depression has already led to the development of more precisely targeted antidepressant medications that boost serotonin to normal levels (see Chapter 2). Certain other antidepressants, such as venlafaxine (Effexor) and bupropion (Wellbutrin or Zyban), are believed to work by increasing norepinephrine and its precursor, dopamine. Benzodiazepines—anti-anxiety agents—stimulate the inhibitory neurotransmitter, called GABA, causing a person to be less anxious or tense. During the next decade, neuropsychiatric research may yield a new generation of breakthrough medications for an ever-growing number of mental disorders.

The Potential Benefits of Psychiatric Medications

A college student with schizophrenia, once so agitated that his nonstop shuffling would wear out the soles of his shoes in a matter of days, can sit quietly and study. A saleswoman who had lived in constant dread of terrifying panic attacks feels in control. A teacher whose obsessive rituals consumed hours of his day can devote his energies to his work and family. A nurse whose depression had sapped her stamina and energy feels like her "old" competent and confident self again.

Medications that alter brain chemistry and relieve psychiatric symptoms have brought great hope and help to millions of people like these. Thanks to the development of a new generation of more precise and effective psychiatric drugs, the success rates for treating many common and disabling disorders—depression, panic disorder, obsessive-compulsive disorder, schizophrenia, and others—have soared. Often used in conjunction with psychotherapy and sometimes used as the primary or the only treatment, these medications have revolutionized mental-health care.

Yet many who could benefit from drug therapy are not receiving it. In part, this is because many psychiatric conditions are underdiagnosed, and people are unaware of what is wrong with them and what can be done to help. Many individuals are reluctant to take mind/mood medications, either because of the stigma attached to them or to the condition for which they are prescribed or because of negative things they've read or heard about highly publicized drugs like fluoxetine (Prozac) or triazolam (Halcion).

Mental disorders are indeed complex problems, and drugs may not be the best or the only solution for some of them. Moreover, like all medications, mind/mood drugs have side effects and must be used with care. When taken appropriately, however, these agents can alleviate tremendous suffering. They can also reduce the financial and personal costs of mental illness by lessening the need for hospitalization for acute problems and by restoring an individual's ability to live up to his or her potential, to work, to relate to others, and to contribute to society.

Understanding Mind/Mood Medications

Mind/mood medications can affect every aspect of a person's physical, mental, and emotional functioning, including alertness, attention, coordination, energy, judgment, sleep patterns, and interpersonal relationships. Some of these medications take effect at once, others take time to act, and some continue to exert their effects long after an individual discontinues their use.

In prescribing these medications, physicians must consider many factors, including the person's general health, history, allergies, and lifestyle. Age can also be an important consideration because older individuals may metabolize certain drugs more slowly or be more susceptible to side effects. A thorough history, including the presence of any mental disorders in other family members, and an assessment of the person's general medical condition to rule out any illnesses that might be causing psychiatric symptoms, is essential. Individuals who have not had a recent full medical evaluation may have to undergo a complete physical examination and a variety of blood and laboratory tests.

The prescribing physician must also weigh the benefits and risks of specific medications. Although many psychiatric drugs are not habit-forming, others can be addictive and must be prescribed and taken with appropriate caution. Many can cause side effects that range from mildly irritating (such as dry mouth) to more bothersome (constipation) to potentially hazardous (dizziness) to life-threatening (seizures or arrhythmias). In general, side effects tend to be most common and troubling when the drugs are first taken, and most diminish or disappear after a few weeks. However, the long-term use of certain types of drugs, such as conventional antipsychotic medications, can lead to serious adverse reactions, such as a chronic neuromuscular condition called tardive dyskinesia (see Glossary).

Most prescriptions for psychiatric drugs are written not by psychiatrists but by primary-care physicians. Those who are not experienced or up to date in psychopharmacology may not prescribe the most effective or appropriate medication, may select an agent solely because it is simple to take and requires little monitoring, may prescribe lower dosages than needed, or may not continue therapy for an adequate period. Determining the right drug in the right dose for any individual requires expertise in treating mental disorders, in-depth understanding of the latest advances in psychopharmacology, and close cooperation between the individual, the physician, and often with the family as well.

Adequate information about psychiatric drugs can help individuals and family members make wise decisions, comply with medical instructions, and handle possible side effects. To be fully informed, consumers should ask these questions before beginning drug therapy:

- Why is this medication necessary?

- What specific symptoms will it relieve?

- What are the other possible benefits?

- What are the possible side effects and risks?

- What are the risks of *not* taking this medication?

- How long will it be before the medication begins to help?

- How often must the drug be taken?

- Is there a preferred time of day or night for taking it?

- Do I have to avoid eating before or after taking it?

- Should it be taken with food?

- Will the medication affect my ability to drive or operate machinery?

- Will it affect my ability to work?

- What is the initial dosage?

- How can I tell if the drug is working?

- Should I call my physician if any particular side effects develop?

- Is there any danger from skipping a dose? From taking a double dose?

- What are the risks of overdosing?

- Does this medicine interact with any other medications?

- Can I drink alcohol while taking this medication?

- Are there any foods or beverages I should avoid?

- How long will I have to take this medication?

- Is there a danger that I'll become addicted?

- What are the alternatives to using this drug?

- What are the odds that this medicine will help me?

- What if this drug doesn't work?

As a rule, only physicians can write prescriptions. Non-medical therapists (such as psychologists, social workers, and psychiatric nurses) who are treating persons who may require a mind/mood medication often work closely with psychiatrists. The individual continues psychotherapy with the therapist but also consults a psychiatrist, who determines the need for medication, prescribes the appropriate dosage, ensures that it is working, and monitors for side effects or medical complications.

If a particular psychiatric drug does not help, there are alternatives and, if necessary, alternatives to the alternatives. No one should become discouraged if the initial medication, or even the second or third one, does not produce the desired results. Almost always, psychiatrists with expertise in pharmacotherapy can ultimately recommend a medication or a combination of medications that *will* work. Indeed, the failure of a particular drug may provide some insight into the way an individual's illness will respond to treatment, increasing the likelihood that the next drug will be more effective.

In some cases, psychiatrists prescribe a combination of medications. For example, depressed individuals who respond only partially after treatment with a single antidepressant may take an additional agent, such as lithium or a thyroid supplement, to boost their chances for complete recovery. The use of combined medications requires clinical expertise and close supervision to ensure maximal benefits and minimal complications.

If the cost of a medication is a concern, talk to your physician about the possibility of using less expensive generic equivalents. When medications are approved by the FDA, the pharmaceutical company that owns the medication is granted a period of time whereby the medication may be manufactured and sold exclusively by the company, using a brand name that the company has selected. This period of time is called the patent life of the medication. After this period expires, other pharmaceutical companies may manufacture the same medication without using the original brand name but by using the name of its generic equivalent. For instance, Upjohn originally developed and marketed the benzodiazepine alprazolam under the trade name Xanax. After the expiration of Xanax's patent life, other companies began to manufacture this medication and market it under its generic name, alprazolam.

When a medication's patent life expires and other companies begin to produce it, the cost of the medication drops substantially. Unfortunately, in some cases the quality of the generic medication may also fall, since the manufacturing guidelines are less stringent. One measure of quality is the medication's bioequivalence, or how much medication gets into your bloodstream in comparison to the branded drug. Also, different non-active ingredients may be used in the manufacturing of the pill or capsule, which may produce unexpected side effects that differ from the branded version. For instance, someone may respond quite well clinically to the brand form of clomipramine, Anafranil, but may respond less well to, require a different dose of, or experience other side effects from a generic form of clomipramine produced by a different company. In some cases, there is no reason not to use generic agents; in others the brand-name medication may be far more reliable and effective and produce fewer side effects. Whichever form you take, it is essential to get precise instructions about doses, timing, and other details related to correct use of the medication (see the list of questions about medication on pages 18–19).

Since many Americans now belong to health maintenance organizations (HMOs) and since pharmacy costs have been rising rapidly, HMOs encourage physicians who treat patients enrolled in their plan to use generic medications because their costs are much lower than brand-name drugs. Some plans also encourage patients to use generics by charging them a lower copayment, the amount of money they must pay the pharmacist when they have the prescription filled.

If you responded well to the brand name of a medication but you have been switched to a generic form and are not responding as well or are experiencing more bothersome side effects, talk to your physician about prescribing the original branded medication. If you begin to feel better again or experience fewer side effects with the brand form, it is likely that you experienced side effects or had a less favorable clinical response based on the generic form of the medication.

If your primary-care physician has prescribed a psychiatric medication for depression or an anxiety disorder and you have not noticed significant improvement within two months, ask about a consultation with a psychiatrist. Increasingly, many insurance and health-care plans are discouraging primary-care physicians from referring patients to specialists, including psychiatrists. However, if you are not feeling better or if improvement is only slight, insist on seeing someone who is skilled in determining whether the problem might be the illness, the drug, the dose, or a need for a different or additional form of medication or therapy.

CHAPTER 2

The Antidepressants

To learn general information about this class of medications and the disorders they treat, read the first part of the chapter. To read about a specific antidepressant, turn to the page indicated below.

AN OVERVIEW OF MOOD DISORDERS

Depressive Disorders

Comparing everyday "blues" to a depressive disorder is like comparing a cold to pneumonia. Major depression can destroy a person's joy for living. Food, friends, sex, or any form of pleasure no longer appeals. It is impossible to concentrate on work and responsibilities. Unable to escape a sense of utter hopelessness, depressed individuals may fight back tears throughout the day and toss and turn through long, empty nights. Thoughts of death or suicide may push into their minds.

But there is good news: Depression is a treatable disease. Psychotherapy is remarkably effective for mild depression. In more serious cases, antidepressant medication can lead to dramatic improvement in 75 to 80 percent of depressed patients.

Major Depression

The simplest definition of major depression is sadness that does not end. It has unique symptoms, which are shown in Table 2-1. The incidence of major depression has soared over the last two decades, especially among young adults.

The National Comorbidity Survey found that major depression is the most widespread mental disorder, affecting 10.3 percent of Americans in any given year. Unfortunately, fewer than 1 out of every 3 depressed people ever seeks treatment.

Table 2-1: Symptoms of Major Depression

CHARACTERISTIC SYMPTOMS OF MAJOR DEPRESSION INCLUDE

Feeling depressed, sad, empty, discouraged, tearful, or
A loss of interest or pleasure in once-enjoyable activities, and

- Eating more or less than usual and either gaining or losing weight
- Having trouble sleeping or sleeping much more than usual
- Feeling slowed down or restless and unable to sit still
- Lack of energy
- Feeling helpless, hopeless, worthless, inadequate
- Difficulty in concentrating, forgetfulness
- Difficulty in thinking clearly or making decisions
- Persistent thoughts of death or suicide
- Withdrawal from others, lack of interest in sex
- Physical symptoms (headaches, digestive problems, aches and pains)

For a diagnosis of major depression, a person must have one or both of the first two symptoms, plus four or more of the remaining symptoms.

Most cases of major depression can be treated successfully, usually with psychotherapy, medication, or both. Psychotherapy alone works in more than half of mild-to-moderate episodes of major depression. Two specific psychotherapies, cognitive-behavioral therapy and interpersonal therapy, have proved as helpful as antidepressant drugs in treating mild cases of depression, although they take longer than medication to achieve results.

Antidepressant medications work for more than half of

those with moderate-to-severe depression and may be useful in treating mild depression in individuals who do not improve with psychotherapy alone. These prescription drugs generally take three or four weeks to produce significant benefits and may not achieve their full impact until up to eight weeks. Combined treatment with psychotherapy and medication helps individuals with severe chronic or recurrent major depression, as well as those who do not fully improve with medication or psychotherapy alone.

In individuals who cannot take antidepressant medications because of medical problems, or who do not improve with psychotherapy or drugs, electroconvulsive therapy (ECT)—the administration of a controlled electrical current through electrodes attached to the scalp—remains the safest and most effective treatment. About 50 percent of depressed individuals who do not get better with antidepressant medication and psychotherapy improve after ECT.

Bipolar Depression

Manic depression, or bipolar disorder, consists of mood swings that may take individuals from manic states of feeling euphoric and energetic to depressive states of utter despair. In episodes of full mania, they may become so impulsive and out of touch with reality that they endanger their careers, relationships, health, or even survival. One percent of the population—about 2 million American adults—suffers from this serious but treatable disorder, which affects both genders and all races equally.

The characteristic symptoms of manic depression include mood swings (from happy to miserable, optimistic to despairing, etc.); changes in thinking (thoughts racing through one's mind, excessive self-confidence, difficulty concentrating, delusions, hallucinations); changes in behavior (sudden immersion in plans and projects, talking very rapidly and much more than usual, excessive spending, impaired judgment, impulsive sexual involvements); and changes in physical condition (less need for sleep, increased energy, fewer health complaints than usual). During "manic" periods, individuals may make grandiose plans or take dangerous risks. But they often plunge from this highest of highs to a terrible low, depressive episode, when they may feel sad, hopeless, and helpless and develop other symptoms of major depression. When you consult a physician, it is important that he or she ask whether you have ever had mood swings or periods of mania, since antidepressant medications may cause a person with bipolar depression to "switch" abruptly from depression to mania.

Other Forms of Depression

In *seasonal affective disorder* (SAD), annual episodes of depression usually begin at the same time each year, most often from the beginning of October through November, and end in March or April, with the coming of spring. January and February, often cloudy and dark, are usually the worst months. According to National Institute of Mental Health (NIMH) estimates, some 10 million Americans have SAD. Although the gloomy gray days of winter can dampen anyone's spirits, these individuals feel helpless, guilt-ridden, and hopeless and have difficulty thinking and making decisions. Typically, they eat more and gain weight. In particular, many crave rich carbohydrates. They spend many more hours asleep, yet feel chronically exhausted.

SAD often improves with a specialized treatment: exposure to bright light, known as phototherapy. Since the first reports on this approach in 1980, numerous studies have confirmed improvement in people with SAD who sit in front of a specially designed light box every day during winter months. For severe forms of seasonal depression, therapists may combine phototherapy with antidepressant medications.

Dysthymia is the clinical term for chronic mild depression. Usually developing in childhood, adolescence, or early adult life, dysthymia occurs equally in boys and girls, but in adults it is more common among women. Individuals with this disorder experience symptoms of depression most of the day, and more days than not, for a period of at least two years. They also may have low self-esteem, eat and sleep more or less than usual, lack energy, have problems concentrating or making decisions, and feel a sense of hopelessness. Their symptoms, however, are less intense than those of major depression. Psychotherapy, antidepressant medication, or a combination of both may be effective in treating dysthymia. Aerobic exercise seems to be an especially helpful form of additional (adjunctive) therapy.

ANTIDEPRESSANTS

Antidepressants are placed in different classes according to either their chemical structure or their mechanism of action. The class called *tricyclic antidepressants* received their name because of their similar three-ring chemical structure. Two subsequently released medications, amoxapine (Asendin) and the now infrequently used maprotiline (Ludiomil), have four-ring structures, hence their class name: *tetracyclics*. A list of the most commonly used tricyclic and tetracyclic antidepressants is shown in Table 2-2.

These antidepressants are thought to work by blocking to varying degrees the reuptake of the neurotransmitters norepinephrine or serotonin (abbreviated 5-HT) in the synapse (the space between neurons), leading to higher levels of these neurotransmitters. The increased levels are believed to result in fewer depressive symptoms. Unfortunately, the tricyclics and tetracyclics also block other

Table 2-2: Tricyclic and Tetracyclic Antidepressants

GENERIC NAME	BRAND NAME
amitriptyline	Elavil, Endep
amoxapine	Asendin
clomipramine	Anafranil
desipramine	Norpramin, Pertofrane
doxepin	Adapin, Sinequan
imipramine	Tofranil and Tofranil-PM (sustained release), Janimine, SK-Pramine
nortriptyline	Aventyl, Pamelor

neurotransmitters' actions that produce many of these drugs' bothersome side effects:

histamine 1 (abbreviated H-1):	sedation and weight gain
acetylcholine (ACH):	dry mouth, constipation, difficulty urinating, blurred vision, confusion
alpha-adrenergic:	orthostatic hypotension (decrease in blood pressure when moving from a lying to a sitting position or from sitting to standing)

Another class of antidepressants are *monoamine oxidase inhibitors* (MAOIs), so named because they block the action of an enzyme called monoamine oxidase (MAO).

This enzyme breaks down neurotransmitters, such as norepinephrine, after they are released into the synaptic space. When MAO is blocked—inhibited—by an MAOI antidepressant, the amount of neurotransmitter in the synapse is increased, leading to both positive effects (less depression) and potentially bad effects (a rise in blood pressure and other side effects). Two currently prescribed MAOIs are phenelzine (Nardil) and tranylcypromine (Parnate).

In the late 1980s, the antidepressant marketplace was revolutionized by the release of a new class of antidepressants that work principally by selectively blocking the reuptake of the neurotransmitter serotonin, hence their class: *selective serotonin reuptake inhibitors* (SSRIs). There are currently five SSRIs available in the United States. They are listed in Table 2-3. This class of antidepressants has fewer side effects and is better tolerated than the older tricyclic antidepressants and the MAOIs.

Table 2-3: Selective Serotonin Reuptake Inhibitors (SSRIs)

GENERIC NAME	BRAND NAME
citalopram	Celexa
fluoxetine	Prozac
fluvoxamine	Luvox
paroxetine	Paxil
sertraline	Zoloft

Another class of antidepressants defined by their mechanism of action are the serotonin (5HT) receptor antagonists (or $5HT_2$ antagonists). They work principally by blocking a specific serotonin neuroreceptor, hence their name, and are also weak serotonin and norepinephrine reuptake inhibitors. The two available $5HT_2$ antagonists are trazodone (Desyrel) and nefazodone (Serzone).

Other new antidepressants have varying mechanisms of

action. All of the newer *atypical antidepressants* are listed
in Table 2-4, along with their mechanism of action.

Table 2-4: New Antidepressants

GENERIC NAME	BRAND NAME	MECHANISM OF ACTION
bupropion and bupropion SR (sustained release)	Wellbutrin, Wellbutrin SR, Zyban	dopamine-norepinephrine reuptake inhibitor
mirtazapine	Remeron	norepinephrine agonist, $5HT_2$ and $5HT_3$ antagonist
nefazodone	Serzone	$5HT_2$ antagonist, weak serotonin and norepinephrine reuptake inhibitor
venlafaxine and venlafaxine-XR (extended release)	Effexor Effexor XR	selective serotonin-norepinephrine reuptake inhibitor

While the antidepressants available today are all effective medications, how well a person responds to a particular drug is an individual matter. About 60 to 70 percent
respond to the first medication prescribed for them. Many
of those who do not respond to the first drug eventually
improve with an alternative one, though it may sometimes
take trials of several drugs to arrive at the one that works.
And combined treatment for depression, which involves
both drug therapy and psychotherapy, has proven most effective of all in both overcoming the depression and lowering relapse rates.

Many medications classified as antidepressants are also
effective for treatment of other mental disorders. For instance, the tricyclics are used to treat panic disorder, posttraumatic stress disorder, generalized anxiety disorder, and
various physical problems, such as chronic pain and mi-

graine headaches. MAO inhibitors are also prescribed for panic disorder and social anxiety disorder. The SSRIs have proved beneficial in treating obsessive-compulsive disorder, anorexia and bulimia nervosa, panic disorder, certain impulse-control disorders, social anxiety disorder, generalized anxiety disorder, and posttraumatic stress disorder.

A PRACTICAL GUIDE TO ANTIDEPRESSANTS

In prescribing an antidepressant, physicians weigh many factors, including the individual's history and current medical status, any history of manic episodes or bipolar disorder (see Chapter 4), previous depressions, prior responses to an antidepressant, and the presence of various symptoms, such as sleep disturbance, weight gain or loss, anxiety or sedation, or psychotic symptoms, such as delusions or hallucinations. It is important for consumers to understand why their doctor recommends a particular medication and to be informed about its possible side effects as well as its potential benefits.

Because individuals vary widely in their responses to different medications, they must work closely with their physicians in choosing and using an antidepressant. In general, starting doses are low and are gradually increased, so it can take several weeks before reaching a full dose. Both the initial dose and the "therapeutic" or effective dose vary from person to person. Younger adults typically need higher doses than older ones.

A critical fact about antidepressant treatment is that it takes time. Although a few individuals may experience some improvement, such as increased energy, by the end of the first week, most do not see significant benefits for three or four weeks. Because doses are increased gradually, five or six weeks may pass from the time a person takes the first pill until symptoms are substantially relieved, and it may take eight weeks or longer for the medication to have its full impact. It is thought that this time is required to either increase or decrease the receptors' ability to bind to selected neurotransmitters.

Doctors need to keep in touch with individuals taking antidepressants to monitor their responses and to make sure that the drugs are having an effect. Within two weeks, many people find they are sleeping better. After about four to eight weeks of treatment, psychiatrists can determine if individuals have experienced a full response, a partial response, or have failed to improve at all. Those with an initial episode of a mild to moderate depression usually continue to take medication for six to twelve months; doses are then tapered off. For those whose depression is more severe or who have had prior depressive episodes, treatment may continue for a longer time. Recent studies have revealed a high rate of recurrence in major depression, and maintenance drug treatment, which can prevent another episode of depression, has become increasingly common.

In general, people have a 50 percent chance of experiencing another depression following their first episode. For individuals with two prior episodes of major depression, the probability of a third episode increases to 70 percent; for those who have had three prior episodes, the risk of recurrence rises to 90 percent.

Individuals who do not improve on one type of antidepressant usually are switched to another type; for example, from a tricyclic to an SSRI or from an SSRI to the atypical bupropion (Wellbutrin or Zyban). Approximately 50 percent of individuals who do not respond to one class of medication will improve with another. In addition, it has also been reported that 50 percent of people who fail to respond to one SSRI will respond to another.

Those with a partial response may benefit from a switch in medication or from augmentation therapy, that is, the addition of other agents to enhance or magnify the beneficial effects of an antidepressant. The agents used for augmentation therapy include the mood stabilizer lithium, thyroid hormone supplements, anticonvulsants (carbamazepine and valproic acid), the anti-anxiety agent buspirone (BuSpar), and stimulants, such as methylphenidate (Ritalin), although there are no scientific guidelines for how long these should be used. If these approaches fail, psychiatrists may try a combination of antidepressants, such as an SSRI along with a tricyclic antidepressant, or electroconvulsive therapy (ECT).

General Precautions

Individuals should give their doctors their complete medical history, and let them know whether they have ever had an allergic reaction to an antidepressant or any other medication, if they are taking any other prescription or nonprescription drugs or vitamins, if they are planning to undergo surgery or any medical tests or procedures in the coming months, and if they have any concurrent or chronic medical conditions, such as a seizure disorder, heart disease or recent heart attack, thyroid problems, or impaired kidney or liver function. It is also important to tell your physician whether you or a family member has ever had a manic episode, because some antidepressants increase the risk for a person with bipolar disorder (manic-depressive illness) to "switch" from depression into mania. All antidepressants may slightly increase the risk for developing seizures; this danger is greater with certain drugs. Another standard—and sound—recommendation is to stop smoking; nicotine lowers the levels of antidepressants in the blood, so may reduce their beneficial effects.

As shown in Tables 2-5, 2-6, 2-7, 2-9, and 2-10, the various classes of antidepressants produce different side effects. Many common side effects, such as dry mouth or nausea, subside after several weeks. Moreover, these reactions do have a positive aspect: They indicate that a drug is working and that blood levels of the drug are rising. Even when side effects are bothersome, it is critical to continue to take the medication long enough for it to be beneficial and to keep increasing the dose as directed until symptoms improve.

For the elderly, dosages must be lower than those for younger persons, and the side effects can be more difficult to tolerate. In women who are pregnant or trying to conceive, the question of initiating or continuing antidepressant treatment is a difficult one. Clinical reports are very limited. Most physicians prefer not to prescribe or continue any medications, including antidepressants, during pregnancy unless they are absolutely essential. The decision to initiate, continue, or stop antidepressants should be a joint one between the woman and her physician. In general, the potential benefits of continuing an antidepressant during pregnancy should greatly outweigh any potential or unknown risks to the fetus.

Individuals taking antidepressants should avoid alcohol, which is itself a depression-producing substance. Alcohol stimulates enzymes that break down antidepressant medication, lowering the amount in the blood and making it more difficult to maintain therapeutic levels. Alcohol depresses the central nervous system and can also enhance the sedating effects of antidepressants that cause drowsiness as a side effect. Individuals who are in maintenance antidepressant drug treatment after their depressive symptoms have ended should also be cautious about alcohol use.

While the danger of overdose is a concern with all medications, regardless of kind, it can be of special concern in depression and certain other mental disorders because of the risk of suicide. Given the risk of suicide in depressed individuals and because tricyclic antidepressants can be fatal in overdose, psychiatrists now tend to prescribe the newer generation of antidepressants, which are less likely to be fatal in overdose. Suicidal thoughts, and sometimes the act itself, can occur in some serious depressions. Most studies indicate that all antidepressants decrease such thoughts. In the early stage of drug treatment, however, they may also paradoxically provoke some individuals to consider suicide itself, perhaps because of an increase in their energy level that impels them to act on their self-destructive impulses. Physicians look for signs that may indicate this, and in some cases may decide to hospitalize the person to prevent a suicide attempt.

Antidepressants should generally not be stopped suddenly; doses must be tapered off gradually. Most people taking antidepressants will experience withdrawal symptoms if they stop the medication abruptly. The most common of these symptoms are insomnia, increased anxiety, a flu-like malaise, diarrhea, and recurrence of depressed mood. Often, a very gradual lowering of the dose can avoid these problems. However, several of the newer antidepressants—nefazodone (Serzone), mirtazapine (Remeron), fluoxetine (Prozac), citalopram (Celexa), and bupropion (Wellbutrin or Zyban)—can be stopped quickly without the risk of withdrawal symptoms.

CLASSES OF ANTIDEPRESSANT DRUGS

Selective Serotonin Reuptake Inhibitors

The SSRIs have become widely used, largely because they cause fewer side effects than other antidepressants and are easy to prescribe and to take (usually in a single dose in the morning). They can be the best choice for depressed individuals who have medical problems, such as heart disease, dementia, or Alzheimer's disease. They are a good option for depressed individuals who have difficulty tolerating any medicine, who are tired or lethargic, or who tend to ruminate or obsess constantly.

The SSRIs are also used to treat obsessive-compulsive disorder, social anxiety disorder, panic disorder, trichotillomania, and bulimia nervosa. Some psychiatrists have used SSRIs to treat depression in individuals with borderline and schizotypal personality disorders. Small clinical studies without control groups have reported significant decreases in symptoms of depression and improvement in difficult characterological traits (such as impulsivity) that may have been aggravated by the depression.

Side Effects

The most common side effects of SSRIs are shown in Table 2-5.

Table 2-5: Common Side Effects of SSRIs	
• Abdominal cramps	• Sexual difficulties
• Agitation	• Sleep disturbance
• Diarrhea	• Sweating
• Headache	• Tremor
• Nausea	• Upset stomach
• Nervousness	• Weight loss or gain
• Sedation	

The SSRIs are usually less sedating than tricyclic antidepressants. They do not lower blood pressure or trigger heart arrhythmias. Some individuals complain of "jitters" or restlessness; because caffeine can contribute to such "hyper" feelings, it is best avoided. Starting with low doses of the drug and increasing gradually can help avert such problems.

The SSRIs can cause sexual dysfunction, in particular retarded ejaculation in men and delayed orgasm in women, or they can intensify a preexisting dysfunction. Because depression itself can cause sexual dysfunction, which often improves as depression lifts, it is not always easy to differentiate between this and a drug side effect. Such side effects occur in about 50 to 60 percent of individuals and may abate with a reduction in dose or a change to a different antidepressant. Most people report a very slight weight loss, a pound or so, although some have reported gaining substantial amounts of weight. The SSRIs usually do not provoke cardiac arrhythmias, but they can increase heart rate and blood pressure. They cause orthostatic hypotension (dizziness from sitting up or standing up suddenly) far less often than the tricyclics, but this problem has occasionally been reported.

Precautions

The SSRIs can increase the blood levels of other medications metabolized in the liver by inhibiting this metabolism. Fluoxetine (Prozac) or paroxetine (Paxil) have been shown to increase levels of warfarin (Coumadin), an anticlotting agent. Sertraline (Zoloft) or citalopram (Celexa), which seem less likely to do so, may serve as alternative medications.

Warnings

Individuals who are taking two or more drugs that boost serotonin levels, such as an SSRI in combination with the serotonin antagonist antidepressant nefazodone (Serzone), may develop an uncommon, potentially deadly condition called serotonin syndrome, which is caused by excessive stimulation of the serotoninergic system. This syndrome can also occasionally occur in those taking a single SSRI, especially at higher doses. Initial symptoms include lethargy, restlessness, confusion, flushing, sweating, tremor, and involuntary muscle jerks. Over time, a small percentage of individuals may develop muscle disorders, hyperthermia, and rigor, which may lead to respiratory problems, increased platelet clotting, destruction of red blood cells by the kidneys and their excretion in urine, and kidney failure. This syndrome requires emergency medical treatment and discontinuation of the serotonin-boosting medications.

None of the SSRIs should ever be used with an MAO

inhibitor; the combination is dangerous. Two weeks should elapse after stopping an MAOI before beginning any other antidepressant. It is also necessary to wait two weeks after stopping an SSRI (and four weeks for the longer-acting fluoxetine [Prozac]) before starting an MAOI. Overdoses with the SSRIs are rarely fatal, but further research is needed for adequate assessment of this danger. The symptoms of a possible overdose include agitation, nausea, and convulsions. Immediate emergency treatment is essential.

Tricyclic and Tetracyclic Antidepressants

Once the agents of first choice in treating depression, these drugs have been largely replaced as first-line drugs by the SSRIs, atypical antidepressants, and nefazodone (Serzone). Tricyclics are now prescribed most often to treat depression complicated by pain or migraine headaches, severe depression that has failed to respond to one of the newer antidepressants, or depression in individuals who have previously responded to them.

Side Effects

For several of the tricyclic antidepressants (imipramine, desipramine, and nortriptyline), monitoring drug levels in the blood helps to ensure the greatest benefits with the fewest side effects. The most common side effects of these medications are summarized in Table 2-6.

Most of these side effects usually abate by the third week of use. In the meantime, practical coping strategies can help. Because these drugs are sedating, taking them before bedtime helps; indeed, the drowsiness can be a plus for those who have trouble sleeping. If coping strategies are not effective and reducing the dosage or trying alternative antidepressants does not help, some physicians pre-

Table 2-6: Common Side Effects of Tricyclic and Tetracyclic Antidepressants

- Blurred vision
- Confusion
- Constipation
- Difficulty urinating
- Dry mouth
- Cardiac arrhythmias
- Nervousness
- Orthostatic hypotension

- Sedation
- Sexual difficulties
- Slowing of electrical impulses through the heart
- Sweating
- Tremor
- Weight gain

scribe medications such as bethanechol chloride to relieve troublesome dry mouth, constipation, and urinary hesitancy and retention.

Weight gain is a common problem; most individuals put on several pounds while taking tricyclics. Particularly among women, this is the most common reason for discontinuing their use. At the beginning of treatment, many people complain of feeling dizzy or "foggy"; this usually lessens over time. However, if individuals become confused or forgetful, their psychiatrists may recommend an antidepressant less likely to produce these effects.

Precautions

Because of the risk for orthostatic (postural) hypotension, especially in those over age sixty-five, individuals should never rise to their feet suddenly, for instance when the telephone or doorbell rings. If they are lying down, they should change to a standing position in two stages, first shifting slowly to a sitting position and then waiting sixty seconds—or longer if they feel light-headed—before slowly standing up.

The tricyclics may aggravate an eye condition called narrow-angle glaucoma and may trigger seizures in susceptible individuals. They can interact with any medications that affect the central nervous system, including antihistamine-type allergy drugs, muscle relaxants, and sleeping pills. Check with a physician before taking any such substances, whether prescription or over-the-counter. Alcohol intensifies sedation and impairs driving ability; it should not be used. The tricyclics should not be discontinued abruptly; this can cause a worsening of the original disorder, or induce headache, restlessness, and flu-like physical symptoms. These drugs' effects may last for up to one to two weeks after they are stopped.

Warnings

The major drawback of the tricyclic antidepressants is the risk of intentional overdose or suicide. Taking a large quantity of any of these medications can be fatal. Because a person with depression is at high risk for suicide, psychiatrists prescribing them often try to minimize the danger of overdose by prescribing no more than one week's supply of the drugs at a time. Frequent visits also allow psychiatrists to provide support and counseling.

Tricyclics slow conduction of electrical impulses through the heart, leading to irregular heartbeats, called arrhythmias, which in some cases may be fatal. Consequently, individuals over the age of fifty should have a routine electrocardiogram (EKG) before starting this class of agents.

The first symptoms of overdose, which typically develop one to four hours after taking the drug, are difficulty in breathing, dangerous changes in heart rhythm, agitation, lowered blood pressure, garbled speech, high fever, confusion, disorientation, and coma. Immediate emergency treatment at a hospital can prevent permanent damage or death.

Monoamine Oxidase Inhibitors

MAO inhibitors, the oldest class of antidepressants, are as effective against depression as tricyclic antidepressants and the SSRIs. However, they are usually not the first drugs of choice for treatment of depression, primarily because of their side effects, their potential for serious adverse effects, and the requirement that individuals taking them avoid certain common foods and beverages. They are prescribed most often for individuals who develop *atypical* depression, which is characterized by oversleeping, overeating, extreme lethargy, great sensitivity to rejection, and highly emotional reactions to life experiences. The MAO inhibitors may also be effective in treating symptoms of panic disorder or specific phobias.

Isocarboxazid (Marplan), a well-known MAO inhibitor, is no longer on the market. A new "reversible" MAO inhibitor, moclobemide, is in use in Canada. It does not require dietary restrictions, but there are questions about its efficacy. It has not been approved for use in the United States.

Side Effects

The most common side effects of MAO inhibitors are shown in Table 2-7. Drowsiness is common, especially early in treatment. Other side effects include blurred vision, weakness, weight gain, sexual dysfunction, a rapid or slow heartbeat, and dry mouth. Less common side effects include constipation, diarrhea, rashes, chest pain, severe headache, chills or shivering, and jaundice.

Precautions

In persons over sixty-five, orthostatic hypotension is a major concern. Individuals taking MAOIs should alert their

Table 2-7: Common Side Effects of MAOIs

- Constipation
- Dangerous hypertension (when combined with certain foods or medications)
- Dry mouth
- Muscle aches
- Nervousness
- Orthostatic hypotension
- Problems in urinating
- Sedation
- Sexual difficulties
- Sleep disturbance
- Weight gain

doctors if they have high blood pressure or heart problems, if they often have severe headaches, or if they expect to be undergoing anesthesia, surgery, or medical testing in the coming months. Anyone using an MAO inhibitor should check with a physician before using *any* drug, including prescription and over-the-counter cold medications, cough syrups, decongestants, nose drops or sprays, treatments for sinus conditions or hay fever, or preparations that suppress appetite or claim to reduce weight. Antihistamines themselves are not a danger unless combined with decongestants.

If surgery is necessary, the anesthesiologist should be informed in advance of the operation that the patient is taking an MAO inhibitor; the medication may have to be discontinued at least ten days before surgery. The use of procaine (Novocain) for dental procedures may be dangerous, and individuals anticipating dental work should consult with their dentist and psychiatrist about potential risks.

Warnings

For individuals taking MAOIs, it is essential (though not always easy) to avoid foods containing tyramine, an amino acid found in many common foods that can interact with the MAO inhibitors and produce potentially toxic effects, including sudden, extremely dangerous surges in blood pressure (hypertensive crisis). This is sometimes called the "cheese reaction" because aged cheeses contain relatively high concentrations of tyramine. The reaction can range from mild to severe, producing symptoms such as sweating, palpitations, headache, and, in extreme cases, a sharp rise in blood pressure and possible bleeding within the brain because of the rupture of cerebral arteries.

Recent studies that measured tyramine in foods have reduced the list of previously banned substances. The primary foods to avoid are avocados, fava beans, cheeses (except cream, cottage, and ricotta), chocolate (in large amounts), overripe bananas and other fruits, sauerkraut, shrimp paste, sour cream, and soy products, including tofu. Beer and ale must not be consumed. Caffeine and some red wines should be used in small amounts only. See Table 2-8 for revised dietary restrictions when taking an MAOI.

Dextromethorphan, a compound frequently included in over-the-counter cold medications, should not be used with MAOIs, since the combination has been reported to cause brief periods of psychosis or bizarre behavior. All illicit or "recreational" drugs should be avoided; cocaine in particular can lead to an extremely dangerous increase in blood pressure.

Individuals taking an MAO inhibitor who develop an extremely painful or unremitting headache should immediately seek medical help, including blood-pressure monitoring. A very high blood-pressure reading may require emergency medical treatment. Persons taking these drugs should carry an identification card or wear a Medic Alert bracelet alerting health-care personnel that if they develop a hypertensive reaction, therapy consists of 2 to 5 mg. of phentolamine (Regitine), and that they should not be given meperidine (Demerol).

Table 2-8: Dietary and Drug Restrictions When Taking MAO Inhibitors

FOODS THAT *MUST* BE AVOIDED

Cheese (except ricotta, cottage cheese, and cream cheese)

Cheese-containing foods (e.g., pizza, fondue, and many Italian dishes)

Fermented or aged foods (especially fermented or aged meats or fish, e.g., corned beef, salami, pepperoni, and sausage)

Liver, beef, chicken, and liverwurst

Broad bean (fava) pods

Meat extracts or yeast extracts, such as Bovril and Marmite (yeast and baked goods containing yeast are safe)

Overripe or spoiled fruits (e.g., bananas, pineapples, avocados, figs, and raisins)

Soy sauce, tofu, fermented bean curd (an ingredient in soybean paste and miso soup)

Sauerkraut

Shrimp paste (shrimp are safe)

Beer and ale (including non-alcoholic varieties)

Vermouth, sherry, cognac

Sour cream

FOODS THAT MAY LEAD TO MEDICAL COMPLICATIONS IF CONSUMED IN LARGE AMOUNTS

Coffee, caffeine

Chocolate

Red wine (especially Chianti)

Yogurt

FOODS THAT ARE NOW CONSIDERED SAFE

Pickled herring (brine is unsafe)

Smoked salmon, smoked whitefish

Yogurt (unless unfresh; check expiration date)

DRUGS THAT *MUST* BE AVOIDED

Cold medications (e.g., Dristan, Contac)

Nasal decongestants and sinus medications

Asthma inhalants

Allergy and hay-fever medications with decongestants

Demerol

Cocaine

Amphetamines

Anti-appetite (diet) preparations

Local anesthetics with epinephrine

Levodopa for Parkinsonism

Dopamine

These restrictions should be followed from one day before to two weeks after taking an MAO inhibitor.

Persons who have not been helped by an MAO inhibitor must wait two weeks after discontinuing these drugs before starting another antidepressant, including another MAO inhibitor, or before using any foods, beverages, or drugs containing tyramine. MAO inhibitors should not be discontinued without consulting a physician, and use should be gradually reduced to avoid withdrawal symptoms. After discontinuation, individuals must follow the dietary restrictions for at least two weeks to avoid possible toxic reactions. They must also wait at least two weeks after stopping an antidepressant other than an MAOI (four weeks for fluoxetine—Prozac—because of its long half-life), before beginning an MAOI.

The symptoms of an overdose with an MAOI include drowsiness, low blood pressure, difficulty breathing, convulsions, coma, and hypertensive crisis. Immediate emergency treatment is essential.

Serotonin Receptor Antagonists

Trazodone (Desyrel) is one of the most sedating antidepressants, so it can help those who have difficulty in falling asleep. Often a bedtime dose is prescribed as a sleep aid for individuals taking SSRIs. Trazodone has been reported to produce priapism at a rate of 1 in 6,000 men. Nefazodone (Serzone) produces less sedation than trazodone. In contrast to the SSRIs, nefazodone does not produce sexual problems and does not cause anxiety or insomnia.

Side Effects

Common side effects of trazodone (Desyrel) and nefazodone (Serzone) are shown in Table 2-9.

Side effects of nefazodone (Serzone) include dizziness, dry mouth, blurred vision, constipation, and urinary retention. These side effects are experienced less often and are less pronounced in lower doses. In those over age sixty-five,

Table 2-9: Common Side Effects of Trazodone (Desyrel) and Nefazodone (Serzone)

TRAZODONE AND NEFAZODONE

- Dizziness
- Headaches
- Nausea
- Upset stomach

TRAZODONE

- Orthostatic hypotension
- Sustained erections (priapism)

NEFAZODONE

- Visual afterimage

orthostatic hypotension is possible. When used in combination with an SSRI, nefazodone may enhance sexual interest and orgasmic functioning, especially in women with sexual dysfunction caused by the SSRI.

Warnings

A very small number of men taking trazodone (Desyrel) (about 1 in 6,000) may develop prolonged and painful erections (priapism), a condition that may require emergency surgery that can lead to permanent impotence. This problem does not occur with nefazodone (Serzone). The risk for lethal overdose is much lower than with the tricyclic antidepressants and is similar to the SSRIs.

Newer Antidepressants

Venlafaxine (Effexor) has shown promise in helping individuals who do not improve with other antidepressants. It recently was approved by the FDA to treat generalized anxiety disorder. At high doses, it is very activating; at higher doses it may increase blood pressure. It does not cause cardiac arrhythmias, but, like the SSRIs, it produces sexual dysfunction. Venlafaxine (Effexor) should *never* be taken with an MAOI.

Mirtazapine (Remeron) is quite sedating and produces an appreciable weight gain of five to ten pounds. It does not produce sexual dysfunction and is safe to use in people with heart disease or who have experienced a heart attack. It should *never* be taken with an SSRI.

Bupropion (Wellbutrin or Zyban) is non-sedating and causes fewer side effects than the tricyclics and MAO inhibitors. It does not make users drowsy, does not cause weight gain, does not affect the heart, and does not cause postural hypotension. It does not produce sexual dysfunction.

Bupropion does pose a risk for seizures, which develop in about 4 of every 1,000 individuals (0.4 percent) taking these medications. To put this risk in perspective, 1 of every 1,000 people *not* taking any medication develops seizures. Daily doses of bupropion higher than 450 mg. in the regular-release form or 400 mg. in the sustained-release (SR) form should not be taken, since the risk of seizures increases dramatically. Individuals with bulimia nervosa should not take high doses of this medication because they are likely to develop seizures. Like the SSRIs, bupropion cannot be used in combination with an MAO inhibitor.

Side Effects

The side effects of venlafaxine (Effexor), bupropion (Wellbutrin or Zyban), and mirtazapine (Remeron) are shown in Table 2-10.

Table 2-10: Common Side Effects of Newer Antidepressants

GENERIC NAME	BRAND NAME	COMMON SIDE EFFECTS
bupropion	Wellbutrin	agitation, sleep
bupropion, sustained-release	Wellbutrin SR Zyban	disturbance, nausea, headache, weight loss, dry mouth
mirtazapine	Remeron	weight gain, increased appetite, dry mouth, sedation, constipation
venlafaxine	Effexor	nausea, sedation, sleep
venlafaxine, sustained-release	Effexor XR	disturbance, sexual difficulties, nervousness, diarrhea, headache, sweating, agitation, hypertension at higher doses

 Generic name: **AMITRIPTYLINE**

 Available in generic form: Yes

 Brand name: Elavil, Endep

 Drug class: Tricyclic antidepressant

Prescribed for: Major depressive disorder, dysthymia (chronic mild to moderate depression), bipolar depression, panic disorder, posttraumatic stress disorder, generalized anxiety disorder, social anxiety disorder, pain symptoms, migraine and tension headaches, insomnia.

General information: One of the older antidepressants, amitriptyline produces many bothersome side effects and is potentially lethal if taken in overdose. It is believed to work by increasing the amount of norepinephrine and, to a lesser extent, serotonin available in the central nervous system. Physical medicine specialists and orthopedic surgeons may prescribe it as an additional medication to treat various chronic pain syndromes. Primary-care physicians may prescribe it to treat insomnia. Generally, amitriptyline takes six to eight weeks at therapeutic levels before working completely. After three to four weeks, there is usually some relief of symptoms, with more complete relief after six to eight weeks. In some cases, amitriptyline may take as long as twelve weeks to achieve maximum benefit.

Dosing information: This medication is available in tablets of various doses: 10, 25, 50, 75, 100, and 150 mg. The usual daily therapeutic dose in healthy adults is between 150 and 200 mg., although some patients may require doses up to 300 mg. Because of the kinds of side effects the drug produces, many people do not tolerate the high-dose ranges. A usual starting dose may be 25 to 50 mg. at bedtime, with weekly increases of 25 to 50 mg. until a daily dose of 150 to 200 mg. is reached. If depressive symptoms persist after eight weeks, the physician may increase the dose up to 300 mg. per day, the usual maximum dose.

Common side effects: Amitriptyline produces significant anticholinergic side effects (see Glossary), including drowsiness, dry mouth, blurred vision, constipation, esophageal reflux (heartburn), urinary retention or difficulty urinating, and orthostatic hypotension. Other side effects include sexual dysfunction (impotence, decreased desire), weight gain, cardiac arrhythmias, and tremor.

Precautions: Men with an enlarged prostate should use this drug with caution, since it may cause them difficulty in urinating. Because all antidepressants may increase the risk of seizures, persons who are taking medications to prevent seizures and who are prescribed amitriptyline for depression may need to have their anti-seizure medication carefully monitored and possibly increased in dose. To cope with dry mouth, those taking amitriptyline should drink water throughout the day or suck on sugarless candy. (Candy with sugar should be avoided, since the anticholinergic effects of this drug increase the possibility of tooth decay.) Exercise and high-fiber foods can lessen the risk of constipation. Some people may need to take a stool softener, such as Colace, or a bulk-forming agent, such as Metamucil, to counteract the constipating effects. Amitriptyline should not be stopped suddenly because of the risk of severe withdrawal symptoms, such as increased anxiety, flu-like symptoms, depression, jitteriness, and agitation. It should be gradually tapered off over a period of several weeks to a month or more.

Warnings: Persons who have recently suffered a heart attack generally should not take amitriptyline or another tricyclic antidepressant because of the increased risk of sudden death, probably related to the production of irregular heartbeats (arrhythmias).

Amitriptyline should *never* be taken with monoamine oxidase inhibitor (MAOI) antidepressants, since this combination may produce severe hypertension, seizures, fever, and even death. Individuals must wait at least two weeks after stopping amitriptyline before beginning an MAOI, and wait two weeks after stopping an MAOI before beginning amitriptyline.

Alcohol: People should not drink alcohol if they are taking antidepressants, since alcohol may produce depressive-like symptoms, and may increase the rate of metabolism of the antidepressant and lower its blood levels.

Food and beverages: No restrictions. If taking amitriptyline on an empty stomach upsets your stomach, try it with food or immediately after eating.

Possible drug interactions: Amitriptyline should not be used with the SSRIs because these drugs inhibit its metabolism, leading to very high blood levels and increasing the likelihood of seizures, arrhythmias (irregular heartbeats), confusion, and dizziness. Because of amitriptyline's sedating effects, avoid other medications that produce sedation, such as the benzodiazepines (Valium, Ativan, and others), antihistamines, and pain medication. Because it can lower blood pressure, amitriptyline should be used with caution when taken with antihypertensive medication.

Use in pregnancy and breast-feeding:
Pregnancy Category D
In general, tricyclic antidepressants are not recommended during pregnancy because their use has not been systematically studied. It is not known whether they increase birth defects or spontaneous miscarriages. If they stop antidepressants during pregnancy, some women may experience a recurrence of their depression. In these circumstances, the physician should discuss the need to restart amitriptyline or seek an alternative medication or treatment. Women should always consult with their physician if they are contemplating pregnancy or if they become pregnant while taking amitriptyline. Amitriptyline should be taken during pregnancy only if the benefits to the mother greatly outweigh any potential or unknown risks to the fetus. Women who are taking a tricyclic antidepressant should not breast-feed, since small amounts will pass into the breast milk and be absorbed into the baby's bloodstream,

leading to possible sedation and affecting the child's developing nervous system.

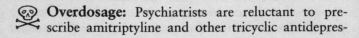 **Use in children:** While tricyclic antidepressants are sometimes prescribed in children for the treatment of bed-wetting, attention deficit hyperactivity disorder (ADHD), and depression, amitriptyline is usually not prescribed. In general, Norpramin, Tofranil, or Pamelor (a metabolite of amitriptyline) is usually used if the physician selects a drug in the tricyclic class. However, because of several recent reports of deaths in young children taking tricyclic antidepressants, this class of antidepressants should be prescribed only by a child psychiatrist or a pediatrician skilled in the use of psychiatric medications and only if other classes of medication have been unsuccessful.

Use in seniors: In general, lower doses of amitriptyline are prescribed in seniors, usually in the range of 75 to 150 mg. a day. Its blood-pressure-lowering effects and the risk of orthostatic hypotension (dangerously low blood pressure) and confusion are greater in older persons. In addition, its adverse effects on the heart increase the risk of cardiac arrhythmias and even of death. People over age fifty should have a baseline electrocardiogram (EKG) before taking amitriptyline, since it prolongs the transmission of electrical impulses through the heart, an effect that may result in potentially life-threatening irregular heartbeats. Because amitriptyline lowers blood pressure, especially when going from a lying or sitting position to standing, seniors should be careful to avoid falling. Its anticholinergic effects may produce confusion and disorientation, especially in seniors or in those in the early stages of Alzheimer's disease.

Overdosage: Psychiatrists are reluctant to prescribe amitriptyline and other tricyclic antidepressants in patients who are at risk for suicide because the risk of fatal overdose is high. If overdose is suspected, bring the bottle of medication to the emergency room with the person, since the date when the medication was prescribed and the number of pills remaining in the bottle can provide helpful information to the treating physician.

Special considerations: Avoid taking amitriptyline in the combination forms Triavil and Limbitrol. Triavil is a combination of amitriptyline and perphenazine (Trilafon), an antipsychotic medication (see page 304). While people with psychotic depression (characterized by depression and delusions and hallucinations) may require antipsychotic medications, most psychiatrists prescribe a separate antipsychotic agent in varying doses and for a limited period of time. Limbitrol is a combination of amitriptyline and chlordiazepoxide (Librium), a benzodiazepine (see page 174). Physicians today rarely prescribe chlordiazepoxide, except in the treatment of alcohol withdrawal.

Patients with bipolar disorder (manic-depressive illness) usually develop depression in addition to mania at some time during the course of their illness. Amitriptyline and other tricyclic antidepressants may produce "switching," a clinical process whereby a person goes from the depressive phase of manic-depressive illness to the manic phase. Prior to starting an antidepressant, people with bipolar disorder should take a mood stabilizer, such as lithium or divalproex (Depakote) (see Chapter 4). However, because even with a mood stabilizer, they may experience switching when placed on a heterocyclic antidepressant, many physicians choose one of the newer antidepressants, such as an SSRI, bupropion (Wellbutrin or Zyban), or nefazodone (Serzone), which are less likely to produce this effect.

Most psychiatrists prescribe amitriptyline infrequently. The preferred alternative is nortriptyline (Pamelor) (see page 110), a metabolite of amitriptyline that produces fewer bothersome anticholinergic side effects (dry mouth, blurred vision, constipation, confusion, urinary retention, and hypotension).

 ## Generic name: AMOXAPINE

 Available in generic form: Yes

 Brand name: Asendin

 Drug class: Tetracyclic antidepressant

Prescribed for: Major depressive disorder, dysthymia (chronic mild to moderate depression), bipolar depression, panic disorder, posttraumatic stress disorder, generalized anxiety disorder, social anxiety disorder, pain symptoms, migraine and tension headaches, insomnia.

General information: One of the older antidepressants, amoxapine produces many bothersome side effects and may be potentially lethal if taken in overdose. It is believed to work by increasing the amount of norepinephrine and, to a lesser extent, serotonin available in the central nervous system. Physical medicine specialists and orthopedic surgeons may prescribe it as an additional medication to treat chronic pain syndromes. Primary-care physicians may prescribe it to treat insomnia. Generally, it takes six to eight weeks at therapeutic levels before amoxapine works completely. After three to four weeks, there is usually some relief of symptoms, with more complete relief after six to eight weeks. In some cases, amoxapine may take as long as twelve weeks to achieve maximum benefit.

Amoxapine is structurally quite similar to the antipsychotic medication loxapine (Loxitane); consequently, some investigators believe it may be particularly effective for people with severe depression with psychosis (delusions and hallucinations). In such cases, most psychiatrists prescribe an antipsychotic agent (see Chapter 6) in addition to amoxapine. Because of its structure, amoxapine has been reported to produce a number of side effects associated with loxapine and other antipsychotic agents, such as motor restlessness, stiffness, tremor, etc. (see page 289).

Dosing Information: Amoxapine is available in tablets of various doses: 25, 50, 100, and 150 mg. The usual initial dose is 100 to 150 mg. at bedtime, with an increase on a weekly basis of 50 to 100 mg. The usual therapeutic dose is between 200 and 300 mg., although some people may require doses up to 400 mg. If the total daily dose is more than 300 mg., it should be given in divided doses, two times a day or more.

Common side effects: Amoxapine produces less sedation and fewer bothersome anticholinergic effects (dry mouth, blurred vision, constipation, urinary retention or difficulty urinating, confusion, etc.) than amitriptyline (Elavil), doxepin (Sinequan), or imipramine (Tofranil), although some of these symptoms may occur.

Precautions: Men with an enlarged prostate should use this drug with caution since it may cause them difficulty in urinating. All antidepressants may increase the risk of seizures, but this risk may be greater for people taking amoxapine. Consequently, persons who are taking medications to prevent seizures and who are prescribed amoxapine for depression may need to have their antiseizure medication carefully monitored and possibly increased in dose. To cope with dry mouth, those taking amoxapine should drink water throughout the day or suck on sugarless candy. (Candy with sugar should be avoided, since the anticholinergic effects of this drug increase the possibility of tooth decay.) Exercise and high-fiber foods can lessen the risk of constipation. Some people may need to take a stool softener, such as Colace, or a bulk-forming agent, such as Metamucil, to counteract amoxapine's constipating effects. Amoxapine should not be stopped suddenly because of severe withdrawal symptoms, such as increased anxiety, flu-like symptoms, depression, jitteriness, and agitation. It should be gradually tapered off over a period of several weeks to a month or more.

Warnings: People who have recently had a heart attack or who have a history of arrhythmias (irregular heartbeats) should not take this medication because of the increased risk of dangerous, irregular heartbeats and sudden death. Amoxapine should *never* be taken with monoamine oxidase inhibitor (MAOI) antidepressants, since this combination may produce severe hypertension, seizures, fever, and even death. Individuals must wait at least two weeks after stopping amoxapine before beginning an MAOI and wait two weeks after stopping an MAOI before beginning amoxapine.

Alcohol: People should not drink alcohol if they are taking antidepressants since alcohol produces depressive-like symptoms, and may increase the metabolic rate of the antidepressant and lower its blood levels.

Food and beverages: No restrictions. If taking amoxapine on an empty stomach upsets your stomach, try it with food or immediately after eating.

Possible drug interactions: This medication should generally not be used with the SSRIs because these drugs inhibit the metabolism of amoxapine, leading to very high blood levels and increasing the likelihood of seizures, arrhythmias (irregular heartbeats), confusion, and dizziness. Because of amoxapine's sedating effects, other medications that produce sedation, such as the benzodiazepines, antihistamines, and pain medication, should be avoided. Because it can lower blood pressure, amoxapine should be used with caution when taken with antihypertensive medications.

Use in pregnancy and breast-feeding: Pregnancy Category C

In general, amoxapine is not recommended during pregnancy, although it is not known whether it increases birth defects or spontaneous miscarriages, because use of this drug in pregnancy has not been systematically studied. If they stop taking amoxapine during pregnancy, some pregnant women may experience a recurrence of depression. In these circumstances, the physician should discuss the need to restart amoxapine or seek an alternative medication or treatment. Women taking a tricyclic antidepressant should avoid breast-feeding, since small amounts will pass into the breast milk and be absorbed into the baby's bloodstream, affecting the child's developing nervous system.

Use in children: Amoxapine is usually not prescribed in children. Tricyclic antidepressants—desipramine (Norpramin), imipramine (Tofranil), or nortriptyline (Pamelor)—are sometimes prescribed for children to treat bed-wetting, attention deficit hyperactivity disorder (ADHD), and depression. However, because of several recent reports of sudden deaths in young children taking tricyclic antidepressants, amoxapine, a tetracyclic, should be used with caution and prescribed only by a child psychiatrist or a pediatrician skilled in the use of psychiatric medications and only if other classes of medication have been unsuccessful.

Use in seniors: In general, lower doses of amoxapine are prescribed in seniors, usually in the range of 100 to 200 mg. a day. Its blood-pressure-lowering effects and the risk of orthostatic hypotension and confusion are greater in older persons. In addition, its adverse effects on the heart increase the risk of irregular heartbeats (arrhythmias) and even of death.

☠ **Overdosage:** Psychiatrists are reluctant to prescribe amoxapine and other heterocyclic antidepressants in patients who are at risk for suicide, since the risk of fatal overdose is high. If overdose is suspected, bring the bottle of medication to the emergency room with the person, since the date when the medication was prescribed and the number of pills remaining in the bottle can provide helpful information to the treating physician.

✍ **Special considerations:** A very small percentage of people who have taken amoxapine have been reported to develop tardive dyskinesia, an irreversible neurologic syndrome that consists of involuntary movements of the lips, face, and upper extremities. This may occur because of the drug's similarity in chemical structure to the antipsychotic agent loxapine (Loxitane). The risk of tardive dyskinesia increases with the length of treatment and the cumulative dosage of medication and is greater in the elderly.

Persons with bipolar disorder (manic-depressive illness) usually develop depression in addition to mania at some point in the course of their illness. Amoxapine and other heterocyclic antidepressants may produce "switching," a clinical process whereby a person goes from the depressive phase of manic-depressive illness to the manic phase. Prior to starting an antidepressant, people with bipolar disorder should first take a mood stabilizer, such as lithium or divalproex (Depakote). However, because even with a mood stabilizer some of these persons may experience switching when placed on a heterocyclic antidepressant, many psychiatrists select one of the newer antidepressants, such as an SSRI, bupropion (Wellbutrin or Zyban), or nefazodone (Serzone), which are less likely to produce this effect.

Generic name: **BUPROPION**

 Available in generic form: No

 Brand name: Wellbutrin, Wellbutrin SR, Zyban

 Drug class: norepinephrine and dopamine reuptake inhibitor

 Prescribed for: Depression, nicotine addiction, and attention deficit hyperactivity disorder (ADHD).

General information: Bupropion is an effective antidepressant that is particularly beneficial in treating depression characterized by lethargy, tiredness, excessive sleeping, and weight gain. It is somewhat stimulating and may produce mild weight loss. In contrast to the serotonin-type antidepressants, bupropion is not effective in treating panic disorder, obsessive-compulsive disorder, anxiety disorders, and eating disorders.

It is still unclear how this drug works, but it is believed to increase the amount of norepinephrine and, at higher doses, dopamine in the brain. These effects are believed to relieve depression.

The risk of seizures is approximately 4 in 1,000 people in doses of up to 450 mg. a day of the immediate-release form, a rate approximately four times that of the other antidepressants. This is not a problem for most people as long as they take bupropion as prescribed. However, those with a history of head trauma or seizure disorder and those taking another medication that may increase their risk for seizures generally should not take bupropion; if they are prescribed bupropion, their anti-seizure medication should be carefully monitored.

More recently, Wellbutrin SR (the sustained-release

form) has been marketed under another name, Zyban, to treat nicotine addiction. Although Zyban is the only drug to receive FDA approval for this purpose, all the antidepressants are believed to be effective to varying degrees in reducing the craving associated with nicotine withdrawal. However, Zyban is probably the most effective agent.

Dosing information: Bupropion is available in an immediate-release form in 75- and 100-mg. tablets. Bupropion also has a sustained-release formulation, called Wellbutrin SR and Zyban, which is available in 100- and 150-mg. tablets. Most physicians prescribe bupropion in the SR form. The usual starting dose of the SR version is 150 mg. once a day for a week, then increasing to 150 mg. twice a day. The maximum recommended dose of the SR form is 200 mg. twice a day. The advantage of this form is that in higher doses the patient has to take the medication only twice a day.

To decrease the risk of seizures, there should be at least four to six hours between doses; the maximum single dose should not exceed 150 mg. of the regular form of bupropion or 200 mg. of the SR form (Wellbutrin SR or Zyban) (i.e., two 100-mg. tablets twice a day).

Common side effects: The most common side effects are dry mouth, agitation, headache, sleep disturbance, and decreased appetite or weight loss. Sleep disturbance is believed to occur less than with the SSRIs.

Most significantly, in contrast to the SSRIs, tricyclic and tetracyclic antidepressants, MAO inhibitors, and venlafaxine (Effexor), bupropion generally does not produce sexual dysfunction (i.e., decreased desire, retarded ejaculation, or delayed orgasm). Along with nefazodone (Serzone) and mirtazapine (Remeron), bupropion is a good alternative for persons who develop sexual dysfunction with other agents.

To decrease the likelihood of sleep disturbance, patients should take their second dose of medication (or their third dose if they are taking the immediate-release form) no later than with their evening meal. Bupropion should not be taken at bedtime.

Precautions: Persons with eating disorders such as bulimia nervosa or anorexia nervosa should not take this medication because of the increased risk of seizures. In addition, those with significant anxiety or an anxiety disorder such as panic disorder, social anxiety disorder, or posttraumatic stress disorder should generally not take bupropion because it is not effective in treating these other conditions. A serotonin-boosting agent, such as an SSRI or nefazodone (Serzone), or a tricyclic antidepressant, such as desipramine (Norpramin), is usually preferable in treating anxiety disorders. People who do not wish to lose weight should not take bupropion, since 25 to 30 percent may experience decreased appetite and a weight loss of more than five pounds. In bipolar individuals who are depressed, bupropion may pose less risk of rapid switching from depression to mania than other drugs, such as tricyclic antidepressants and even the SSRIs, although this latter effect has not been definitively proven. People with bipolar depression should first be placed on a mood stabilizer (lithium or divalproex [Depakote]) before taking buproprion.

Warnings: As stated previously, a major concern is the possible development of seizures. Individuals may reduce this risk by limiting a single dose of the medication to a maximum of 200 mg. of the SR form and 150 mg. of the immediate-release form and allowing a minimum of six hours between doses.

Like most other antidepressants, bupropion should *never* be taken with a monoamine oxidase inhibitor (MAOI), since this combination may produce severe hypertension, seizures, fever, and even death. Individuals should wait at least two weeks after stopping an MAOI before switching to bupropion, and wait two weeks after stopping bupropion before beginning an MAOI.

Alcohol: People should not drink alcohol if they are taking antidepressants, since alcohol produces depressive-like symptoms and may increase the rate of metabolism of the antidepressant and lower its blood levels.

Food and beverages: No restrictions. If taking bupropion on an empty stomach upsets your stomach, try it with food or immediately after eating.

Possible drug interactions: Carbamazepine (Tegretol) reduces the blood levels of bupropion, resulting in a loss of antidepressant activity. Drugs that may affect the liver, such as cimetidine (Tagamet), phenobarbital, phenytoin (Dilantin), and others, should be used cautiously with bupropion. Because bupropion works on the norepinephrine and dopamine systems, those taking levodopa or carbidopa (Sinemet), medications that increase dopamine levels in the brain to treat Parkinson's disease, should use it with caution. The combination of these drugs may increase side effects such as hallucinations.

Use in pregnancy and breast-feeding: Pregnancy Category B

Bupropion is not recommended in women who are pregnant or contemplating pregnancy, since its effect on the fetus is not known. If they stop antidepressants during pregnancy, some women may experience a recurrence of their depression. In these circumstances, the physician should discuss the need to restart the medication or seek an alternative medication or treatment. Women should always consult with their physician if they are contemplating pregnancy or if they become pregnant while taking bupropion. Bupropion should be taken during pregnancy only if the benefits to the mother greatly outweigh any potential or unknown risks to the fetus. Women who are taking bupropion should not breast-feed, since small amounts of the drug will pass into the breast milk and be absorbed into the baby's bloodstream, leading to possible sedation and affecting the child's developing nervous system.

♀ **Use in children:** Small controlled clinical trials have found bupropion to be effective in treating attention deficit hyperactivity disorder (ADHD). It may possibly be effective in treating conduct disorder in children and residual symptoms of attention deficit hyperactivity disorder (ADHD) in adults. Because of its effects on the norepinephrine system, bupropion is considered a possible alternative to methylphenidate (Ritalin) or dextroamphetamine (see pages 364 and 352). The usual starting dose in children is 37.5 mg. twice a day of the immediate-release form (the 75-mg. tablet can be cut in half) and 50 mg. (half of the 100 mg. tablet) twice a day of the sustained-release form. The usual maximum dose in children is 250 mg. a day, and it is 400 mg. a day in adolescents.

🏠 **Use in seniors:** Bupropion is well tolerated by seniors; no special cautions or restrictions are indicated.

☠ **Overdosage:** The greatest risk of an overdose of bupropion is seizures. Individuals should be taken immediately to the emergency room so they can be carefully monitored. Other symptoms of overdose are hallucinations, delusions, and confusion. If overdose is suspected, bring the bottle of medication to the emergency room with the person, since the date when the medication was prescribed and the number of pills remaining in the bottle can provide helpful information to the treating physician.

Special considerations: Bupropion is an effective antidepressant that does not produce blood-pressure changes or electrocardiogram (EKG) changes at normal therapeutic doses. Consequently, it may be safely used in people with heart disease or in those recovering from a heart attack. Its primary drawback is an increased risk of seizures, a problem found largely in high-risk patients (i.e., those with a seizure disorder or who have experienced head trauma). It is not as effective as most other antidepressants in treating depression complicated by an anxiety disorder or eating disorders. Bupropion may be abruptly stopped without the risk of withdrawal symptoms.

 Generic name: CITALOPRAM

 Available in generic form: No

 Brand name: Celexa

Drug class: Selective serotonin reuptake inhibitor (SSRI)

Prescribed for: Depression (major depressive disorder, dysthymia, bipolar depression, and others), premenstrual dysphoric disorder, anorexia nervosa, bulimia nervosa, panic disorder, obsessive-compulsive disorder, borderline personality disorder, posttraumatic stress disorder, social anxiety disorder, generalized anxiety disorder, and selected impulse-control disorders. This drug was approved for the treatment of depression in 1998. Its usefulness in treating other mental disorders has not been firmly established. However, because other SSRIs have been shown to help people suffering from these conditions, citalopram is expected to be effective for them as well.

General information: Citalopram works similarly to the other SSRIs—fluoxetine (Prozac), sertraline (Zoloft), paroxetine (Paxil), and fluvoxamine (Luvox)—by blocking serotonin uptake and increasing the amount of serotonin available in the brain. As with all other antidepressant medications, citalopram takes from six to eight weeks to achieve maximum benefit. People with obsessive-compulsive disorder may not feel better for as long as twelve to sixteen weeks. The major advantages of this medication, like the other SSRIs, are safety, minimal side effects, and relative ease of administration.

Dosing information: Citalopram is available in 20- and 40-mg. scored tablets. The usual starting dose is 20 mg. once a day in the morning. After one to two weeks, the dose may be increased to 40 mg. The usual effective dose is between 20 and 40 mg. a day. Some persons may require doses up to 60 mg. a day, especially those suffering from obsessive-compulsive disorder.

Although its use in panic disorder has not been systematically studied, people with this condition should probably start with a dose of 10 mg. a day, then increase in 10-mg. increments weekly to a dose of 40 mg. a day. Some individuals may require an increase to 60 mg. a day; the additional dose should be taken in 10-mg. increments every two to four weeks.

Common side effects: The most common side effects reported in controlled clinical trials were dry mouth, increased sweating, nausea, tiredness, insomnia, diarrhea, and tremor. These trials indicated that the rate of sexual dysfunction with citalopram might be lower than that currently reported with other SSRIs; however, subsequent experience has revealed that the actual rates are similar to other SSRIs, in the 40 to 60 percent range. The primary sexual complaint to date has been ejaculatory delay or delayed orgasm. Some people may experience decreased desire or a lack of interest in sexual activity. In the clinical trials, patients experienced either no weight gain or slight weight loss.

Precautions: Like other antidepressants, citalopram may lower the seizure threshold, although the risk is believed to be lower than that of the tricyclic antidepressants and bupropion (Wellbutrin or Zyban). People with bipolar depression should first be placed on a mood stabilizer (such as lithium or divalproex [Depakote]), since citalopram may cause rapid "switching" from depression to mania. However, this occurs less often in people taking citalopram and other SSRIs than in those taking tricyclic antidepressants. Citalopram may be abruptly stopped without the risk of withdrawal symptoms, such as anxiety, depression, flu-like symptoms, and temperature elevation.

Warnings: Citalopram should *never* be taken with monoamine oxidase inhibitor (MAOI) antidepressants, since this combination may produce severe hypertension, seizures, fever, and even death. Individuals should wait at least two weeks after stopping citalopram before beginning an MAOI, and should wait at least two weeks after stopping an MAOI before beginning citalopram. Individuals who are taking two or more drugs that boost serotonin levels, such as an SSRI in combination with the serotonin antagonist antidepressant nefazodone (Serzone), may develop an uncommon, potentially deadly condition called serotonin syndrome, caused by excessive stimulation of the serotoninergic system. This syndrome can also occasionally occur in those taking a single SSRI, especially at higher doses. Initial symptoms include lethargy, restlessness, confusion, flushing, sweating, tremor, and involuntary muscle jerks. Over time, a small percentage of persons may develop muscle disorders, hyperthermia, and rigor, which may lead to respiratory problems, increased platelet clotting, destruction of red blood cells by the kidneys and their excretion in urine, and kidney failure. This syndrome requires emergency medical treatment and discontinuation of the serotonin-boosting medications.

Alcohol: People should not drink alcohol if they are taking antidepressants, since alcohol produces depressive-like symptoms and may increase the rate of metabolism of the antidepressant and lower its blood levels.

Food and beverages: No restrictions. If taking citalopram on an empty stomach upsets your stomach, try it with food or immediately after eating.

Possible drug interactions: In contrast to several of the other SSRIs, citalopram taken in combination with tricyclic antidepressants should generally *not* increase blood levels of the tricyclics. Possible exceptions are imipramine (Tofranil) and desipramine (Norpramin), so caution is essential in combining citalopram with these drugs.

Use in pregnancy and breast-feeding:
Pregnancy Category C

The effects of citalopram on the developing fetus in pregnant women are unknown. If they stop antidepressants during pregnancy, some women may experience a recurrence of their depression. In these circumstances, the physician should discuss the need to restart the medication or seek an alternative medication or treatment. Women should always consult with their physician if they are contemplating pregnancy or if they become pregnant while taking citalopram. Citalopram should be taken during pregnancy only if the benefits to the mother greatly outweigh any potential or unknown risks to the fetus. Women taking citalopram should not breast-feed, since small amounts of the drug will pass into the breast milk and be absorbed into the baby's bloodstream, leading to possible sedation and affecting the child's developing nervous system.

Use in children: This medication has not been studied in children. Because it has only recently been approved by the FDA for use in the United States, more information on its effectiveness in children should become available over the next several years.

Use in seniors: Citalopram has been shown to be effective in seniors. Because the liver of an older person metabolizes most drugs less well, lower doses, in the range of 20 to 40 mg. a day, may be prescribed. Seniors should begin with a dose of 10 mg. and increase it in 10-mg. increments weekly, as needed. Since many seniors take multiple medications, the effect of citalopram on the blood levels of their other drugs requires careful consideration. Citalopram has been reported to produce insomnia and because many older persons suffer sleep disturbances, its use should be monitored closely.

Overdosage: Two deaths have been reported in persons who took extremely high doses of citalopram. However, in contrast to the tricyclic antidepressants, overdoses of citalopram and the other SSRIs are generally less dangerous. This may not be the case when individuals overdose with multiple medications; other drugs can increase the risk of more serious complications. If an overdose is suspected, bring the bottle of medication to the emergency room with the person, since the date when the medication was prescribed and the number of pills remaining in the bottle can provide helpful information to the treating physician.

Special considerations: Because citalopram is less activating than fluoxetine (Prozac), those with depression and associated anxiety symptoms may tolerate it better than those with melancholic depression. Citalopram and the other SSRIs alone do not produce any cardiac side effects, so they are recommended for individuals with heart disease and those who develop depression following a heart attack, rather than a tricyclic antidepressant. Because citalopram is a relatively new drug, more clinical information is needed over the next several years to understand more fully its relative advantages and disadvantages.

 Generic name: CLOMIPRAMINE

 Available in generic form: Yes

 Brand name: Anafranil

Drug class: Tricyclic antidepressant

 Prescribed for: Obsessive-compulsive disorder, major depressive disorder, dysthymia (chronic mild to moderate depression), bipolar depression, panic disorder, insomnia.

General information: This is the newest of the tricyclic antidepressants. It is believed to work principally by increasing the amount of serotonin available in the central nervous system. Although clomipramine is approved by the FDA only for the treatment of obsessive-compulsive disorder, physicians also use it to treat refractory depression, panic disorder, and other conditions, as indicated above. In general it takes six to eight weeks at therapeutic dosage levels before clomipramine becomes fully effective. For obsessive-compulsive disorder, people may not experience significant symptom relief until after twelve to sixteen weeks of treatment, usually at higher doses than normally used to treat depression.

Dosing information: Clomipramine is available in 25-, 50-, and 75-mg. capsules. The usual starting dose is 25 to 50 mg., with 25- to 50-mg. increases on a weekly basis. The usual therapeutic dose in healthy adults is between 150 and 250 mg. daily. Because of its anticholinergic side effects, many people do not tolerate the high-dose ranges well. The daily dose of 250 mg. should not be exceeded because of the increased risk for seizures.

Common side effects: Clomipramine produces somewhat fewer anticholinergic side effects (see Glossary) than the tricyclic antidepressant amitriptyline (Elavil), but it does cause some of these effects, including drowsiness, dry mouth, blurred vision, constipation, esophageal reflux (heartburn), urinary retention, difficulty urinating, and orthostatic hypotension. Other side effects include sexual dysfunction (impotence, decreased desire), weight gain, irregular heartbeat (arrhythmias), and tremor.

Precautions: Men with an enlarged prostate should use this drug with caution because it may cause them difficulty in urinating. All antidepressants may increase the risk of seizures, but the risk may be greater for people taking clomipramine. Persons who are taking medications to prevent seizures and are prescribed clomipramine for depression may need to have their antiseizure medication carefully monitored and possibly increased in dose. To cope with dry mouth, they should drink water throughout the day or suck on sugarless candy. (Candy with sugar should be avoided, since the anticholinergic effects of this drug increase the possibility of tooth decay.) Exercise and high-fiber foods can lessen the risk of constipation. Some people may need to take a stool softener, such as Colace, or a bulk-forming agent, such as Metamucil, to counteract the constipating effects. Clomipramine should not be stopped suddenly because of the risk of severe withdrawal symptoms, such as increased anxiety, flu-like symptoms, depression, jitteriness, and agitation. It should be gradually tapered off over a period of several weeks to a month or more.

Warnings: People who have recently had a heart attack or who have a history of arrhythmias (irregular heartbeat) should not take clomipramine or other tricyclic antidepressants because of the increased risk of dangerous arrhythmias and sudden death. Clomipramine should *never* be taken with monoamine oxidase inhibitor (MAOI) antidepressants, since this combination may produce severe hypertension, seizures, fever, and even death. Individuals must wait at least two weeks after stopping clomipramine before beginning an MAOI, and wait two weeks after stopping an MAOI before beginning clomipramine.

Alcohol: People should not drink alcohol if they are taking antidepressants, since alcohol produces depressive-like symptoms and may increase the rate of metabolism of the antidepressant and lower its blood levels.

Food and beverages: No restrictions. If taking clomipramine on an empty stomach upsets your stomach, try it with food or immediately after eating.

Possible drug interactions: Clomipramine should not be used with the SSRIs, since these drugs, with the possible exception of citalopram, inhibit its metabolism, leading to very high blood levels and increasing the likelihood of seizures, arrhythmias (irregular heartbeats), confusion, and dizziness. Because of clomipramine's sedating effects, avoid other medications that may produce sedation, such as the benzodiazepines, antihistamines, and pain medications. Because it can lower blood pressure, clomipramine should be used with caution when taken with antihypertensive medications.

Use in pregnancy and breast-feeding: Pregnancy Category C

In general, tricyclic antidepressants are not recommended during pregnancy because their use in pregnancy has not been systematically studied. It is not known whether they increase birth defects or spontaneous miscarriages. If they stop taking clomipramine during pregnancy, some women may experience a recurrence of obsessive-compulsive symptoms or depression. In these circumstances, the physician should discuss the need to restart clomipramine or seek an alternative medication or treatment. Women should always consult with their physician if they are contemplating pregnancy or become pregnant while taking clomipramine. Women taking a tricyclic antidepressant should not breast-feed, since small amounts will pass into the breast milk and be absorbed into the baby's bloodstream, leading to possible sedation and affecting the child's developing nervous system.

Use in children:
Clomipramine has been studied as a treatment for obsessive-compulsive disorder in children over the age of ten and in adolescents. The safety and effectiveness of clomipramine in children under the age of ten have not been established. A starting dose of 25 mg. is generally recommended, with 25-mg. increases weekly, up to a maximum of 200 mg. a day, depending on body mass. The side effects experienced by children between ages ten to seventeen are similar to those in adults.

Use in seniors:
Lower doses of clomipramine are generally prescribed in seniors, usually in the range of 75 to 150 mg. a day. Its blood-pressure-lowering effects and the risk of orthostatic hypotension are greater in older people. Many older men also suffer from prostatic hypertrophy (enlarged prostate); they should avoid this medication because clomipramine may cause them difficulty in urinating. People over age fifty should have a baseline elec-

trocardiogram (EKG) before taking clomipramine, since it
prolongs the transmission of electrical impulses through
the heart, an effect that may result in potentially life-
threatening irregular heartbeats. Its anticholinergic effects
may produce confusion and disorientation, especially
in seniors or in those in the early stages of Alzheimer's
disease.

Overdosage: Psychiatrists are reluctant to prescribe clomipramine and other tricyclic antidepressants in persons who are at risk for suicide, since the
possibility of fatal overdose is high. If an overdose is suspected, bring the bottle of medication to the emergency
room with the person, since the date the medication was
prescribed and the number of pills remaining in the bottle
can provide helpful information to the treating physician.

Special considerations: Persons with bipolar disorder (manic-depressive illness) usually develop depression as well as mania at some time during the course
of their illness. Clomipramine and other tricyclic antidepressants may produce "switching," a clinical process
whereby a person goes rapidly from the depressive phase
of manic-depressive illness to the manic phase. Prior to
starting an antidepressant, individuals with bipolar disorder should take a mood stabilizer such as lithium or divalproex (Depakote). However, because even with a mood
stabilizer they may still experience switching when placed
on a tricyclic antidepressant, many physicians choose one
of the newer antidepressants, such as an SSRI, bupropion
(Wellbutrin or Zyban), or nefazodone (Serzone), which are
less likely to produce this effect.

Generic name: **DESIPRAMINE**

 Available in generic form: Yes

 Brand name: Norpramin, Pertofrane

 Drug class: Tricyclic antidepressant

Prescribed for: Major depressive disorder, dysthymia (chronic mild to moderate depression), bipolar depression, panic disorder, posttraumatic stress disorder, generalized anxiety disorder, social anxiety disorder, pain symptoms, migraine and tension headaches, insomnia.

General information: One of the older antidepressants, desipramine is a metabolite or by-product of imipramine (Tofranil) (see page 96). It is believed to work by increasing the amount of norepinephrine and, to a lesser extent, serotonin available in the central nervous system. Desipramine produces many bothersome side effects and may be potentially lethal if taken in overdose. Physical medicine specialists and orthopedic surgeons may prescribe it as an additional medication to treat various chronic pain syndromes. Primary-care physicians may prescribe it to treat insomnia. In general, it takes six to eight weeks at therapeutic dosage levels before desipramine becomes fully effective. After three to four weeks, there is usually some relief of symptoms, with more complete relief after six to eight weeks. In some cases, it may take as long as twelve weeks to achieve maximum benefit.

Dosing information: Desipramine is available in 10-, 25-, 50-, 75-, 100-, and 150-mg. tablets. It also comes in a 25- and 50-mg. capsule. Medication is usually begun at doses of 50 to 75 mg. at bedtime, and increased weekly in increments of 25 to 50 mg. until a daily dose of 150 to 200 mg. is reached. If depressive symptoms persist after eight weeks, the physician may increase the dose to 300 mg. per day, the usual maximum dose. For individuals with panic disorder, physicians prescribe 10 mg. a day and increase the dose in weekly increments of 10 mg. to prevent the onset or worsening of panic symptoms.

Common side effects: Desipramine is one of the most energizing or activating of the tricyclic antidepressants and produces fewer anticholinergic side effects (see Glossary). Other side effects include sweating, sexual dysfunction (impotence, decreased desire), weight gain, irregular heartbeats (arrhythmias), and tremor.

Precautions: Men with an enlarged prostate should use this drug with caution because desipramine may cause them difficulty in urinating. All antidepressants may increase the risk of seizures. Persons who are taking medications to prevent seizures and are prescribed desipramine for depression may need to have their anti-seizure medication carefully monitored and possibly increased in dose. To cope with dry mouth, individuals should drink water throughout the day or suck on sugarless candy. (Candy with sugar should be avoided, since the anticholinergic effects of this drug increase the possibility of tooth decay.) Exercise and high-fiber foods can lessen the risk of constipation. Some people may need to take a stool softener, such as Colace, or a bulk-forming agent, such as Metamucil, to counteract the constipating effects. Desipramine should not be stopped suddenly because of the risk of severe withdrawal symptoms, such as increased anxiety, flulike symptoms, depression, jitteriness, and agitation. It should be gradually tapered off over a period of several weeks to a month or more.

Warnings: Patients who become depressed following a heart attack should not take desipramine or other tricyclic antidepressants because of the increased risk of dangerous arrhythmias and sudden death. Desipramine should *never* be taken with monoamine oxidase inhibitor (MAOI) antidepressants, since this combination may produce severe hypertension, seizures, fever, and even death. Individuals must wait at least two weeks after stopping desipramine before beginning an MAOI, and wait two weeks after stopping an MAOI before beginning desipramine.

Alcohol: People should not drink alcohol if they are taking antidepressants, since alcohol produces depressive-like symptoms and may increase the rate of metabolism of the antidepressant and lower its blood levels.

Food and beverages: No restrictions. If taking desipramine on an empty stomach upsets your stomach, try it with food or immediately after eating.

Possible drug interactions: Desipramine should not be used with the SSRIs, since these drugs inhibit its metabolism, leading to very high blood levels and increasing the likelihood of seizures, arrhythmias (irregular heartbeats), confusion, and dizziness. Because of desipramine's sedating effects, avoid other medications that may produce sedation, such as the benzodiazepines, antihistamines, and pain medications. Because it can lower blood pressure, desipramine should be used with caution when taken with antihypertensive medication.

Use in pregnancy and breast-feeding:
Pregnancy Category C
In general, tricyclic antidepressants are not recommended during pregnancy because their use in pregnancy has not been systematically studied. It is not known whether they increase birth defects or spontaneous miscarriages. If they

stop taking antidepressants during pregnancy, some women may experience a recurrence of their depression. In these circumstances, the physician should discuss the need to restart the medication or seek an alternative medication or treatment. Women should always consult with their physician if they are contemplating pregnancy or if they become pregnant while taking desipramine. This drug should be taken during pregnancy only if the benefits to the mother greatly outweigh any potential or unknown risks to the fetus. Women taking a tricyclic antidepressant should not breast-feed, since small amounts will pass into the breast milk and be absorbed into the baby's bloodstream, leading to possible sedation and affecting the child's developing nervous system.

Use in children: Tricyclic antidepressants such as desipramine are sometimes prescribed in children for the treatment of bed-wetting, attention deficit hyperactivity disorder (ADHD), and depression. The usual recommended dose of desipramine is between 1 and 5 mg. per kilogram (approximately 2.2 pounds) of body weight per day. Because of recent reports of sudden death in young children taking tricyclic antidepressants, desipramine should be prescribed only by a child psychiatrist or a pediatrician skilled in the use of psychiatric medications and only if other medications have been unsuccessful.

Use in seniors: Lower doses of desipramine are prescribed in seniors, usually in the range of 100 to 150 mg. a day. Its blood-pressure-lowering effects and the risk of orthostatic hypotension and confusion are greater in older people. In addition, desipramine's adverse effects on the heart increase the risk of irregular heartbeats (arrhythmias) and even of death. People over age fifty should have a baseline electrocardiogram (EKG) before taking desipramine, since it prolongs the transmission of electrical impulses through the heart, an effect that may result in potentially life-threatening irregular heartbeats. Its anti-cholinergic effects may produce confusion and disorientation, especially in seniors or in those in early stages of Alzheimer's disease.

☠ **Overdosage:** Psychiatrists are reluctant to prescribe desipramine and other tricyclic antidepressants in persons at risk for suicide, since the possibility of fatal overdose is high. If overdose is suspected, bring the bottle of medication to the emergency room with the person, since the date when the medication was prescribed and the number of pills remaining in the bottle can provide helpful information to the treating physician.

✍ **Special considerations:** Since all antidepressants increase the risk of seizures, persons taking medications to prevent seizures who require antidepressant medication need careful monitoring and a possible increase in their anti-seizure medication.

Individuals with bipolar disorder (manic-depressive illness) usually develop depression as well as mania at some time during the course of their illness. Desipramine and other tricyclic antidepressants may produce "switching," a clinical process whereby a person goes from the depressive phase of manic-depressive illness to the manic phase. Prior to starting an antidepressant, individuals with bipolar disorder should take a mood stabilizer, such as lithium or divalproex (Depakote). However, because even with a mood stabilizer some people may still experience switching when placed on a tricyclic antidepressant, many psychiatrists select one of the newer antidepressants, such as an SSRI, bupropion (Wellbutrin or Zyban), or nefazodone (Serzone), which are less likely to produce this effect.

The major active metabolite of imipramine (Tofranil) is desipramine (Norpramin). Because desipramine produces fewer anticholinergic side effects (dry mouth, blurred vision, constipation, confusion, urinary retention) than imipramine, desipramine is preferred over imipramine by many psychiatrists.

 Generic name: **DOXEPIN**

 Available in generic form: Yes

 Brand name: Sinequan

 Drug class: Tricyclic antidepressant

Prescribed for: Major depressive disorder, dysthymia (chronic mild to moderate depression), bipolar depression, panic disorder, posttraumatic stress disorder, generalized anxiety disorder, social anxiety disorder, pain symptoms, migraine and tension headaches, insomnia.

General information: One of the older antidepressants, doxepin is believed to work by increasing the amount of norepinephrine and, to a lesser extent, serotonin, available in the central nervous system. Doxepin produces many bothersome side effects and may be potentially lethal if taken in overdose. Physical medicine specialists and orthopedic surgeons may prescribe it as an additional medication to treat various chronic pain syndromes. Primary-care physicians may prescribe it to treat insomnia. Psychiatrists may prescribe it to treat nausea or sleep disturbance in people taking SSRIs. In general, it takes six to eight weeks at therapeutic dosage levels before doxepin becomes fully effective. After three to four weeks, there is usually some relief of symptoms, with more complete relief after six to eight weeks. In some cases, it may take as long as twelve weeks to achieve maximum benefit.

Dosing information: Doxepin is available in 10-, 25-, 50-, 75-, 100-, and 150-mg. capsules and in oral concentrate. The usual initial dose is 50 to 75 mg. at bedtime, with 50- to 75-mg. increases weekly until a daily dose of 150 to 200 mg. is reached. If depressive symptoms persist after eight weeks, the physician may increase the dose up to 300 mg. per day.

Common side effects: Doxepin produces significant anticholinergic side effects (see Glossary), including drowsiness, dry mouth, blurred vision, constipation, esophageal reflux (heartburn), urinary retention or difficulty in urinating, and orthostatic hypotension. Other side effects include sexual dysfunction (impotence, decreased desire), weight gain, irregular heartbeats (arrhythmias), and tremor.

Precautions: Men with an enlarged prostate should use this drug with caution because doxepin may cause them difficulty in urinating. All antidepressants may increase the risk of seizures. Persons who are taking medications to prevent seizures and are prescribed doxepin for depression may need to have their anti-seizure medication carefully monitored and possibly increased in dose. To cope with dry mouth, individuals should drink water throughout the day or suck on sugarless candy. (Candy with sugar should be avoided, since the anticholinergic effects of this drug increase the possibility of tooth decay.) Exercise and high-fiber foods can lessen the risk of constipation. Some people may need to take a stool softener, such as Colace, or a bulk-forming agent, such as Metamucil, to counteract the constipating effects. Doxepin should not be stopped suddenly because of severe withdrawal symptoms, such as increased anxiety, flu-like symptoms, depression, jitteriness, and agitation. It should be gradually tapered off over a period of several weeks to a month or more.

Warnings: People who become depressed following a heart attack or who have a history of arrhythmias (irregular heartbeat) should not take doxepin because of the increased risk of dangerous, irregular heartbeats and sudden death. Doxepin should *never* be taken with monoamine oxidase inhibitor (MAOI) antidepressants since this combination may produce severe hypertension, seizures, fever, and even death. Individuals must wait at least two weeks after stopping doxepin before beginning an MAOI, and wait two weeks after stopping an MAOI before beginning doxepin.

Alcohol: People should not drink alcohol if they are taking antidepressants, since alcohol produces depressive-like symptoms and may increase the rate of metabolism of the antidepressant and lower its blood levels.

Food and beverages: No restrictions. If taking doxepin on an empty stomach upsets your stomach, try it with food or immediately after eating.

Possible drug interactions: Doxepin should not be used with the selective serotonin reuptake inhibitors since the SSRIs inhibit its metabolism, leading to very high blood levels and increasing the likelihood of seizures, arrhythmias (irregular heartbeats), confusion, and dizziness. Because of doxepin's sedating effects, other medications that may produce sedation, such as the benzodiazepines, antihistamines, and pain medications, should be avoided. Because it can lower blood pressure, doxepin should be used with caution when taken with antihypertensive medication.

**Use in pregnancy and breast-feeding:
Pregnancy Category C**
Doxepin is not recommended during pregnancy because its use in pregnancy has not been systematically studied. It

is not known whether it increases birth defects or spontaneous miscarriages. If they stop taking antidepressants during pregnancy, some women may experience a recurrence of their depression. In these circumstances, the physician should discuss the need to restart the medication or seek an alternative medication or treatment. Women should always consult with their physician if they are contemplating pregnancy or if they become pregnant while taking doxepin. Women who are taking a tricyclic antidepressant should not breast-feed, since small amounts will pass into the breast milk and be absorbed into the baby's bloodstream, leading to possible sedation and affecting the child's developing nervous system.

Use in children: Doxepin is usually not prescribed in children. Other tricyclic antidepressants, such as desipramine (Norpramin), imipramine (Tofranil), or nortriptyline (Pamelor), are sometimes used for the treatment of bed-wetting, attention deficit hyperactivity disorder (ADHD), and depression. Because of recent reports of deaths in young children taking tricyclic antidepressants, this class of antidepressants should be prescribed only by a child psychiatrist or a pediatrician skilled in the use of psychiatric medications and only if other medications have been unsuccessful.

Use in seniors: In general, lower doses of doxepin are prescribed for seniors, usually in the range of 75 to 150 mg. a day. Its blood-pressure-lowering effects and the risk of orthostatic hypotension and confusion are greater in older people. In addition, doxepin's adverse effects on the heart increase the risk of irregular heartbeats (arrhythmias) and even of death. People over age fifty should have a baseline electrocardiogram (EKG) before taking doxepin, since it prolongs the transmission of electrical impulses through the heart, an effect that may result in potentially life-threatening irregular heartbeats. Its anticholinergic effects may produce confusion and disorientation, especially in seniors or in those in early stages of Alzheimer's disease.

Overdosage: Psychiatrists are reluctant to prescribe doxepin and other tricyclic antidepressants in persons at risk for suicide, since the risk of fatal overdose is high. If overdose is suspected, bring the bottle of medication to the emergency room with the person, since the date when the medication was prescribed and the number of pills remaining in the bottle can provide helpful information to the treating physician.

Special considerations: Individuals with bipolar disorder (manic-depressive illness) usually develop depression in addition to mania at some time during the course of their illness. Doxepin and other tricyclic antidepressants may produce "switching," a clinical process whereby a person goes from the depressive phase of manic-depressive illness to the manic phase. Prior to starting an antidepressant, people with bipolar disorder should take a mood stabilizer such as lithium or divalproex (Depakote). However, because even with a mood stabilizer some patients may still experience switching when placed on a tricyclic antidepressant, many psychiatrists select one of the newer antidepressants, such as an SSRI, bupropion (Wellbutrin or Zyban), or nefazodone (Serzone), since these agents are less likely to have this effect.

 Generic name: FLUOXETINE

 Available in generic form: No

 Brand name: Prozac

Drug class: Selective serotonin reuptake inhibitor (SSRI)

Prescribed for: Depression (major depressive disorder, dysthymia [chronic mild to moderate depression], bipolar depression, and others), premenstrual dysphoric disorder, anorexia nervosa, bulimia nervosa, panic disorder, obsessive-compulsive disorder, borderline personality disorder, posttraumatic stress disorder, social anxiety disorder, generalized anxiety disorder, selected impulse control disorders. Although originally approved only for the treatment of depression, fluoxetine is now used clinically to treat a wide range of psychiatric conditions.

General information: Fluoxetine was the first of the antidepressants approved by the FDA that increase the amount of serotonin available in the brain by blocking its reuptake. As with other antidepressant medications, it takes from six to eight weeks to produce maximum benefit. People with obsessive-compulsive disorder may not feel better for as long as twelve to sixteen weeks. The major advantages of fluoxetine like the other SSRIs, are safety, minimal side effects, and relative ease of administration.

Dosing information: Fluoxetine is available in 10- and 20-mg. capsules, a scored 10-mg. tablet that can easily be broken in half, and an elixir (liquid form) at a strength of 20 mg. per 5 cc. of liquid. The usual starting dose is 10 mg. After one week to ten days, the dose is increased to 20 mg. The usual effective dose is between 20 and 40 mg. a day. For people with obsessive-compulsive disorder, the daily dose is usually in the 40- to 80-mg. range. Doses greater than 80 mg. are generally not necessary. Fluoxetine is usually taken in the morning in a single dose, although some people taking doses of 40 mg. or more prefer to take it twice a day to decrease temporary side effects such as nausea and agitation.

For panic disorder, physicians usually prescribe an initial dose of 5 mg. (one-half of a 10-mg. tablet) a day and increase the dosage slowly to the same therapeutic dose range as required to treat depression. A lower dose is used initially to decrease the likelihood of the medication triggering a panic attack.

Common side effects: The most common side effects reported in controlled clinical trials were nervousness, agitation, headache, tremor, dry mouth, nausea, gastrointestinal symptoms (diarrhea or cramping), and tremor. Individuals may also experience insomnia early in treatment, a symptom that sometimes persists. Some people report daytime sedation, without insomnia or as a result of insomnia. If insomnia persists, the physician may prescribe an additional medication for sleep, for instance, a sedating antidepressant such as trazodone (Desyrel) (see page 137); a benzodiazepine, such as temazepam (Restoril) (see page 263), or the nonbenzodiazepine hypnotic agent zolpidem (Ambien) (see page 276).

Similar to the other SSRIs, fluoxetine produces a relatively high rate of sexual dysfunction, affecting 40 to 60 percent of those taking the drug. The most frequent types are delayed orgasm in women and retarded ejaculation in men. Some experience decreased desire or lack of interest in sexual activity. Some people who have been on fluoxetine for a long period of time report weight gain. The cause of this side effect is unclear.

Precautions: As with other antidepressants, SSRIs may increase the likelihood of seizures, although the risk is believed to be lower than with the tricyclic antidepressants and bupropion (Wellbutrin or Zyban). People with bipolar depression should first be placed on a mood stabilizer, such as lithium or divalproex (Depakote), since fluoxetine may cause rapid "switching" from depression to mania. This occurs less often in people taking fluoxetine and other SSRIs than in those taking tricyclic antidepressants. Fluoxetine is the only SSRI that can be stopped abruptly without withdrawal symptoms (anxiety, depression, elevated temperature, restlessness, and flu-like symptoms). This is because of its long half-life of several weeks to a month (see Glossary), and its slow elimination from the body.

Warnings: A small percentage of people (1 to 4 percent) may develop a rash and associated aches, joint pain, and elevated temperature. If you do, stop the medication immediately and contact your physician. Generally, those who develop a rash with fluoxetine are switched to another SSRI or an antidepressant in a different drug class. Rarely, a small percentage of individuals may experience an increase in bleeding, which is believed to be due to the effect of fluoxetine on platelets. Fluoxetine should *never* be taken with monoamine oxidase inhibitors (MAOIs), since this combination may produce severe hypertension, seizures, fever, and even death. Individuals should wait at least four weeks after stopping fluoxetine before beginning an MAOI and wait at least two weeks after stopping an MAOI before beginning fluoxetine. Individuals who are taking two or more drugs that boost serotonin levels, such as an SSRI in combination with the serotonin antagonist antidepressant nefazodone (Serzone), may develop an uncommon, potentially deadly condition called serotonin syndrome, caused by excessive stimulation of the serotoninergic system. This syndrome can also occasionally occur in those taking a single SSRI, especially at higher doses. Initial symptoms include lethargy, restlessness, confusion, flushing, sweating, tremor, and involuntary muscle jerks. Over time, a small percentage of persons may develop muscle disorders, hyperthermia, and rigor, which may lead to respiratory problems, increased platelet clotting, destruction of red blood cells by the kidneys and their excretion in urine, and kidney failure. This syndrome requires emergency medical treatment and discontinuation of the serotonin-boosting medications.

Alcohol: People should not drink alcohol if they are taking antidepressants, since alcohol produces depressive-like symptoms and may increase the rate of metabolism of the antidepressant and lower its blood levels.

Food and beverages: No restrictions. If taking fluoxetine on an empty stomach upsets your stomach, try it with food or immediately after eating.

Possible drug interactions: Fluoxetine has been reported to increase blood levels of phenytoin (Dilantin), an anti-seizure medication, certain antipsychotic medications, including haloperidol (Haldol), clozapine (Clozaril), and pimozide (Orap), selected benzodiazepines, including alprazolam (Xanax) and diazepam (Valium), and lithium. When used with the anticoagulant warfarin (Coumadin), fluoxetine may significantly prolong bleeding time. Fluoxetine may also increase blood levels of the antihypertensive agent propranolol (Inderal), slowing the heart considerably and producing dizziness, tiredness, and arrhythmias.

The combination of fluoxetine and tricyclic antidepressants requires extreme caution because fluoxetine significantly increases the blood levels of the tricyclic, leading to possible cardiac arrhythmias and other serious adverse side effects.

Use in pregnancy and breast-feeding:
Pregnancy Category C

There is an extensive database on the use of fluoxetine in women during pregnancy, and it is believed that there is no increased risk to them or the fetus if they take fluoxetine during pregnancy. However, women should always consult with their physician if they are contemplating pregnancy or if they become pregnant while taking fluoxetine, since its effects on the developing fetus have not been conclusively established. Women taking fluoxetine should not breast-feed, since small amounts of the drug will pass into the breast milk and be absorbed into the baby's bloodstream, leading to possible sedation and other unknown effects on the child's developing nervous system.

Use in children: Although its use has not been systematically studied in children, fluoxetine is prescribed to treat obsessive-compulsive disorder, depression, eating disorders, and attention deficit hyperactivity disorder (ADHD) in children. The dosage ranges reported in the literature are similar to those used in adults.

Use in seniors: Fluoxetine has been shown to be effective in treating obsessive-compulsive disorder and depression in seniors. Because the liver of an older person does not metabolize most drugs as well as in earlier years, slightly lower doses may be prescribed. Most seniors respond well to a 20-mg. dose, although some with obsessive-compulsive disorder may require a dose of 40 mg. Since many seniors take multiple medications, the effect of fluoxetine on the blood levels of other medications must be carefully monitored. Because many older persons suffer sleep disturbances, fluoxetine should be monitored closely, since it has been reported to increase insomnia.

Overdosage: In contrast to the tricyclic antidepressants, overdoses of fluoxetine and the other SSRIs are generally much less dangerous, especially when taken alone. There have been two deaths reported from a massive overdose of fluoxetine; in both cases, the drug was combined with other medications. More often individuals overdose with multiple medications, and the other drugs may increase the risk of more serious complications. If overdose is suspected, bring the bottle of medication to the emergency room with the person, since the date when the medication was prescribed and the number of pills remaining in the bottle can provide helpful information to the treating physician.

 Special considerations: Because fluoxetine is the most activating of the SSRIs, individuals with depression and associated anxiety symptoms often tolerate it less well than those with melancholic depression. Fluoxetine and the other SSRIs alone do not produce any cardiac side effects and are recommended for persons with heart disease or who develop depression following a heart attack, rather than a tricyclic antidepressant.

 Generic name: **FLUVOXAMINE**

 Available in generic form: No

 Brand name: Luvox

Drug class: Selective serotonin reuptake inhibitor (SSRI)

Prescribed for: Fluvoxamine was approved by the FDA only for the treatment of obsessive-compulsive disorder; consequently, its usefulness in treating other mental disorders has not been firmly established. However, it is believed to be effective in treating the same disorders as the other SSRIs: depression (major depressive disorder, dysthymia, bipolar depression, and others), premenstrual dysphoric disorder, anorexia nervosa, bulimia nervosa, panic disorder, borderline personality disorder, posttraumatic stress disorder, social anxiety disorder, generalized anxiety disorder, selected impulse control disorders.

General information: Fluvoxamine and other SSRIs increase the amount of serotonin available in the brain by blocking its reuptake. As with other antidepressants, fluvoxamine and other SSRIs take from six to eight weeks to produce maximum benefit. Those with obsessive-compulsive disorder may not feel better for as long as twelve to sixteen weeks. The major advantages of this medication, like the other SSRIs, are safety, minimal side effects, and relative ease of administration.

Dosing information: Fluvoxamine is available in 25-, 50-, and 100-mg. tablets. The usual starting dose is 50 mg. of fluvoxamine at bedtime; the dose is increased 50 mg. weekly. The usual therapeutic dose is between 100 and 200 mg. a day, although some people may require up to 300 mg. Because fluvoxamine has a relatively short half-life (see Glossary), when doses are greater than 100 mg. it is usually prescribed in two equal doses, taken once during the day and once at night. However, fluvoxamine is quite sedating, so a larger dose may be taken at bedtime if the person experiences daytime sedation.

Common side effects: The most common side effects are daytime sedation, dizziness, headache, weakness, nausea, various gastrointestinal symptoms (diarrhea, constipation, cramping), tremors, and excessive sweating. Insomnia, though it occurs, is less common than with the other SSRIs.

Similar to other SSRIs, fluvoxamine produces a relatively high rate of sexual dysfunction, affecting 40 to 60 percent of those taking the drug. The most frequent types are delayed orgasm in women and retarded ejaculation in men. Some people may experience decreased desire or lack of interest in sexual activity. Another recently reported side effect is increased weight gain in people who have been on fluvoxamine for a long period of time (a year or more). The cause of this side effect is unclear.

Precautions: As with other antidepressants, fluvoxamine may increase the likelihood of seizures, although the risk is believed to be lower than that of the tricyclic antidepressants and bupropion (Wellbutrin or Zyban). Individuals with bipolar depression should first be placed on a mood stabilizer, such as lithium or divalproex (Depakote), since fluvoxamine may cause rapid "switching" from depression to mania. This occurs less often in those taking fluvoxamine and other SSRIs than in those taking tricyclic antidepressants. Fluvoxamine should not be stopped suddenly because of the risk of severe withdrawal symptoms, such as anxiety, depression, flu-like symptoms, and temperature elevation. Fluvoxamine should be tapered off over a period of several weeks to a month or more.

Warnings: Fluvoxamine should *never* be taken with monoamine oxidase inhibitors (MAOIs), since this combination may produce severe hypertension, seizures, fever, and even death. Individuals should wait at least two weeks after stopping fluvoxamine before beginning an MAOI and wait two weeks after stopping an MAOI before beginning fluvoxamine. Individuals who are taking two or more drugs that boost serotonin levels, such as an SSRI in combination with the serotonin antagonist antidepressant nefazodone (Serzone), may develop an uncommon, potentially deadly condition called serotonin syndrome, caused by excessive stimulation of the serotoninergic system. This syndrome can also occasionally occur in those taking a single SSRI, especially at higher doses. Initial symptoms include lethargy, restlessness, confusion, flushing, sweating, tremor, and involuntary muscle jerks. Over time, a small percentage of persons may develop muscle disorders, hyperthermia, and rigor, which may lead to respiratory problems, increased platelet clotting, destruction of red blood cells by the kidneys and their excretion in urine, and kidney failure. This syndrome requires emergency medical treatment and discontinuation of the serotonin-boosting medications.

⏳ **Alcohol:** People should not drink alcohol if they are taking antidepressants, since alcohol produces depressive-like symptoms and may increase the rate of metabolism of the antidepressant and lower its blood levels.

🍽 **Food and beverages:** No restrictions. If taking fluvoxamine on an empty stomach upsets your stomach, try it with food or immediately after eating.

💊 **Possible drug interactions:** Fluvoxamine may increase the blood levels of the antihistamine astemizole (Hismanal) and the anti-heartburn agent cisapride (Propulsid). These drugs should not be used with fluvoxamine because at high doses they may produce irregular heartbeats (arrhythmias) and death. Fluvoxamine may increase blood levels of the benzodiazepines alprazolam (Xanax) and diazepam (Valium), leading to excessive sedation and lack of coordination. Fluvoxamine may increase blood levels of the decongestant theophylline, leading to increased nervousness or anxiety. When used with the anticoagulant warfarin (Coumadin), fluvoxamine may significantly prolong bleeding time. Fluvoxamine may decrease the blood levels of the antihypertensive agent propanolol (Inderal), slowing the heart considerably and leading to dizziness, tiredness, and arrhythmias. Because of its sedating effects, other medications that produce sedation, such as the benzodiazepines, antihistamines, and pain medications, should be avoided.

If fluvoxamine is combined with tricyclic antidepressants, it may increase blood levels of the tricyclic drugs, leading to possible cardiac arrhythmias and conduction abnormalities in the heart (although much less than with the other SSRIs). Used alone, fluvoxamine and the other SSRIs do not produce any cardiac side effects and are recommended for persons who develop depression following a heart attack.

Use in pregnancy and breast-feeding: Pregnancy Category C

The effects of fluvoxamine on the developing fetus in pregnant women are unknown. If they stop antidepressants during pregnancy, some women may experience a recurrence of their depression. In these circumstances, the physician should discuss the need to restart the medication or seek an alternative medication or treatment. Women should always consult with their physician if they are contemplating pregnancy or if they become pregnant while taking fluvoxamine. It should be taken during pregnancy only if the benefits to the mother greatly outweigh any potential unknown risks to the fetus. Women taking fluvoxamine should not breast-feed, since small amounts of the drug will pass into the breast milk and be absorbed into the baby's bloodstream, leading to possible sedation and other unknown effects on the child's developing nervous system.

Use in children: Fluvoxamine was studied in children between the ages of eight and seventeen to treat obsessive-compulsive disorder and found to be effective. Child psychiatrists may also use fluvoxamine in children to treat depression and attention deficit hyperactivity disorder (ADHD). The dosage for children is similar to that in adults, 50 to 200 mg. a day, usually given in two equal doses.

Use in seniors: Fluvoxamine is believed to be effective in treating depression, obsessive-compulsive disorder, and other anxiety disorders in seniors. Because the liver of an older person does not metabolize most drugs as well as in earlier years, slightly lower doses (50 to 100 mg.) may be prescribed. Since many seniors take multiple medications, the effect of fluvoxamine on the blood levels of other medications must be carefully monitored.

Overdosage: In contrast to the tricyclic antidepressants, fluvoxamine, the other SSRIs, and other newer antidepressants are generally much safer in overdose, especially when taken alone. However, individuals often overdose with multiple medications, and other drugs may increase the risk of more serious complications. If overdose occurs, bring the bottle of medication to the emergency room with the person, since the date when the medication was prescribed and the number of pills remaining in the bottle can provide helpful information to the treating physician.

 Special considerations: Because fluvoxamine is the most sedating of the SSRIs, physicians generally prescribe it for those individuals with significant anxiety or sleep disturbance. Fluvoxamine and the other SSRIs alone do not produce any cardiac side effects and are recommended for persons with heart disease or who develop depression following a heart attack, rather than a tricyclic antidepressant.

 Generic name: **IMIPRAMINE IMIPRAMINE PAMOATE**

 Available in generic form: Yes

 Brand name: Tofranil, Tofranil-PM (sustained-release), SK-Pramine, and Janimine

Drug class: Tricyclic antidepressant

Prescribed for: Major depressive disorder, dysthymia (chronic mild to moderate depression), bipolar depression, panic disorder, posttraumatic stress disorder, generalized anxiety disorder, social anxiety disorder, pain symptoms, migraine and tension headaches, insomnia.

General information: One of the older antidepressants, imipramine is believed to work by increasing the amount of norepinephrine and, to a lesser extent, serotonin available in the central nervous system. Imipramine produces many bothersome side effects and may be potentially lethal if taken in overdose. Physical medicine specialists and orthopedic surgeons may prescribe it as an additional medication to treat chronic pain syndromes. Primary-care physicians may prescribe it to treat insomnia. In general, it takes six to eight weeks at therapeutic dosage levels before imipramine becomes fully effective. After three to four weeks, there is usually some relief of symptoms, with more complete relief after six to eight weeks. In some cases, it may take as long as twelve weeks to achieve maximum benefit. Imipramine is viewed as the "gold standard" medication against which newer antidepressants are usually compared, particularly when a pharmaceutical company is seeking FDA approval of a new antidepressant. One of imipramine's metabolites or by-products is desipramine (Norpramin).

Dosing information: Imipramine is available in 10-, 25-, and 50-mg. tablets and 25- and 50-mg. capsules. Tofranil-PM comes in 75-, 100-, 125-, and 150-mg. tablets. Medication is usually begun at doses of 50 to 75 mg. at bedtime, with an increase weekly in 25- to 50-mg. increments. The usual therapeutic dose is between 150 and 200 mg. a day. If depressive symptoms persist after eight weeks, the physician may increase the dose to 300 mg. For individuals with panic disorder, the initial dose is usually 10 to 25 mg. a day, with an increase in 10- to 25-mg. increments weekly. This is done to prevent the onset or worsening of panic symptoms, since imipramine is activating or energizing and may worsen anxiety or panic symptoms if it is begun at too high a dose.

Common side effects: Imipramine produces significant anticholinergic side effects (see Glossary), including drowsiness, dry mouth, blurred vision, constipation, esophageal reflux (heartburn), urinary retention or difficulty in urinating, and orthostatic hypotension. Other side effects include sexual dysfunction (impotence, decreased desire), weight gain, irregular heartbeats (arrhythmias), and tremor.

Precautions: Men with an enlarged prostate should use this drug with caution because it may cause them difficulty in urinating. All antidepressants may increase the risk of seizures. Persons who are taking medications to prevent seizures and are prescribed imipramine for depression may need to have their anti-seizure medication carefully monitored and possibly increased in dose.

To cope with dry mouth, individuals should drink water throughout the day or suck on sugarless candy. (Candy with sugar should be avoided, since the anticholinergic effects of this drug increase the possibility of tooth decay.) Exercise and high-fiber foods can lessen the risk of constipation. Some people may need to take a stool softener, such as Colace, or a bulk-forming agent, such as Metamucil, to counteract the constipating effects. Imipramine should not be stopped suddenly because of severe withdrawal symptoms, such as increased anxiety, flu-like symptoms, depression, jitteriness, and agitation. It should be gradually tapered off over a period of several weeks to a month or more.

Warnings: People who become depressed following a heart attack or who have a history of arrhythmias (irregular heartbeats) should not take imipramine because of the increased risk of dangerous, irregular heartbeats and sudden death. Imipramine should *never* be taken with monoamine oxidase inhibitor (MAOI) antidepressants, since this combination may produce severe hypertension, seizures, fever, and even death. Individuals must wait at least two weeks after stopping imipramine before beginning an MAOI, and wait two weeks after stopping an MAOI before beginning imipramine.

Alcohol: People should not drink alcohol if they are taking antidepressants, since alcohol produces depressive-like symptoms and may increase the rate of metabolism of the antidepressant and lower its blood level.

Food and beverages: No restrictions. If taking imipramine on an empty stomach upsets your stomach, try it with food or immediately after eating.

Possible drug interactions: Imipramine should not be used with the selective serotonin reuptake inhibitors, since the SSRIs inhibit its metabolism, leading to very high blood levels and increasing likelihood of seizures, arrhythmias (irregular heartbeats), confusion, and dizziness. Because of imipramine's sedating effects, other medications that may produce sedation, such as the benzodiazepines, antihistamines, and pain medications, should be avoided. Because it can lower blood pressure, imipramine should be used with caution if taken with antihypertensive medication.

Use in pregnancy and breast-feeding: Pregnancy Category B

In general, imipramine is not recommended during pregnancy because its use in pregnancy has not been systematically studied. It is not known whether it increases birth defects or spontaneous miscarriages. If they stop taking imipramine during pregnancy, some women may experience a recurrence of their depression. In these circumstances, the physician should discuss the need to restart imipramine. Women should always consult with their physician if they are contemplating pregnancy or if they become pregnant while taking imipramine. Women taking a tricyclic antidepressant should not breast-feed, since small amounts will pass into the breast milk and be absorbed into the baby's bloodstream, leading to possible sedation and affecting the child's developing nervous system.

Use in children: Tricyclic antidepressants such as imipramine are sometimes prescribed in children for the treatment of bed-wetting, attention deficit hyperactivity disorder (ADHD), and depression. The usual recommended dose is between 1 and 5 mg. per kilogram (approximately 2.2 pounds) of body weight per day, and the FDA recommends not exceeding this dose. Because of recent reports of sudden death in young children taking tricyclic antidepressants, imipramine should be prescribed only by a child psychiatrist or a pediatrician skilled in the use of psychiatric medications and only if trials of other medications have been unsuccessful.

Use in seniors: In general, lower doses of imipramine are prescribed for seniors, usually in the range of 75 to 150 mg. a day. Its blood-pressure-lowering effects and the risk of orthostatic hypotension and possible confusion are greater in older people. In addition, imipramine's adverse effects on the heart increase the risk of irregular heartbeats (arrhythmias) and even death. People over age fifty should have a baseline electrocardiogram (EKG) before taking imipramine, since it prolongs the transmission of electrical impulses through the heart, an effect that may result in potentially life-threatening irregular heartbeats. Its anticholinergic effects may produce confusion and disorientation, especially in seniors or in those in early stages of Alzheimer's disease.

☠ **Overdosage:** Psychiatrists are reluctant to prescribe imipramine and other tricyclic antidepressants in persons at risk for suicide, since the risk of fatal overdose is high. If overdose is suspected, bring the bottle of medication to the emergency room with the person, since the date when the medication was prescribed and the number of pills remaining in the bottle can provide helpful information to the treating physician.

♔ **Special considerations:** Persons who become depressed following a heart attack should not take imipramine or another tricyclic antidepressant because of the increased risk of sudden death, probably related to the possibility of irregular heartbeats (arrhythmias).

Individuals with bipolar disorder (manic-depressive illness) usually develop depression as well as mania at some time during the course of their illness. Imipramine and other tricyclic antidepressants may produce "switching," a clinical process whereby a person goes from the depressive phase of manic-depressive illness to the manic phase. Prior to starting an antidepressant, people with bipolar disorder should take a mood stabilizer, such as lithium or divalproex (Depakote). However, because even with a mood stabilizer some people may still experience switching when placed on a tricyclic antidepressant, many psychiatrists select one of the newer antidepressants, such as an SSRI, bupropion (Wellbutrin or Zyban), or nefazodone (Serzone), which are less likely to produce this effect.

The major active metabolite of imipramine is desipramine (Norpramin). Because desipramine produces fewer anticholinergic side effects (dry mouth, blurred vision, constipation, confusion, urinary retention) than imipramine, desipramine is preferred over imipramine by many psychiatrists.

Generic name: **MIRTAZAPINE**

 Available in generic form: No

 Brand name: Remeron

 Drug class: (alpha₂) receptor antagonist and 5-HT₂ and 5-HT₃ antagonist

 Prescribed for: Depression, panic disorder, post-traumatic stress disorder, insomnia.

General information: Mirtazapine, one of the newest antidepressants to become available in the United States, blocks two serotonin receptor subtypes, the 5-HT₂ and 5-HT₃ receptors. When stimulated, these receptors are believed to produce nausea, vomiting, gastrointestinal distress, anxiety, and sexual dysfunction, symptoms that often occur with other antidepressants. Consequently, people taking mirtazapine generally do not develop these symptoms. Through its effect on the norepinephrine system, mirtazapine increases the amount of norepinephrine available in the central nervous system, producing its antidepressant effects. Because it is quite sedating, it may have limited use in persons with "retarded" depression, which is characterized by lethargy, tiredness, and excessive sleeping, but it may be especially well tolerated in people with depression complicated by anxiety or in those with depression and significant insomnia.

Dosing information: Mirtazapine is available in 15-, 30-, and 45-mg. scored tablets. Generally, the initial dose is 15 mg. at bedtime, with an increase after a week to 30 mg. Paradoxically, the 30-mg. dose is reported to produce less sedation than the 15-mg. dose, possibly because of the increased effects on norepinephrine at 30 mg., which is associated with greater energy and alertness. The usual effective dose is between 30 and 45 mg. at bedtime, although some people may require doses up to 60 mg., the usual maximum dose.

Common side effects: The most common side effects of mirtazapine are sedation, dry mouth, constipation, dizziness, increased appetite, and weight gain. Like bupropion (Wellbutrin or Zyban) and nefazodone (Serzone), mirtazapine does not produce sexual dysfunction, so is a good alternative for persons who develop this problem with other antidepressants.

Precautions: Because most people taking mirtazapine gain weight even during early stages of treatment and are unable to lose it, it should be used cautiously in individuals who are overweight or who want to lose weight. Although mirtazapine has rarely been associated with the production of rapid switching from depression to mania in bipolar individuals, persons with bipolar depression should be placed on a mood stabilizer, either lithium or divalproex (Depakote), prior to beginning mirtazapine. As with other antidepressants, mirtazapine may increase the risk of seizures, although this risk is believed to be quite low.

Warnings: There have been reports of a slight increase in liver-function test abnormalities with mirtazapine and an increase in non-fasting cholesterol and triglyceride levels. During clinical trials, two cases of agranulocytosis (no production of white blood cells) and one case of neutropenia (a reduction in white-blood-cell production) were reported. The individuals recovered after discontinuing mirtazapine. Anyone who develops sore throat and fever along with a reduced white-blood-cell count should discontinue mirtazapine and be carefully followed up by a physician.

Alcohol: People should not drink alcohol if they are taking antidepressants, since alcohol produces depressive-like symptoms and may increase the rate of metabolism of the antidepressant and lower its blood levels.

Food and beverages: No restrictions. If taking mirtazapine on an empty stomach upsets your stomach, try it with food or immediately after eating.

Possible drug interactions: Like most antidepressants, mirtazapine should *never* be taken with monoamine oxidase inhibitors (MAOIs), since this combination may produce severe hypertension, high fevers, seizures, and even death. Individuals should wait at least two weeks after stopping an MAOI before switching to mirtazapine, and wait two weeks after stopping mirtazapine before switching to an MAOI. Because of mirtazapine's sedating effects, other medications that produce sedation, such as the benzodiazepines, antihistamines, and pain medications, should be avoided. Because of mirtazapine's potential effect on the liver, periodic tests of liver function, triglycerides, and cholesterol levels may be indicated.

Use in pregnancy and breast-feeding: Pregnancy Category C

As with many other antidepressants, the effects of mirtazapine on the developing fetus are unknown. Women should always consult their physician if they are taking mirtazapine and either are contemplating pregnancy or become pregnant. The medication should be taken during pregnancy only if its benefits for the woman outweigh any potential unknown risks to the fetus. Women taking mirtazapine should not breast-feed, since small amounts of the drug will pass into breast milk and be absorbed into the baby's bloodstream, leading to possible sedation and other unknown effects on the child's developing nervous system.

Use in children: There is little information concerning mirtazapine's use in children. Its safety and general effectiveness in children and adolescents have not been established.

Use in seniors: Mirtazapine is reported to be as effective in older people as in healthy young adults. Because of its sedating effects, a slightly lower starting dose of 7.5 to 15 mg. is advised. The usual effective dose in seniors is 30 mg.

Overdosage: In contrast to the tricyclic antidepressants, mirtazapine is much safer in overdose, especially when taken alone. More often, individuals overdose with multiple medications, and other drugs may increase the risk of more serious complications. Significant sedation is the most common effect of an overdose with mirtazapine. If overdose is suspected, bring the bottle of medication to the emergency room with the person, since the date when the medication was prescribed and the number of pills remaining in the bottle can provide helpful information to the treating physician.

Special considerations: Mirtazapine may be an effective alternative for persons who develop sexual dysfunction or sleep disturbance on SSRIs, venlafaxine (Effexor), tricyclic antidepressants, or MAO inhibitors. In addition, mirtazapine may be beneficial for persons with depression and a chronic medical illness who have lost considerable weight because of their illness or its treatment (e.g., cancer patients undergoing chemotherapy). Mirtaza-pine can be stopped abruptly without withdrawal symptoms.

Generic name: NEFAZODONE

 Available in generic form: No

 Brand name: Serzone

 Drug class: 5-HT$_2$ antagonist

Prescribed for: Depression (especially when complicated by anxiety or insomnia), panic disorder, generalized anxiety disorder, posttraumatic stress disorder, social anxiety disorder, migraine headaches.

General information: In addition to being a serotonin reuptake inhibitor, nefazodone blocks a specific serotonin (5-HT) receptor subtype, the 5-HT$_2$ receptor. It is also thought to be a weak inhibitor of norepinephrine reuptake. Nefazodone is as effective as the SSRIs and the older antidepressants, tricyclics, and MAOIs, and may be especially effective in the treatment of posttraumatic stress disorder and depression complicated by insomnia, anxiety, and migraine headaches.

Dosing information: Nefazodone is available in 50-, 100-, 150-, 200-, and 250-mg. tablets. The usual starting dose is 50 mg. twice a day, with increases weekly in 100-mg. increments. The usual therapeutic dose is between 400 and 600 mg. a day, either in equal doses in the morning and at bedtime or, if light-headedness or sedation occur during the day, a larger amount or the entire dose at bedtime. The medication may be abruptly stopped without the risk of withdrawal reactions.

Common side effects: The most common side effects are sedation, light-headedness, dizziness, visual trails (an afterimage in peripheral vision when tracking objects), and, as with the other serotonin-type antidepressants, nausea, dry mouth, headaches, and occasional restlessness.

Like mirtazapine (Remeron) and bupropion (Wellbutrin or Zyban), nefazodone does not produce sexual dysfunction, so it is a good alternative for persons who develop this problem with other antidepressants. In addition, nefazodone does not interfere with sleep, and may even improve sleep in persons with depression complicated by insomnia.

Precautions: For people with liver disease, the metabolism of the drug may be reduced. Consequently, lower doses should be taken by these people. Also, although nefazodone usually does not lower blood pressure, it should be taken with caution by people on antihypertensive medications, since it produces dizziness and light-headedness.

Warnings: Certain drugs should be avoided because of interactions. Nefazodone should *never* be taken with a monoamine oxidase inhibitor (MAOI), since this combination may produce severe hypertension, seizures, fever, and even death. Individuals must wait at least two weeks after stopping nefazodone before beginning an MAOI, and wait two weeks after stopping an MAOI before beginning nefazodone. There have been two reports of liver failure in persons taking nefazodone, but this is believed to be rare. Unlike the 5-HT$_2$ antagonist trazodone (Desyrel), nefazodone has not been reported to produce priapisms (prolonged or painful erections).

 Alcohol: People should not drink alcohol if they are taking antidepressants because alcohol produces depressive-like symptoms and may increase the rate of metabolism of the antidepressant and lower its blood levels.

Food and beverages: No restrictions; however, food may decrease its absorption. If taking nefazodone on an empty stomach upsets your stomach, try it with food or immediately after eating.

Possible drug interactions: Nefazodone is metabolized somewhat differently from the tricyclic antidepressants and some of the SSRIs. Caution must be taken when nefazodone is prescribed with alprazolam (Xanax) or triazolam (Halcion), since it increases the blood levels of both. In addition, nefazodone should not be taken with the antihistamines terfenadine (Seldane), which was recently removed from the market, and astemizole (Hismanal), the antibiotic erythromycin, the antifungal agent ketoconazole (Nizoral), and the heartburn medication cisapride (Propulsid) because of the increased risk of irregular heartbeats (arrhythmias). With the exception of fluoxetine (Prozac), persons switching from an SSRI to nefazodone should wait two weeks to avoid a drug interaction that can cause agitation and anxiety. Because of its long half-life, individuals who have been taking fluoxetine (Prozac) should be off this medication for four weeks prior to beginning nefazodone.

Use in pregnancy and breast-feeding: Pregnancy Category C

Nefazodone has not been studied in pregnant women, and the effects of nefazodone on the developing fetus are unknown. Women should always consult with their physician if they are taking nefazodone and are contemplating pregnancy or become pregnant. Although there is no evidence to suggest that nefazodone may increase the risk of miscarriage or fetal malformations, it should be used only if the benefits to the mother outweigh any potential risk to the fetus. Women taking nefazodone should not breast-feed, since small amounts of the drug will pass into the breast milk and be absorbed into the baby's bloodstream, leading to possible sedation and other unknown effects on the child's developing nervous system.

Use in children: Nefazodone has not been systematically studied in children or adolescents under the age of eighteen, and there are few reports on its use in depression in this age range. The side effects are reported to be similar to those in adults. In general, the SSRIs are prescribed to treat depression in children.

Use in seniors: In general, the effective daily dose for seniors may be slightly less than for younger individuals, in the 200- to 400-mg. range. A usual starting dose may be 50 mg. at bedtime, with 50-mg. increases every four days to a week, until the total daily dose is between 200 and 400 mg. Although nefazodone generally does not trigger blood-pressure changes, seniors should be aware that dizziness and light-headedness may increase their risk of falls.

Overdosage: There have been few reported serious or life-threatening consequences of overdoses. Nefazodone's risks are similar to those of the SSRIs. However, individuals often overdose with multiple medications, and other drugs may increase the risk of more serious complications. Bring the bottle of medication to the emergency room with the person, since the date when the medication was prescribed and the number of pills remaining in the bottle can provide helpful information to the treating physician.

Special considerations: Nefazodone may be an effective alternative for persons who develop sexual dysfunction on SSRIs, venlafaxine (Effexor), tricyclic antidepressants, or MAO inhibitors, and for those who develop significant sleep disturbance or anxiety while on SSRIs, especially the more activating fluoxetine (Prozac).

 Generic name: **NORTRIPTYLINE**

 Available in generic form: Yes

 Brand name: Pamelor, Aventyl HCI

 Drug class: Tricyclic antidepressant

Prescribed for: Major depressive disorder, dysthymia (chronic mild to moderate depression), bipolar depression, panic disorder, posttraumatic stress disorder, generalized anxiety disorder, social anxiety disorder, pain symptoms, migraine and tension headaches, insomnia.

General information: One of the older antidepressants, nortriptyline is believed to work by increasing the amount of norepinephrine and, to a lesser extent, serotonin available in the central nervous system. Nortriptyline produces many bothersome side effects and may be potentially lethal if taken in overdose. Physical medicine specialists and orthopedic surgeons may prescribe it as an additional medication to treat chronic pain syndromes. Primary-care physicians may prescribe it to treat insomnia. In general, it takes six to eight weeks at therapeutic dosage levels before nortriptyline becomes fully effective. After three to four weeks, there is usually some relief of symptoms, with more complete relief after six to eight weeks. In some cases, it may take as long as twelve weeks to achieve maximum benefit.

Nortriptyline is the only antidepressant for which regular tests of blood levels may be necessary because there is a "therapeutic window," a blood-level range within which individuals usually obtain the maximum potential benefit. For this reason, the person may have to go to a laboratory to have blood drawn in the morning following the bedtime dose of nortriptyline. Nortriptyline is a major metabolite of amitriptyline (Elavil).

Dosing information: Nortriptyline is available in 10-, 25-, 50 , and 75-mg. capsules and oral concentrate. The usual initial dose is between 25 and 50 mg. a day, with an increase weekly in 25- to 50-mg. increments. The usual therapeutic dose is between 75 and 150 mg. a day. The usual maximum dose is 150 mg. a day. This medication may be given in divided doses during the day or taken in a single dose at bedtime.

Common side effects: Nortriptyline produces significant anticholinergic side effects (see Glossary), including drowsiness, dry mouth, blurred vision, constipation, esophageal reflux (heartburn), urinary retention or difficulty in urinating, and orthostatic hypotension. Other side effects include sexual difficulties (impotence, decreased desire), weight gain, irregular heartbeats (arrhythmias), and tremor.

Precautions: Men with an enlarged prostate should use this drug with caution because it may cause them difficulty in urinating. All antidepressants may increase the risk of seizures. Persons who are taking medications to prevent seizures and are prescribed nortriptyline for depression may need to have their anti-seizure medication carefully monitored and possibly increased in dose.

To cope with dry mouth, individuals should drink water throughout the day or suck on sugarless candy. (Candy with sugar should be avoided, since the anticholinergic effects of this drug increase the possibility of tooth decay.) Exercise and high-fiber foods can lessen the risk of constipation. Some people may need to take a stool softener, such as Colace, or a bulk-forming agent, such as Metamucil, to counteract the constipating effects. Nortriptyline should not be stopped suddenly because of the risk of severe withdrawal symptoms, such as increased anxiety, flu-like symptoms, depression, jitteriness, and agitation. It should be gradually tapered off over a period of several weeks to a month or more.

Warnings: People who become depressed following a heart attack or who have a history of arrhythmias (irregular heartbeats) should not take nortriptyline because of the increased risk of dangerous, irregular heartbeats and sudden death. Nortriptyline should *never* be taken with monoamine oxidase inhibitor (MAOI) antidepressants, since this combination may produce severe hypertension, seizures, fever, and even death. Individuals must wait at least two weeks after stopping nortriptyline before beginning an MAOI, and wait two weeks after stopping an MAOI before beginning nortriptyline.

Alcohol: People should not drink alcohol if they are taking antidepressants, since alcohol produces depressive-like symptoms and may increase the rate of metabolism of the antidepressant and lower its blood levels.

Food and beverages: No restrictions. If taking nortriptyline on an empty stomach upsets your stomach, try it with food or immediately after eating.

Possible drug interactions: Nortriptyline should generally not be used with the selective serotonin reuptake inhibitors, since the SSRIs inhibit its metabolism, leading to very high blood levels and increasing the likelihood of seizures, arrhythmias (irregular heartbeats), confusion, and dizziness. Because of nortriptyline's sedating effects, other medications that may produce sedation, such as the benzodiazepines, antihistamines, and pain medications, should be avoided. Because it can lower blood pressure, nortriptyline should be used with caution when taken with antihypertensive medication.

Use in pregnancy and breast-feeding: Pregnancy Category D

In general, nortriptyline is not recommended during pregnancy because its use in pregnancy has not been systematically studied. It is not known whether it increases birth defects or spontaneous miscarriages. If they stop taking nortriptyline during pregnancy, some women may experience a recurrence of their depression. In these circumstances, the physician should discuss the need to restart nortriptyline. Women should always consult with their physician if they are contemplating pregnancy or if they become pregnant while taking nortriptyline. Women taking a tricyclic antidepressant should not breast-feed, since small amounts will pass into the breast milk and be absorbed into the baby's bloodstream, leading to possible sedation and affecting the child's developing nervous system.

Use in children:

Tricyclic antidepressants such as nortriptyline are sometimes prescribed in children for the treatment of bed-wetting, attention deficit hyperactivity disorder (ADHD), and depression. The usual recommended dose is between 0.5 and 2 mg. per kilogram (approximately 2.2 pounds) of body weight per day. Because of recent reports of sudden death in young children taking tricyclic antidepressants, nortriptyline should be prescribed only by a child psychiatrist or a pediatrician skilled in the use of psychiatric medications and only if other medications have been unsuccessful.

Use in seniors:

Lower doses of nortriptyline are prescribed in seniors, usually in the range of 50 to 75 mg. a day. Its blood-pressure-lowering effects and the risk of orthostatic hypotension and confusion are greater in older people. In addition, nortriptyline increases the risk of irregular heartbeats (arrhythmias) and even of death. People over age fifty should have a baseline electrocardiogram (EKG) before taking nortriptyline, since it prolongs the transmission of electrical impulses through the heart, an effect that may result in potentially life-threatening irregular heartbeats. Its anticholinergic effects may produce confusion and disorientation, especially in seniors or in those in early stages of Alzheimer's disease.

Overdosage: Psychiatrists are reluctant to prescribe nortriptyline and other tricyclic antidepressants in persons at risk for suicide, since the risk of fatal overdose is high. If overdose is suspected, bring the bottle of medication to the emergency room with the person, since the date when the medication was prescribed and the number of pills remaining in the bottle can provide helpful information to the treating physician.

Special considerations: Persons who become depressed following a heart attack should not take nortriptyline or another tricyclic antidepressant because of the increased risk of sudden death, probably related to the production of irregular heartbeats (arrhythmias).

Persons with bipolar disorder (manic-depressive illness) usually develop depression as well as mania at some time during the course of their illness. Nortriptyline and other tricyclic antidepressants may produce "switching," a clinical process whereby a person goes from the depressive phase of manic-depressive illness to the manic phase. Prior to starting an antidepressant, people with bipolar disorder should take a mood stabilizer, such as lithium or divalproex (Depakote). However, because even with a mood stabilizer some patients may still experience switching when placed on a tricyclic antidepressant, many psychiatrists select one of the newer antidepressants, such as an

SSRI, bupropion (Wellbutrin or Zyban), or nefazodone (Serzone), which are less likely to produce this effect.

Nortriptyline is the major active metabolite of amitriptyline (Elavil). Because nortriptyline produces fewer anticholinergic side effects (dry mouth, blurred vision, constipation, confusion, urinary retention) than amitriptyline (Elavil), nortriptyline is preferred over amitriptyline by many psychiatrists.

 Generic name: **PAROXETINE**

 Available in generic form: No

 Brand name: Paxil

 Drug class: Selective serotonin reuptake inhibitor (SSRI)

Prescribed for: Depression (major depressive disorder, dysthymia, and others), premenstrual dysphoric disorder, anorexia nervosa, bulimia nervosa, panic disorder, obsessive-compulsive disorder, borderline personality disorder, posttraumatic stress disorder and social anxiety disorder, generalized anxiety disorder, selected impulse-control disorders.

General information: Paroxetine works similarly to other SSRIs by increasing the amount of serotonin available in the brain by blocking its reuptake. It was originally approved only for the treatment of depression; however, like the other SSRIs, it is now used to treat a wide range of psychiatric conditions. As with other antidepressant medications, paroxetine takes from six to eight weeks to produce maximum benefit. Those with obsessive-compulsive disorder may not feel better for as long as twelve to sixteen weeks. The major advantages of this medication, and the other SSRIs, are safety, minimal side effects, and relative ease of administration.

Dosing information: Paroxetine is available in 10-, 20-, 30-, and 40-mg. tablets and in an oral suspension at a strength of 10 mg. per 5 cc. of liquid. A scored 20-mg. tablet can easily be divided in two. The usual starting dose is 10 mg., increased in 10-mg. increments weekly. The usual therapeutic dose for treatment of depression is between 30 and 50 mg., although persons with obsessive-compulsive disorder may require higher doses, up to 60 mg. The usual maximum dose is 60 mg. Because sedation is a common side effect, paroxetine is sometimes taken in the evening in a single dose. However, most people prefer to take it in the morning or in divided doses in the morning or afternoon because although it produces sedation, it frequently interferes with sleep. The sedation is attributed to the anticholinergic side effects, and the insomnia is believed to result from the increase in serotonin.

Common side effects: Paroxetine produces more anticholinergic side effects (see Glossary) than the other SSRIs. These include dry mouth, constipation, tiredness, and blurred vision. Like other SSRIs, it may produce nausea, headache, insomnia, daytime sedation, sleep disturbance, tremors, and gastrointestinal symptoms (diarrhea or cramping).

Similar to the other SSRIs, paroxetine produces a relatively high rate of sexual dysfunction, affecting 40 to 60 percent of those taking the drug. The most frequent types are delayed orgasm in women and retarded ejaculation in men. Some people may experience decreased desire or lack of interest in sexual activity. Another, more recently reported, side effect is increased weight gain in people who have been on paroxetine for a long period of time (a year or more). The cause of this side effect is unclear.

Precautions: As with other antidepressants, paroxetine may increase the likelihood of seizures, although the risk is believed to be less than with the tricyclic antidepressants and bupropion (Wellbutrin or Zyban). Persons with bipolar disorder should first be placed on a mood stabilizer such as lithium or divalproex (Depakote), since paroxetine may cause rapid "switching" from depression to mania. This occurs less often in people taking paroxetine and other SSRIs than in those taking tricyclic antidepressants. Paroxetine should not be stopped abruptly because of the risk of severe withdrawal symptoms such as anxiety, depression, flu-like symptoms, and temperature elevation. Paroxetine should be tapered off gradually over a period of several weeks to a month or more.

Warnings: Paroxetine should *never* be taken with monoamine oxidase inhibitors (MAOIs), since this combination may produce severe hypertension, seizures, fever, and even death. Individuals should wait at least two weeks after stopping paroxetine before beginning an MAOI and wait two weeks after stopping an MAOI before beginning paroxetine. Individuals who are taking two or more drugs that boost serotonin levels, such as an SSRI in combination with the serotonin antagonist antidepressant nefazodone (Serzone), may develop an uncommon, potentially deadly condition called serotonin syndrome, caused by excessive stimulation of the serotoninergic system. This syndrome can also occasionally occur in those taking a single SSRI, especially at higher doses. Initial symptoms include lethargy, restlessness, confusion, flushing, sweating, tremor, and involuntary muscle jerks. Over time, a small percentage of individuals may develop muscle disorders, hyperthermia, and rigor, which may lead to respiratory problems, increased platelet clotting, destruction of red blood cells by the kidneys and their excretion in urine, and kidney failure. This syndrome requires emergency medical treatment and discontinuation of the serotonin-boosting medications.

Alcohol: People should not drink alcohol if they are taking antidepressants, since alcohol produces depressive-like symptoms and may increase the rate of metabolism of the antidepressant and lower its blood levels.

Food and beverages: No restrictions. If taking paroxetine on an empty stomach upsets your stomach, try it with food or immediately after eating.

Possible drug interactions: Paroxetine has been reported to increase blood levels of medications containing the decongestant theophylline, which is frequently found in asthma or cold medications. It may potentially prolong bleeding time when used with anticoagulants such as warfarin (Coumadin). When paroxetine is given with the anti-ulcer drug cimetidine (Tagamet), blood levels of paroxetine may be substantially increased.

The combination of paroxetine and tricyclic antidepressants can be dangerous, since paroxetine significantly increases blood levels of tricyclics, leading to possible irregular heartbeats (arrhythmias) and other serious adverse side effects.

Use in pregnancy and breast-feeding:
Pregnancy Category C

The effects of paroxetine on the developing fetus are unknown. If they stop antidepressants during pregnancy, some women may experience a recurrence of their depression. In these circumstances, the physician should discuss the need to restart the medication or seek an alternative medication or treatment. Women should always consult with their physician if they are contemplating pregnancy or if they become pregnant while taking paroxetine. Paroxetine should be taken during pregnancy only if the benefits to the mother greatly outweigh any potential unknown risks to the fetus. Women taking paroxetine should not breast-feed, since small amounts of the drug will pass into the breast milk and be absorbed into the baby's bloodstream, leading to possible sedation and other unknown effects on the child's developing nervous system.

Use in children: Although paroxetine has not been systematically studied in children, it sometimes is used in children to treat depression, obsessive-compulsive disorder, and attention deficit hyperactivity disorder (ADHD). The dosage used in children is similar to adults.

Use in seniors: Paroxetine has been shown to be effective in seniors. Because the liver of an older person does not metabolize most drugs as well as in earlier years, lower doses (20 to 30 mg.) may be prescribed. Seniors should routinely begin with a dose of 10 mg., with increases in 10-mg. increments weekly, as needed. Since many seniors take multiple medications, the effect of paroxetine on the blood levels of other drugs must be carefully monitored. Because many older persons suffer sleep disturbances, paroxetine should be monitored closely because it has been reported to increase insomnia.

Overdosage: In contrast to the tricyclic antidepressants, paroxetine, the other SSRIs, and other newer antidepressants are generally much safer in overdose, especially when taken alone. However, individuals often overdose with multiple medications, and other drugs may increase the risk of more serious complications. If an overdose is suspected, bring the bottle of medication to the emergency room with the person, since the date when the medication was prescribed and the number of pills remaining in the bottle can provide helpful information to the treating physician.

Special considerations: Because paroxetine is more sedating than fluoxetine (Prozac), citalopram (Celexa), or sertraline (Zoloft), individuals with depression and associated anxiety symptoms may tolerate it better than those with melancholic depression. Because paroxetine and the other SSRIs alone do not produce any cardiac side effects, they are recommended for those with heart disease or who develop depression following a heart attack, rather than a tricyclic antidepressant.

Generic name: PHENELZINE

 Available in generic form: Yes

Brand name: Nardil

Drug class: Monoamine oxidase inhibitor (MAOI)

Prescribed for: Depression (especially unresponsive to other antidepressants), panic disorder, social anxiety disorder, migraine headaches, posttraumatic stress disorder.

General information: MAOIs work by preventing monoamine oxidase (MAO), a scavenger enzyme found in the central nervous system, from breaking down the neurotransmitters norepinephrine and serotonin, thereby increasing the amount of their availability. MAOIs are particularly effective in treating "atypical" forms of depression, in which patients exhibit self-pity, sensitivity to rejection by others, severe tiredness, a need for increased sleep, increased appetite, and a worsening of mood in the evening.

 Dosing information: Phenelzine is available in 15-mg. tablets. The initial dose in treating depression is 15 mg., with an increase weekly in 15-mg. increments to the usual therapeutic dose of between 45 and 60 mg. Some individuals may require doses of up to 90 mg. a day. Similar dosages are generally used for the anxiety disorders (panic disorder, social anxiety disorder, posttraumatic stress disorder). Phenelzine is usually taken at night because it produces drowsiness. However, because it may also produce insomnia, some people prefer to take all or part of the medication during the day.

Common side effects: Drowsiness is common, especially early in treatment. Other common side effects are muscle aches, nervousness, dry mouth, orthostatic hypotension, problems in urinating, sedation, sexual difficulties, sleep disturbance, and weight gain. Less common side effects include constipation, diarrhea, rashes, chest pain, severe headaches, chills or shivering, and jaundice. Phenelzine also may produce insomnia, resulting in daytime fatigue. Muscle aches, tension, twitches and jerks, and sensory numbness may be caused by the tendency of MAOIs to reduce pyridoxine (vitamin B_6) in the body. Taking a 100-mg. vitamin B_6 supplement daily should correct this deficiency. The most common sexual difficulties are anorgasmia and impotence; these symptoms are more common with phenelzine than the MAOI tranylcypromine (Parnate).

Precautions: Individuals taking MAOIs should alert their doctors if they have high blood pressure or heart problems, if they often have severe headaches, or if they expect to be undergoing anesthesia, surgery, or medical testing in the coming months. Anyone using an MAO inhibitor should check with a physician before using *any* drug, including prescription and over-the-counter cold medications, cough syrups, decongestants, nose drops or sprays, treatments for sinus conditions or hay fever, or preparations that suppress appetite or claim to reduce weight. Antihistamines themselves are not a danger unless combined with decongestants.

If surgery is necessary, the anesthesiologist should be informed in advance of the operation that the patient is taking an MAO inhibitor; the medication may have to be discontinued at least ten days before surgery. The use of procaine (Novocain) for dental procedures may be dangerous, and individuals anticipating dental work should consult with their dentist and psychiatrist about potential risks.

Warnings: For individuals taking these drugs, it is essential (though not always easy) to avoid tyramine, an amino acid found in many common foods, which can interact with the MAO inhibitors and produce potentially toxic effects, including sudden, extremely dangerous surges in blood pressure (hypertensive crisis). This is sometimes called the "cheese reaction" because aged cheeses contain relatively high concentrations of tyramine. It can range from mild to severe, producing symptoms such as sweating, palpitations, headache, and, in extreme cases, a sharp rise in blood pressure and possible bleeding within the brain because of the rupture of cerebral arteries.

Recent studies that measured tyramine in foods have reduced the list of previously banned substances. The primary foods to avoid are avocados, fava beans, cheeses (except cream, cottage, and ricotta), chocolate (in large amounts), overripe bananas and other fruits, sauerkraut, shrimp paste, sour cream, and soy products, including tofu. Caffeine and some red wines should be used in small amounts only. (See Table 2-8 for dietary restrictions when taking an MAOI.) MAO inhibitors can also interact harmfully with certain over-the-counter and prescription medications and with illegal drugs, especially cocaine.

Individuals taking an MAO inhibitor who develop extremely painful or unremitting headaches should immediately seek medical help, including blood-pressure monitoring. A very high blood-pressure reading may require emergency medical treatment. Persons taking MAO inhibitors should carry an identification card or wear a Medic Alert bracelet alerting health-care personnel that if they develop a hypertensive crisis, therapy consists of 2 to 5 mg. of phentolamine (Regitine), and that they should not be given meperidine (Demerol).

Persons who have not been helped by an MAO inhibitor must wait fourteen days after discontinuing these drugs before starting another antidepressant, including another MAO inhibitor, or using any foods, beverages, or drugs containing tyramine. MAO inhibitors should not be discontinued without consulting a physician, and use should be gradually reduced to avoid withdrawal symptoms. After discontinuation, individuals must continue to follow the dietary restrictions for at least two weeks to avoid possible toxic reactions.

$\triangledown$ **Alcohol:** See Warnings (page 44) and Table 2-8. Beer and ale must not be consumed because taking these beverages may lead to potentially toxic effects, including sudden, extremely dangerous surges in blood pressure (hypertensive crisis). Red wine (especially Chianti), when consumed in large amounts, may also produce similar effects.

Food and beverages: See Warnings (page 44) and Table 2-8.

Possible drug interactions: A host of medications must never be used when taking phenelzine or another MAOI. These include cold medications, cough preparations containing dextromethorphan (DM), nasal decongestants and sinus medications, asthma inhalants, allergy and hay fever medications, meperidine (Demerol), cocaine, amphetamines, diet suppressants, local anesthetics that contain epinephrine, levodopa and dopamine (used to treat Parkinson's disease). Other antidepressants or another MAOI should not be taken with phenelzine. These include *all* the antidepressants: tricyclic antidepressants, SSRIs, venlafaxine (Effexor), mirtazapine (Remeron), bupropion (Wellbutrin or Zyban), and nefazodone (Serzone). The only possible exception is trazodone (Desyrel). The anti-anxiety agent buspirone (BuSpar) should not be taken with MAOIs. At least two weeks should elapse after stopping phenelzine before beginning another antidepressant. At least two weeks should elapse after stopping an antidepressant before starting phenelzine; fluoxetine (Prozac) requires a wait of four weeks. As a rule, an MAOI is not combined with a tricyclic antidepressant, although there are times when a skilled psychiatrist may begin treatment with a tricyclic antidepressant and an MAOI together or may gradually add an MAOI to an existing tricyclic antidepressant regimen.

Use in pregnancy and breast-feeding: Pregnancy Category C

Phenelzine is not recommended during pregnancy because of the risk of hypertensive crisis. It is not known whether it increases birth defects or spontaneous miscarriages because its use in pregnancy has not been systemically studied. Women should always consult their physician if they are taking phenelzine and are contemplating pregnancy or become pregnant. MAOIs cannot be combined with medications, such as terbutaline, which are used to stop premature labor. Some pregnant women who had been taking phenelzine prior to pregnancy may experience a recurrence of their depression if they discontinue it. In these circumstances, the physician should discuss the need to restart phenelzine. Women taking phenelzine should not breastfeed, since small amounts will pass into the breast milk and be absorbed into the baby's bloodstream, affecting the child's developing nervous system.

⚕ **Use in children:** Phenelzine and the other MAOIs are not recommended for children and adolescents because of the need for dietary precautions and the availability of other safe and effective antidepressants.

🏠 **Use in seniors:** Because of the high rate of orthostatic hypotension, the risk of falls associated with such blood-pressure changes, and the need for careful dietary controls, MAOIs are usually not prescribed for older persons until several other classes of antidepressants have not proved effective. In addition, because seniors often take multiple medications, the risk of drug interactions is much greater.

☠ **Overdosage:** When MAOIs are taken in overdose, the most common adverse effects are drowsiness, low blood pressure, difficulty breathing, convulsions, coma, and hypertensive crisis, which require aggressive hospital treatment to prevent strokes and other serious complications. Persons who take an overdose of phenelzine should be taken immediately to the emergency room for evaluation and treatment. Bring the bottle of medication to the emergency room with the person, since the date when the medication was prescribed and the number of pills remaining in the bottle can provide helpful information to the treating physician.

✍ **Special considerations:** It is advisable to carry an identification card or a Medic Alert bracelet alerting health care personnel that you are taking an MAO inhibitor. In addition, carry a wallet-sized list of foods high in tyramine and medications that you should avoid.

Prior to any dental procedure or surgical procedure, inform your dentist or physician that you are taking an MAO inhibitor because of the great potential for interactions with anesthetic agents.

In general, the newer antidepressants—SSRIs, nefazodone (Serzone), bupropion (Wellbutrin and Zyban), venlafaxine (Effexor), and mirtazapine (Remeron)—have replaced the MAO inhibitors as preferred medications. There are, however, some individuals for whom the only effective treatment will be MAOIs. Phenelzine is less stimulating and more sedating than tranylcypromine (Parnate). Consequently, if a person cannot tolerate tranylcypromine (Parnate) because of its stimulating effects and needs to take an MAOI, phenelzine is a reasonable alternative.

 ## Generic name: SERTRALINE

 Available in generic form: No

 Brand name: Zoloft

 Drug class: Selective serotonin reuptake inhibitor (SSRI)

Prescribed for: Depression (major depressive disorder, dysthymia, and others), premenstrual dysphoric disorder, anorexia nervosa, bulimia nervosa, panic disorder, obsessive-compulsive disorder, borderline personality disorder, posttraumatic stress disorder, social anxiety disorder, generalized anxiety disorder, selected impulse control disorders.

General information: Sertraline and other SSRIs increase the amount of serotonin available in the brain by blocking its reuptake. It was originally approved only for the treatment of depression; however, like other SSRIs, it is now used to treat a wide range of psychiatric conditions. As with other antidepressant medications, sertraline takes from six to eight weeks to produce maximum benefit. Those with obsessive-compulsive disorder may not feel better for as long as twelve to sixteen weeks. The major advantages of this medication, like the other SSRIs, are safety, minimal side effects, and relative ease of administration.

Dosing information: Sertraline is available in 25-, 50-, and 100-mg. tablets. The usual starting dose for most people with depression is 25 or 50 mg. a day. The dose is increased in 25- to 50-mg. increments weekly. The usual therapeutic dose is between 100 and 200 mg. a day, though some people may respond to doses as low as 50 mg. Individuals with panic disorder often cannot tolerate a 50-mg. initial dose, so the initial dose is generally 25 mg., with increases in 25-mg. increments every week to ten days until a therapeutic dose of 100 to 200 mg. is reached. Sertraline is usually taken in a single dose in the morning.

Common side effects: Like other SSRIs, sertraline may cause nervousness, agitation, headache, tremor, nausea, various gastrointestinal symptoms (diarrhea, constipation, or cramping), and tremors. Some people experience insomnia early in treatment, a symptom that sometimes persists. Others report daytime sedation, without insomnia or as a result of insomnia. If insomnia persists, the physician may prescribe an additional medication for sleep; for instance, a sedating antidepressant such as trazodone (Desyrel) (see page 137), a benzodiazepine such as temazepam (Restoril) (see page 263), or the nonbenzodiazepine hypnotic agent zolpidem (Ambien) (see page 276). Sertraline generally produces more gastrointestinal side effects, especially diarrhea and abdominal cramping, than the other SSRIs.

Similar to the other SSRIs, sertraline produces a relatively high rate of sexual dysfunction, affecting 40 to 60 percent of those taking the drug. The most frequent types are delayed orgasm in women and retarded ejaculation in men. Some experience decreased desire or lack of interest in sexual activity. Some people who have been taking sertraline for a long period of time report weight gain. The cause of this side effect is unclear.

Precautions: As with other antidepressants, SSRIs may increase the likelihood of seizures, although the risk is believed to be lower than with the tricyclic antidepressants and bupropion (Wellbutrin or Zyban). People with bipolar depression should first be placed on a mood stabilizer such as lithium or divalproex (Depakote), since sertraline may cause rapid "switching" from depression to mania. This occurs less often in people taking sertraline and other SSRIs than in those taking tricyclic antidepressants.

Sertraline should not be stopped suddenly because of withdrawal symptoms such as anxiety, nervousness, depression, flu-like symptoms, and temperature elevation. Withdrawal symptoms occur less frequently in sertraline than with other short-acting SSRIs, such as paroxetine (Paxil) or fluvoxamine (Luvox), although they do sometimes occur. Sertraline should be tapered off over a period of several weeks to a month or more.

Warnings: Sertraline should *never* be taken with monoamine oxidase inhibitor (MAOI) antidepressants, since this combination may produce severe hypertension, seizures, fever, and even death. Individuals should wait at least two weeks after stopping an MAOI before beginning sertraline and wait two weeks after stopping sertraline before beginning an MAOI. Individuals who are taking two or more drugs that boost serotonin levels, such as an SSRI in combination with the serotonin antagonist antidepressant nefazodone (Serzone), may develop an uncommon, potentially deadly condition called serotonin syndrome, caused by excessive stimulation of the serotoninergic system. This syndrome can also occasionally occur in those taking a single SSRI, especially at higher doses. Initial symptoms include lethargy, restlessness, confusion, flushing, sweating, tremor, and involuntary muscle jerks. Over time, a small percentage of persons may develop muscle disorders, hyperthermia, and rigor, which may lead to respiratory problems, increased platelet clotting, destruction of red blood cells by the kidneys and their excretion in urine, and kidney failure. This syndrome requires emergency medical treatment and discontinuation of the serotonin-boosting medications.

Alcohol: People should not drink alcohol if they are taking antidepressants, since alcohol produces depressive-like symptoms and may increase the rate of metabolism of the antidepressant and lower its blood levels.

Food and beverages: When taken with food, sertraline's absorption into the bloodstream may be increased rather than decreased. For this reason, it is advisable to take it on an empty stomach or an hour before or two hours after eating.

Possible drug interactions: Sertraline may prolong bleeding time when combined with warfarin (Coumadin). It may lower electrolytes (sodium, potassium, and others) in the blood when combined with a diuretic, such as furosemide (Lasix). Sertraline potentially may increase blood levels of diazepam (Valium) and the anti-seizure medication phenytoin (Dilantin). It may also increase levels of the antipsychotic medications haloperidol (Haldol), clozapine (Clozaril), and pimozide (Orap). Sertraline may also increase blood levels of the antihypertensive agent propranolol (Inderal), slowing the heart considerably and producing dizziness, tiredness, and arrhythmias.

The combination of sertraline and tricyclic antidepressants requires extreme caution because sertraline significantly increases blood levels of the tricyclic, leading to

possible cardiac arrhythmias and other serious adverse
side effects.

Use in pregnancy and breast-feeding:
Pregnancy Category C

The effects of sertraline on the developing fetus in pregnant women are unknown. Women should always consult
their physician if they are taking sertraline and are contemplating pregnancy or become pregnant. Sertraline
should be taken during pregnancy only if the benefits to
the mother outweigh any potential unknown risks to the
fetus. Women taking sertraline should not breast-feed,
since small amounts of the drug will pass into the breast
milk and be absorbed into the baby's bloodstream, leading
to possible sedation and other unknown effects on the
child's developing nervous system.

Use in children: Although its use has not been systematically studied in children, sertraline is sometimes prescribed to treat depression, obsessive-compulsive
disorder, eating disorders, and attention deficit hyperactivity disorder (ADHD). The dosage ranges used in children
are similar to those used in adults.

Use in seniors: Sertraline has been shown to be effective in seniors. Because the liver of an older person does not metabolize most drugs as well as in earlier
years, lower doses may be prescribed, such as 50 to 100 mg.
Since many seniors take multiple medications, the effect of
sertraline on the blood levels of other medications must be
carefully monitored. Because many older people suffer
sleep disturbances, sertraline should be monitored closely,
since it has been reported to increase insomnia.

Overdosage: In contrast to the tricyclic antidepressants, overdoses of sertraline and the other SSRIs
are generally much less dangerous, especially when taken

alone. More often, persons overdose with multiple medications, and the other drugs may increase the risk of more serious complications. If an overdose is suspected, bring the bottle of medication to the emergency room with the person, since the date when the medication was prescribed and the number of pills remaining in the bottle can provide helpful information to the treating physician.

Special considerations: Sertraline and the other SSRIs alone do not produce any cardiac side effects and are recommended for persons with heart disease or who develop depression following a heart attack, rather than a tricyclic antidepressant. Because sertraline is more activating than paroxetine (Paxil) and fluvoxamine (Luvox)—though less so than fluoxetine (Prozac)—individuals with depression and associated anxiety symptoms may initially tolerate it less well than those who have melancholic depression. Consequently, lower initial doses are generally used in people with depression and associated anxiety.

 Generic name: **TRANYLCYPROMINE**

 Available in generic form: Yes

 Brand name: Parnate

 Drug class: Monoamine oxidase inhibitor (MAOI)

Prescribed for: Depression (especially unresponsive to other antidepressants), panic disorder, social anxiety disorder, migraine headaches, posttraumatic stress disorder.

General information: MAOIs work by preventing monoamine oxidase (MAO), a scavenger enzyme found in the central nervous system, from breaking down the neurotransmitters norepinephrine and serotonin, thereby increasing their availability. MAOIs are particularly effective in treating "atypical" forms of depression, where persons exhibit self-pity, sensitivity to rejection by others, severe tiredness, a need for increased sleep, increased appetite, and a worsening of mood in the evening.

Dosing information: Tranylcypromine is available in 10-mg. tablets. The initial dose is generally 10 mg. a day, with an increase weekly in 10-mg. increments. The usual therapeutic dose is between 30 and 50 mg. a day, and the usual maximum dose is 60 mg. Because tranylcypromine is quite stimulating and frequently causes insomnia, it is usually taken during the day.

Common side effects: Drowsiness is common, especially early in treatment. Other common side effects are muscle aches, nervousness, dry mouth, orthostatic hypotension, problems in urinating, sedation, sexual difficulties, sleep disturbance, and weight gain. Less common side effects include constipation, diarrhea, rashes, chest pain, severe headaches, chills or shivering, and jaundice. Tranylcypromine is quite stimulating, often resulting in insomnia. Muscle aches, tension, twitches and jerks, and sensory numbness may be caused by the tendency of MAOIs to reduce pyridoxine (vitamin B_6) in the body. Taking a 100-mg. vitamin B_6 supplement daily should correct this deficiency. The most common sexual difficulties are anorgasmia and impotence, although these symptoms are less common with tranylcypromine than with the MAOI phenelzine (Nardil).

Precautions: Individuals taking MAOIs should alert their doctors if they have high blood pressure or heart problems, if they often have severe headaches, or if they expect to be undergoing anesthesia, surgery, or medical testing in coming months. Anyone using an MAO inhibitor should check with a physician before using *any* drug, including prescription and over-the-counter cold medications, cough syrups, decongestants, nose drops or sprays, treatments for sinus conditions or hay fever, or preparations that suppress appetite or claim to reduce weight. Antihistamines themselves are not a danger unless combined with decongestants.

If surgery is necessary, the anesthesiologist should be informed in advance of the operation that the patient is taking an MAO inhibitor; the medication may have to be discontinued at least ten days before surgery. The use of procaine (Novocain) for dental procedures may be dangerous, and individuals anticipating dental work should consult with their dentist and psychiatrist about potential risks.

⨂ **Warnings:** For individuals taking these drugs, it is essential (though not always easy) to avoid tyramine, an amino acid found in many common foods that can interact with the MAO inhibitors and produce potentially toxic effects, including sudden, extremely dangerous surges in blood pressure (hypertensive crisis). This is sometimes called the "cheese reaction" because aged cheeses contain relatively high concentrations of tyramine. It can range from mild to severe, producing symptoms such as sweating, palpitations, headache, and, in extreme cases, a sharp rise in blood pressure and possible bleeding within the brain because of the rupture of cerebral arteries.

Recent studies that measured tyramine in foods have reduced the list of previously banned substances. The primary foods to avoid are avocados, fava beans, cheeses (except cream, cottage, and ricotta), chocolate (in large amounts), overripe bananas and other fruits, sauerkraut, shrimp paste, sour cream, and soy products, including tofu. Caffeine and some red wines should be used in small amounts only. (See Table 2-8 for revised dietary restrictions when taking an MAOI.) MAO inhibitors can also interact harmfully with certain over-the-counter and prescription medications and with illegal drugs, especially cocaine. All illicit or "recreational" drugs should be avoided. The use of cocaine can lead to an extremely dangerous increase in blood pressure.

Individuals taking an MAO inhibitor who develop an extremely painful or unremitting headache should immediately seek medical help, including blood-pressure monitoring. A very high blood-pressure reading may require emergency medical treatment. Persons taking MAO inhibitors should carry an identification card or wear a Medic Alert bracelet instructing health-care personnel that if they develop a hypertensive crisis, therapy consists of 2 to 5 mg. of phentolamine (Regitine), and that they should not be given meperidine (Demerol).

Persons who have not been helped by an MAO inhibitor must wait fourteen days after discontinuing these drugs before starting another antidepressant, including another MAO inhibitor, and before using any foods, beverages, or drugs containing tyramine. MAO inhibitors should not be discontinued without consulting a physician, and use should be gradually reduced to avoid withdrawal symptoms. After discontinuation, individuals must continue to follow the dietary restrictions for at least two weeks to avoid possible toxic reactions.

Alcohol: See Warnings (pages 133–134) and Table 2-8. Beer and ale must not be consumed because taking these beverages may lead to potentially toxic effects, including sudden, extremely dangerous surges in blood pressure (hypertensive crisis). Red wine (especially Chianti), when consumed in large amounts, may also produce similar effects.

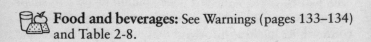 **Food and beverages:** See Warnings (pages 133–134) and Table 2-8.

Possible drug interactions: A host of medications must never be taken when using tranylcypromine or another MAOI. These include cold medications, cough preparations containing dextromethorphan (DM), nasal decongestants and sinus medications, asthma inhalants, allergy and hay fever medications; meperidine (Demerol), cocaine, amphetamines, diet suppressants, local anesthetics that contain epinephrine, and levodopa and dopamine (used to treat Parkinson's disease). Other antidepressants or another MAOI should not be taken with tranylcypromine. This includes *all* the antidepressants: tricyclic antidepressants, SSRIs, venlafaxine (Effexor), mirtazapine (Remeron), bupropion (Wellbutrin or Zyban), and nefazodone (Serzone). Wait at least two weeks after stopping tranylcypromine before beginning another antidepressant, or after stopping an antidepressant before starting tranylcypromine; fluoxetine (Prozac) requires a wait of four weeks. As a rule, an MAOI is not combined with a tricyclic antidepressant, although there are times when a skilled psychiatrist may prescribe a tricyclic antidepressant and an MAOI together or may gradually add an MAOI to an existing tricyclic antidepressant regimen.

**Use in pregnancy and breast-feeding:
Pregnancy Category C**

Tranylcypromine is not recommended during pregnancy because of the risk of hypertensive crisis. It is not known whether it increases birth defects or spontaneous miscarriages because its use in pregnancy has not been systemically studied. Women should always consult their physician if they are taking tranylcypromine and are contemplating pregnancy or become pregnant. MAOIs cannot be combined with medications, such as terbutaline, which are used to stop premature labor. Some pregnant women who had been taking tranylcypromine prior to pregnancy may experience a recurrence of their depression if they discontinue it. In these circumstances, the physician should discuss the need to restart tranylcypromine. Women taking tranylcypromine should not breast-feed, since small amounts will pass into the breast milk and be absorbed into the baby's bloodstream, affecting the child's developing nervous system.

Use in children: Tranylcypromine and the other MAOIs are not recommended for children or adolescents because of the need for dietary precautions and the availability of other safe and effective antidepressants.

Use in seniors: Because of the high rates of hypotension, the risk of falls associated with such blood-pressure changes, and the need for careful dietary controls, MAOIs are usually not prescribed for older persons until several other classes of antidepressants have not proved effective. In addition, because many seniors require multiple medications, the risk of drug interactions is much greater.

Overdosage: When MAOIs are taken in overdose, the most common adverse effects are drowsiness, low blood pressure, difficulty breathing, convulsions, coma, and hypertensive crisis, which require aggressive hospital treatment to prevent strokes and other serious complications. Persons who take an overdose of tranylcypromine should be taken immediately to the emergency room for evaluation and treatment. Bring the bottle of medication to the emergency room with the person, since the date when the medication was prescribed and the number of pills remaining in the bottle can provide helpful information to the treating physician.

Special considerations: It is advisable to carry an identification card or a Medic Alert bracelet telling health-care personnel that you are taking an MAO inhibitor. In addition, carry a wallet-sized list of foods high in tyramine and medications that you should avoid.

Prior to any dental procedure or surgical procedure, inform your dentist or physician that you are taking an MAO inhibitor because of the risk of potential drug interactions with anesthetic agents.

In general, the newer antidepressants—SSRIs, nefazodone (Serzone), bupropion (Wellbutrin and Zyban), venlafaxine (Effexor), and mirtazapine (Remeron)—have replaced the MAO inhibitors as preferred medications. There are, however, some patients for whom the only effective treatment will be MAOIs. Tranylcypromine is more stimulating and less sedating than phenelzine (Nardil). Consequently, if a person cannot tolerate phenelzine because of its sedating effects and needs to take an MAOI, tranylcypromine is a reasonable alternative.

 Generic name: TRAZODONE

 Available in generic form: Yes

 Brand name: Desyrel

 Drug class: 5-HT$_2$ antagonist

 Prescribed for: Depression (major depression, dysthymia), insomnia, agitation.

General information: In addition to being a weak serotonin reuptake inhibitor, trazodone is believed to block a serotonin receptor subtype, the 5-HT$_2$ receptor. The blocking of this receptor may be important in treating depression, anxiety, and agitation.

Trazodone is used most often to treat sleep disturbances and insomnia, especially in those who are taking an SSRI for depression. It is also used to treat agitation in persons suffering from Alzheimer's disease or other brain disorders. It is unclear whether trazodone itself possesses anti-agitation properties or whether its sedative effects reduce agitation.

Dosing information: Trazodone is available in 50-, 100-, and 150-mg. tablets. The branded form of trazodone, Desyrel, is also available in 150-mg. Dividose tablets that can be divided in 50-mg. segments. However, because of cost restrictions imposed by managed care, the Dividose tablet is less frequently prescribed.

For the treatment of depression, the entire dose of trazodone is generally taken at bedtime. The initial dose is 50 mg., with weekly increases in 50-mg. increments. The usual therapeutic dose to treat depression is between 300 and 400 mg., although some people may require doses up to 600 mg.

For insomnia, trazodone is usually prescribed at a dose of 50 mg. at bedtime. This dose may need to be increased to as much as 150 mg.

For treatment of agitation in elderly persons with Alzheimer's disease, trazodone is usually taken twice a day. The initial starting dose is 50 mg. in the morning and 50 mg. at bedtime, with 50-mg. increases weekly. Therapeutic doses range between 100 and 600 mg., depending upon the severity of the agitation. Trazodone may be stopped abruptly without the risk of withdrawal symptoms.

Common side effects: Side effects include sedation, drowsiness, dry mouth, nausea and vomiting, blurred vision, dizziness, light-headedness, and orthostatic hypotension. This is especially problematic in seniors because of the increased risk of falls.

Precautions: There have been some reports that high doses of trazodone produce irregular heartbeats. Consequently, people who have experienced a recent heart attack, who have a history of irregular heartbeats (arrhythmias), or who are on medications to treat arrhythmias should use this medication with caution. It is not known whether the combination of trazodone with an MAOI produces side effects. It is generally recommended that trazodone not be used with MAOIs, but if there is a need for such a combination, trazodone should be begun at a low dose (50 mg.) and increased gradually.

Warnings: Trazodone has been reported to produce priapism (painful, sustained erections) in men at a rate of 1 in 6,000. Nearly half of persons with priapism require surgery to correct the condition; approximately half of those undergoing surgery become impotent. Although this is a rare side effect, physicians generally caution men about it prior to treatment.

Alcohol: People should not drink alcohol if they are on antidepressants, since alcohol produces depressive-like symptoms and may increase the rate of metabolism of the antidepressant and lower its blood levels.

Food and beverages: No restrictions. If taking trazodone on an empty stomach upsets your stomach, try it with food or immediately after eating.

Possible drug interactions: Trazodone may increase blood levels of digoxin (a cardiac medication) and phenytoin (Dilantin), an anti-seizure medication, and decrease blood levels of warfarin (Coumadin), an anticoagulant.

🐾 Use in pregnancy and breast-feeding:
Pregnancy Category C

The effects of trazodone on the developing fetus are unknown. Women should always consult with their physician if they are taking trazodone and are contemplating pregnancy or become pregnant. The medication should be continued only if its benefits for the woman outweigh any potential risks for the fetus. Women taking trazodone should not breast-feed, since small amounts of the drug and its metabolites will pass into the breast milk and be absorbed into the baby's bloodstream, leading to possible sedation and other unknown effects on the child's developing nervous system.

🜍 Use in children:
Trazodone has not been systematically studied in children and is infrequently prescribed. In general, the SSRIs are used to treat depression in children.

🏠 Use in seniors:
In general, seniors will respond to lower doses of trazodone (200 to 300 mg. a day). Because trazodone produces orthostatic hypotension, the medication should be begun at lower doses, such as 25 to 50 mg., with 25- to 50-mg. increases weekly. In addition, seniors should get up slowly when moving from a lying or sitting position to avoid dizziness, light-headedness, and falls.

☠ Overdosage:
Trazodone overdoses are generally believed less dangerous than those with the MAOIs or the tricyclic antidepressants. Overdoses will cause sedation and dizziness. People who overdose should be taken immediately to an emergency room. Bring the bottle of medication to the emergency room with the person, since the date when the medication was prescribed and the number of pills remaining in the bottle can provide helpful information to the treating physician.

Special considerations: Usually, physicians prescribe nefazodone (Serzone) to treat depression instead of trazodone, since nefazodone produces less orthostatic hypotension and does not cause priapism.

 Generic name: VENLAFAXINE

 Available in generic form: No

 Brand name: Effexor, Effexor XR

Drug class: Combined serotonin and norepinephrine reuptake inhibitor

Prescribed for: Depression (major depressive disorder, dysthymia, bipolar depression, and especially refractory and melancholic depression), depression complicated by anxiety, attention deficit disorder in adults, generalized anxiety disorder. Its usefulness in treating other mental disorders has not been firmly established.

General information: Venlafaxine is both an SSRI and a norepinephrine reuptake inhibitor. Venlafaxine works by increasing not only the amount of serotonin available in the brain, but also the amount of norepinephrine and, at higher doses, dopamine. Because of its side effects, venlafaxine needs to be started at a low dose and gradually adjusted upward. If the initial dose is too high, most people cannot tolerate the resulting anxiety, nervousness, and nausea and may discontinue venlafaxine before it can produce benefits. Psychiatrists generally prescribe venlafaxine when conventional medications do not work.

Dosing information: Venlafaxine is available in 25-, 37.5-, 50-, 75-, and 100-mg. tablets. The new extended-release version, venlafaxine–extended release

(Effexor XR), which psychiatrists usually prescribe, is available in 37.5-, 75-, and 150-mg. tablet sizes. The XR version is preferred because the medication can be taken at a single time, usually in the morning, and because people are better able to tolerate the side effects associated with the XR formulation. Because it may be taken in a single dose, the XR version also improves the likelihood that people will adhere to the recommended dosage. The usual starting dose is 37.5 mg. of the XR form, with an increase in 37.5-mg. increments weekly. Most persons respond to a dose of 150 to 225 mg. a day in both the standard and the extended-release forms. The usual maximum daily dose is 225 mg. of the XR and 375 mg. of the regular form.

Common side effects: The most common side effects are nausea, vomiting, dizziness, anxiety, daytime tiredness, nervousness, insomnia, headache, and dry mouth. Most of these side effects are usually limited in duration. If side effects become intolerable when the dose is increased, reducing the dose for a week or more and then increasing it again may help.

Like the SSRIs, venlafaxine produces sexual dysfunction, principally delayed orgasm in women and ejaculatory delay in men. It also may interfere with sleep. Various strategies can treat sexual dysfunction, or the physician may prescribe a concurrent antidepressant that does not affect normal sexual functioning, such as bupropion (Wellbutrin or Zyban), nefazodone (Serzone), or mirtazapine (Remeron). In contrast to the SSRIs, increasing the dose of venlafaxine may decrease the frequency of sexual dysfunction because of the increased norepinephrine effects at higher doses. For sleep disturbance, physicians may prescribe the antidepressant trazodone (Desyrel), the benzodiazepine hypnotic agent temazepam (Restoril), or the nonbenzodiazepine hypnotic agent zolpidem (Ambien). Venlafaxine should not be stopped suddenly because of severe withdrawal symptoms such as increased anxiety, flu-like symptoms, depression, jitteriness, and agitation. It should be tapered off gradually over a period of several weeks to a month or more.

Precautions: A significant increase in mean blood pressure was noted in original clinical trials in approximately 5 percent of patients. Although very few subjects had to stop venlafaxine because of an increase in blood pressure, venlafaxine should be used cautiously in persons with hypertension. Prior to starting venlafaxine, it is advisable to have the physician obtain a baseline blood pressure, especially in individuals older than fifty or who are on medication to treat high blood pressure. In doses greater than 225 mg., routine monitoring of blood pressure is recommended.

Warnings: Venlafaxine should *never* be taken with monoamine oxidase inhibitors (MAOIs), since this combination may produce severe hypertension, seizures, fever, and even death. Individuals who are taking two or more drugs that boost serotonin levels, such as venlafaxine in combination with an SSRI, may develop an uncommon, potentially deadly condition called serotonin syndrome, which is caused by excessive stimulation of the serotoninergic system. This syndrome can also occasionally occur in those taking a single SSRI, especially at higher doses. Initial symptoms include lethargy, restlessness, confusion, flushing, sweating, tremor, and involuntary muscle jerks. Over time, a small percentage of persons may develop muscle disorders, hyperthermia, and rigor, which may lead to respiratory problems, increased platelet clotting, destruction of red blood cells by the kidneys and their excretion in urine, and kidney failure. This syndrome requires emergency medical treatment and discontinuation of the serotonin-boosting medications.

Alcohol: People should not drink alcohol if they are on antidepressants, since alcohol produces depressive-like symptoms and may increase the rate of metabolism of the antidepressant and lower its blood levels.

Food and beverages: No restrictions. If taking venlafaxine on an empty stomach upsets your stomach, try it with food or immediately after eating.

Possible drug interactions: If venlafaxine is combined with tricyclic antidepressants, it may increase blood levels of the tricyclic drugs, leading to possible cardiac arrhythmias and conduction abnormalities in the heart. Venlafaxine does not produce any cardiac side effects and is recommended for persons who develop depression following a heart attack.

**Use in pregnancy and breast-feeding:
Pregnancy Category C**

As with many antidepressants, the effects of venlafaxine on the developing fetus are unknown. Women should always consult with their physician if they are taking venlafaxine and are contemplating pregnancy or become pregnant. The medication should be taken or continued during pregnancy only if its benefits for the woman outweigh any potential unknown risks for the fetus. Women taking venlafaxine should not breast-feed, since small amounts of the drug will pass into the breast milk and be absorbed into the baby's bloodstream, leading to possible sedation and other unknown effects on the child's developing nervous system.

Use in children: The use of venlafaxine in children has not been systematically studied, and there are few reports on its effectiveness in treating depression.

Use in seniors: Like other antidepressants, venlafaxine generally is prescribed in lower doses in seniors, usually in the 100- to 150-mg. range. They should have a baseline blood-pressure check because of venlafaxine's tendency to increase blood pressure at higher doses.

Overdosage: Like the SSRIs, venlafaxine is not lethal in overdose. However, one reason for concern is a significant increase in blood pressure in persons who have taken a large number of venlafaxine tablets, especially if they have a history of hypertension. People who take an overdose should always be brought to a hospital emergency room. Bring the bottle of medication to the emergency room with the person, since the date when the medication was prescribed and the number of pills remaining in the bottle can provide helpful information to the treating physician.

Special considerations: Venlafaxine is an excellent medication, especially for treating depression that has not responded to other antidepressants. It is usually prescribed by psychiatrists rather than primary-care physicians because it requires close monitoring and a slow increase in dose in order to minimize side effects. If the physician suggests venlafaxine, individuals should request the XR form, since it is more convenient and is better tolerated. Venlafaxine alone does not produce any cardiac side effects and is recommended for individuals with heart disease or who develop depression following a heart attack, rather than a tricyclic antidepressant.

CHAPTER 3

Anti-anxiety Medications (Tranquilizers)

To learn general information about this class of medications and the disorders they treat, read the first part of the chapter. To read about a specific anti-anxiety medication, turn to the page indicated below.

ANXIETY DISORDERS

The most common of mental illnesses, anxiety disorders may involve inordinate fears of certain objects or situations (phobias), episodes of sudden, inexplicable terror (panic attacks), chronic distress (generalized anxiety disorder, or GAD), or persistent, disturbing thoughts and behaviors (obsessive-compulsive disorder). Over a lifetime, according to the National Comorbidity Survey, as many as 1 in 4 Americans may experience an anxiety disorder. Only 1 of every 4 of these individuals is ever correctly diagnosed and treated, yet most who do get treatment, even for severe and disabling problems, improve dramatically.

Phobias

Phobias, the most prevalent type of anxiety disorder, are out-of-the-ordinary, irrational, intense, persistent fears of certain objects or situations. In the course of a lifetime, about 11 percent of adults develop such acute terror that they go to extremes to avoid whatever it is that they fear, even though they realize that these feelings are excessive or unreasonable. There are two types of phobias: specific phobias and social anxiety disorder. The most common specific phobias involve animals, particularly dogs, snakes, insects, and mice; the sight of blood; closed spaces (claustrophobia); heights (acrophobia); air travel; and being in places or situations from which individuals believe it would be difficult or embarrassing to escape (agoraphobia).

The other type of phobia, called social phobia or social anxiety disorder, interferes with a person's ability to work or to form social relationships. When the phobia is not restricted to a particular situation, such as public speaking, but includes all social activities, such as interactions with people at work and during social events, it is called a generalized social anxiety disorder.

For generalized social anxiety disorder, paroxetine (Paxil) or other SSRIs are the usual treatment of choice. For specific phobias, the best approach is behavior therapy, which consists of gradual, systematic exposure to the feared object, a process called systematic desensitization. Numerous studies have proven that exposure—especially in vivo exposure, in which individuals are exposed to the actual source of their fear rather than simply imagining it—is highly effective. Medical hypnosis, the induction of an altered state of consciousness, can also help.

Panic Attacks and Panic Disorder

Individuals who have had panic attacks describe them as the most frightening experiences of their lives (see Table 3-1). Without reason or warning, their hearts race wildly. They may become light-headed or dizzy. Because they can't catch their breath, they may start breathing rapidly and hyperventilate. Parts of their bodies, such as their fingers or toes, may tingle or feel numb. Worst of all is the terrible sense that something dreadful is about to happen: that they will die, lose their minds, or have a heart attack. Most attacks reach peak intensity within ten minutes. Afterward, individuals live in dread of another attack. Panic disorder develops when attacks recur or apprehension

Table 3-1: Symptoms of Panic Disorder

CHARACTERISTIC SYMPTOMS OF PANIC ATTACKS ARE

• Palpitations, pounding heart, or accelerated heart rate	• Feeling dizzy, unsteady, light-headed, or faint
• Sweating	• Feelings of unreality or being detached from oneself
• Trembling or shaking	
• Sensations of shortness of breath or smothering	• Fear of losing control or going crazy
• Feeling of choking	• Fear of dying
• Chest pain or discomfort	• Numbness or tingling sensations
• Nausea or abdominal distress	
	• Chills or hot flashes

about them becomes so intense that the person cannot function normally.

About one-third of all young adults experience at least one panic attack between the ages of fifteen and thirty-five. Full-blown panic disorder, which usually develops before age thirty, occurs in about 1.6 percent of all adults in the course of a lifetime. Women are more than twice as likely as men to experience panic attacks, although no one knows precisely why. Parents, siblings, and children of individuals with panic disorders are also more likely to develop them than are others.

Treatment helps as many as 90 percent of those with panic disorder; they either improve significantly or recover completely, usually within six to eight weeks. The two primary approaches are cognitive-behavioral therapy, which teaches specific strategies for coping with symptoms like rapid breathing, and medication. Individuals who receive both cognitive-behavioral therapy and medication are less likely to suffer relapses than those taking medication alone.

Generalized Anxiety Disorder

The hallmark of a generalized anxiety disorder (GAD) is excessive or unrealistic apprehension that causes physical symptoms and lasts for six months or longer. Unlike fear, which helps us recognize and avoid real danger, GAD is an irrational or unwarranted response to harmless objects or situations of exaggerated danger. The most common symptoms are elevated heart rate, sweating, increased blood pressure, muscle aches, intestinal pains, irritability, sleep problems, and difficulty concentrating.

Chronically anxious individuals worry not just some of the time and not just about the stresses and strains of ordinary life, but constantly and about almost everything: their health, families, finances, marriages, potential dangers. Treatment for GAD may consist of a combination of psychotherapy, behavioral therapy, and anti-anxiety drugs.

Obsessive-Compulsive Disorder

As many as 1 in 40 Americans have a type of anxiety called obsessive-compulsive disorder (OCD). Some of these individuals suffer only from an obsession, a recurring idea, thought, or image that they realize, at least initially, is senseless. The most common obsessions are repetitive thoughts of violence (e.g., killing a child), contamination (becoming infected by shaking hands), and doubt (wondering whether one has performed some act, such as having hurt someone in a traffic accident). Most people with OCD also suffer from a compulsion, that is, a repetitive behavior performed according to certain rules or in a stereotyped fashion. The most common compulsions involve handwashing, cleaning, hoarding useless items, counting, or checking (as in checking to make sure a door is locked dozens of times).

Individuals with OCD realize that their thoughts or behaviors are bizarre, but they cannot resist or control them.

Eventually, the obsessions or compulsions consume a great deal of time and significantly interfere with normal routines, job functioning, or usual social activities or relationships with others. A young woman who must follow a very rigid dressing routine may always be late for class, for example; a student who must count each letter of the alphabet as he types may not be able to complete a term paper.

OCD is believed to have biological roots. It may be a result of gene abnormalities, a head injury, or even an autoimmune reaction after a childhood streptococcus infection. Treatment may consist of cognitive therapy to correct irrational assumptions, behavioral techniques like progressively limiting the amount of time someone obsessed with cleanliness can spend washing and scrubbing, and medication like an SSRI. About 70 to 80 percent of those with OCD improve with treatment.

Posttraumatic Stress Disorder

In the past, posttraumatic stress disorder (PTSD) was viewed as a psychological response to out-of-the-ordinary stressors, such as captivity or combat. However, these are not the only experiences that can forever change the way people view themselves and their world. With the recent surge in violent crime and in natural disasters, thousands of individuals have experienced or witnessed traumatic events. Children, in particular, are likely to develop PTSD symptoms when they live through a traumatic event or witness an assault on a loved one or friend. Sometimes an entire community, such as the residents of a town hit by a devastating flood or hurricane, develops symptoms.

In a survey of more than 400 undergraduates, 84 percent listed at least one traumatic event of sufficient intensity to elicit posttraumatic stress disorder. One-third had experienced four or more such events. The students who had these experiences, which included witnessing violence or death, child abuse, and sexual assault, reported higher levels of depression, anxiety, and other psychological symptoms.

A history of childhood sexual abuse can greatly increase the likelihood of developing PTSD. An episode that repeats the abuse, such as a sexual assault or rape, can trigger an intense reaction as individuals "reexperience" the initial trauma of their youth. Adolescents who are dependent on alcohol also are particularly susceptible to PTSD.

In PTSD, individuals reexperience their terror and helplessness again and again in their dreams or intrusive thoughts. To avoid this psychic pain, they may try to avoid anything associated with the trauma. Some enter a state of emotional numbness and can no longer respond to people and experiences the way they once did, especially when it comes to showing tenderness or affection. Those who have been mugged or raped may be afraid to venture out by themselves.

The sooner trauma survivors receive psychological help, the better they are likely to fare. Often, simply talking about what happened with an empathic person or someone who has shared the experience as soon as possible—preferably before going to sleep on the day of the event—can help an individual begin to deal with what has occurred. Group sessions, ideally beginning soon after the trauma, allow individuals to share views and experiences. Medications and behavioral, cognitive, and psychodynamic therapy can help individuals suffering from PTSD.

EPIDEMIOLOGY

Over a lifetime, according to the National Comorbidity Survey, as many as 25 percent—1 in every 4—of the men and women in the United States may experience an anxiety disorder. More than a third of all individuals who consult mental-health professionals do so because of anxiety disorders. In the past, their complaints were often misunderstood, misdiagnosed, or dismissed as primarily a psychological response to stress or conflict. These views have changed dramatically.

Thanks to breakthroughs in research and understanding, we now know that anxiety disorders, such as panic disorder, are primarily biological illnesses, associated with an underlying genetic vulnerability and alterations in brain chemistry. Stress and conflict can certainly make anxiety disorders worse, but they don't necessarily cause them. In most cases, an interplay of three major factors—biological, psychosocial (including stress), and behavioral—determines the nature and severity of the disorder.

The new insights into the nature of anxiety disorders have led to major advances in treatment. For some problems, such as specific phobias, cognitive-behavioral therapy has proven highly effective. For others, such as panic disorder, medications, particularly in combination with cognitive-behavioral therapy, provide great relief. Self-help techniques, ranging from basics like avoiding caffeine to specialized strategies such as controlled breathing, can also be helpful.

The most important medications for serious anxiety disorders are commonly referred to as "antidepressants." The reason is simple. Their helpfulness in treating depression was discovered several years before scientists realized that these same medications are also highly effective in treating anxiety disorders. However, most antidepressants (see Chapter 2) appear to be just as effective as the benzodiazepines (profiled in this chapter) for individuals with generalized anxiety disorder and for those with symptoms of both an anxiety disorder and depression. Recently, the Food and Drug Administration (FDA) approved venlafaxine (Effexor) to treat GAD and paroxetine (Paxil) to treat social anxiety disorder. The FDA had previously approved paroxetine (Paxil) and sertraline (Zoloft) to treat panic disorder, and both these medications and fluoxetine (Prozac), fluvoxamine (Luvox), and clomipramine (Anafranil) to treat obsessive-compulsive disorder. As physicians become more aware of the effectiveness of antidepressants to treat these conditions, they are expected to prescribe the newer antidepressants for GAD, panic disorder, PTSD, and other anxiety disorders, instead of benzodiazepines. Because antidepressants are discussed in detail in Chapter 2, they are not included here. However, two additional types of medications, benzodiazepines and azapirones, that are also very useful in the treatment of anxiety disorders are discussed in detail below.

The principal medications currently used by primary-care physicians to relieve the symptoms of generalized anxiety disorder are the benzodiazepines, which are among the most widely prescribed of all psychiatric medications (see Table 3-2), and buspirone (BuSpar). Because of their safety, benzodiazepines have largely replaced older anti-anxiety (anxiolytic) medications, such as the barbiturates and meprobamate (Miltown). However, benzodiazepines may produce dependence and thus lead to addiction, so for longer-term treatment of anxiety, buspirone (BuSpar) is frequently preferred.

BENZODIAZEPINES

The benzodiazepines include drugs that are highly effective in relieving anxiety symptoms, such as alprazolam (Xanax), clonazepam (Klonopin), and lorazepam (Ativan), as well as others with different effects. Neuroscientists have located receptors for benzodiazepines in the brains of both animals and humans. These receptors are in close proximity to another receptor, called the GABA receptor. When benzodiazepine receptors are stimulated, they in turn enhance the action of the brain's major inhibitory neurotransmitter, GABA; GABA decreases the excitability of neurons, leading to a decrease in anxiety symptoms.

Table 3-2: Drugs Commonly Used for
Generalized Anxiety Disorder

CLASS AND MEDICATION	BRAND NAME
Short half-life benzodiazepines[a]	
alprazolam	Xanax
clonazepam	Klonopin
lorazepam	Ativan
oxazepam	Serax
Long half-life benzodiazepines[b]	
chlordiazepoxide	Librium
clorazepate	Tranxene
diazepam	Valium
Azapirone	
buspirone	BuSpar

[a]Half-life, 5–20 hours.
[b]Half-life, 20–200 hours.

The more likely a particular benzodiazepine is to bind with the benzodiazepine-GABA receptor complex, the greater its therapeutic effects on anxiety.

The use of certain benzodiazepines that had revolutionized the treatment of anxiety disorders in the 1960s—including diazepam (Valium) and chlordiazepoxide (Librium)—has declined with the development of newer drugs that are equally if not more effective and that may cause fewer side effects.

Benzodiazepines are "cross-tolerant" with alcohol, which means that benzodiazepines produce similar effects upon the brain and the body as alcohol. Consequently, for acute detoxification of persons suffering from alcoholism, physicians prescribe a benzodiazepine, usually a longer-acting agent such as chlordiazepoxide or diazepam, to substitute for the alcohol, given in doses high enough to prevent the onset of withdrawal symptoms from stopping alcohol. These symptoms include tremors, restlessness, anxiety, rapid pulse, elevated blood pressure, sweating, nausea, and vomiting. More severe symptoms of alcohol withdrawal include seizures, hallucinations, and delirium, characterized by confusion and disorientation. For treatment of alcohol withdrawal, patients are usually hospitalized for two or three days and are treated with a benzodiazepine, such as chlordiazepoxide or diazepam, and other medications, such as thiamine, folate, and B_{12}. They also receive careful medical monitoring as the benzodiazepine is rapidly tapered off over several days to a week.

General Precautions

For most people, moderate doses of benzodiazepines for no more than two weeks carry little risk of dependence. However, use beyond this, even for as brief a period as two to four weeks, can induce both physical and psychological dependence. Because the risk of dependence is so high, benzodiazepine use should be supervised and limited. Psychiatrists prescribe these medications with caution, especially in individuals with a family or personal history of alcoholism or substance abuse. Individuals taking benzodiazepines should not drink alcohol, which interacts with these drugs and can lower blood pressure to a dangerous level, decrease the breathing rate, and cause loss of consciousness and possible death. Men and women already dependent on alcohol or drugs may become addicted to benzodiazepines after just one or two doses. People over the age of sixty should not take benzodiazepines, since these medications produce clumsiness, increase their risks for falls, cause memory disturbance and sometimes confusion, and produce sedation.

Interactions between benzodiazepines and other drugs,

such as marijuana, sedatives, and narcotics, are also dangerous and, in some cases, potentially fatal. In addition, many other medications, especially those that affect liver function, can increase the actions and side effects of the benzodiazepines. Among these are birth-control pills; anti-ulcer drugs such as cimetidine (Tagamet); propranolol (Inderal) and other beta-blockers; and disulfiram (Antabuse), which is used to treat alcoholism. Individuals should always consult their physicians before taking any of these medications. The only benzodiazepines that do not interact with these drugs are lorazepam (Ativan), oxazepam (Serax), and temazepam (Restoril), a medication used for treating insomnia (see Chapter 5).

People who take benzodiazepines for three or four weeks or longer and then stop abruptly may experience withdrawal symptoms, including anxiety, irritability, restlessness, insomnia, impaired memory and concentration, and panic attacks. Some of these symptoms are the same ones that led them to take benzodiazepines in the first place. Withdrawal can begin from one to ten days after discontinuation, depending on the particular benzodiazepine. All of the benzodiazepines require slow, carefully supervised tapering off over a period of weeks or months.

The benzodiazepines vary widely in their half-lives and potency, that is, in how long their metabolites remain active in the body and how powerful their impact is (see Table 3.2). Half-life is an especially important consideration for the elderly, who may become drowsy or confused by medications that remain in the body for a long period. Also, longer-acting agents have more of a tendency to build up in the body and produce sedation and confusion. The benzodiazepines with short half-lives, which are eliminated very quickly from the body, are less likely to cause these side effects. However, withdrawal symptoms can be more acute than those of benzodiazepines with longer half-lives.

If your psychiatrist has prescribed a benzodiazepine

take the first dose at home at a time when you do not have to drive or operate machinery; these medications impair coordination and mental alertness. If you drive and are taking a benzodiazepine, leave more space between your vehicle and the one in front of you, since your reflexes will be somewhat impaired. Also, since the benzodiazepines produce sedation, be careful when driving when tired or at night. Women who are hoping to conceive or who are pregnant or nursing should not use benzodiazepines.

Although benzodiazepines are often used in suicide attempts, they rarely cause death unless they are combined with alcohol, sedatives, or narcotics. Signs of overdose include sedation, reduced coordination, slurred speech, poor concentration, decreased breathing rate, confusion, and memory problems. Immediate treatment at the nearest emergency room is critical.

Side Effects

Benzodiazepines can cause drowsiness (particularly in the first few days of use), impaired coordination, memory disturbances, problems in concentration, and muscle weakness. If these effects persist, reducing the dose or switching to another benzodiazepine can minimize some of them. Another option is a change to buspirone (BuSpar), a completely different type of antianxiety agent, or to an antidepressant (see Chapter 2) instead of a benzodiazepine.

Some individuals taking benzodiazepines have paradoxical responses, that is, reactions opposite to those that might be expected. These include a loss of inhibition that can lead to bizarre behavior, intense anger, outbursts of rage or violence, intense feelings of depression, and extreme anxiety or irritability. These reactions may be more likely to occur in the elderly, people with brain damage, and those who have a prior history of hostility, poor impulse control, antisocial or borderline personality disorder, aggression. If a paradoxical reaction develops, the drug should be discontinued, and another agent, such as buspirone (BuSpar), should be used instead.

Alprazolam (Xanax)

The primary advantage of alprazolam (Xanax) is the speed with which it begins to relieve anxiety and panic symptoms—much more quickly than the antidepressants, which can take two or three weeks to begin to produce benefits. However, individuals who stop taking alprazolam often report that their anxiety symptoms return even more intensely than before. Alprazolam can be highly addictive and produces the most severe withdrawal symptoms of any of the benzodiazepines, including seizures, extreme anxiety, psychosis, increased heart rate and blood pressure, memory and concentration disturbance, and hallucinations. This drug should never be discontinued abruptly; doses should be gradually reduced to minimize withdrawal symptoms.

Chlordiazepoxide (Librium)

Introduced in 1960, Librium revolutionized the drug treatment of anxiety. Its use has declined with the development of agents that are equally effective but have shorter half-lives and fewer potential drug interactions. It is now used mainly to treat alcohol withdrawal symptoms.

Clonazepam (Klonopin)

Clonazepam (Klonopin) is used to treat panic disorder and other mild to moderate anxiety disorders and may also be useful in treating mania, tics, tremors, and movement disorders. Many people feel the effects of this medication within the first day or within a few days of treatment. Long-term use can lead to physical and psychological dependence; however, the risk of dependence and the severity of withdrawal symptoms is somewhat less than the other high-potency benzodiazepines, such as alprazolam (Xanax) or lorazepam (Ativan). Some people feel lethargic and less alert or able to concentrate when taking this medication. Clonazepam can also affect physical coordination. For panic disorder, clonazepam generally is prescribed for at least six months to a year. Because panic disorder often recurs, doctors may recommend continuing treatment for a longer period. In general, most psychiatrists prefer treating individuals with panic disorder with an antidepressant, such as an SSRI, rather than with clonazepam or another benzodiazepine because of their concern about dependence and withdrawal reactions when the benzodiazepine is stopped.

Diazepam (Valium)

Once one of the most widely prescribed of all drugs, diazepam (Valium) as a treatment for anxiety has been supplanted by medications that are equally effective but carry fewer risks for physical and psychological dependence and problems of withdrawal. It is now used primarily for alcohol withdrawal, muscle spasms, and epilepsy.

Lorazepam (Ativan)

This agent is used to treat panic disorder and other mild to moderate anxiety disorders. It is often prescribed by physicians in medical settings, for example, by mouth or injection before surgery to relieve apprehension. Because it is metabolized differently from several other benzodiazepines—diazepam (Valium), chlordiazepoxide (Librium), and clonazepam (Klonopin)—it has less effect on the liver and therefore may be a better choice for those taking other medications that can affect liver function, such as birth-control pills, propranolol (Inderal), disulfiram (Antabuse), and anti-ulcer drugs, such as cimetidine (Tagamet).

Oxazepam (Serax)

Like other benzodiazepines, oxazepam (Serax) is used to treat mild to moderate anxiety symptoms; it is also sometimes prescribed for alcohol addiction or withdrawal. Oxazepam is considered a good choice for older persons because it has a gradual onset of action, doesn't produce intense effects such as euphoria, and has a short half-life so that it is cleared from the body reasonably quickly. Because it is metabolized differently from other benzodiazepines and in a manner similar to lorazepam (Ativan), it has less effect on the liver, and therefore may be a better choice for those taking other medications that can affect liver function, such as birth-control pills, propranolol (Inderal), disulfiram (Antabuse), and anti-ulcer drugs, such as cimetidine (Tagamet).

Buspirone (BuSpar)

Buspirone (BuSpar), which belongs to a family of medications called azapirones, may relieve anxiety symptoms primarily by altering serotonin-receptor sensitivity and increasing serotonin activity in the brain. It is used to treat generalized anxiety disorder, social anxiety disorder, and refractory obsessive-compulsive disorder (OCD that is resistant to treatment), usually in combination with an SSRI. It is also a good choice for individuals with a personal or family history of alcohol or substance dependence or abuse. It is especially useful in treating anxiety with associated depressive symptoms. In higher doses, it may be an effective antidepressant.

Although buspirone has a chemical structure completely different from the benzodiazepines, it is equally

effective for most kinds of anxiety disorders, the exception
being panic disorder. When used with other medications,
especially SSRIs, it may be effective in treating residual or
persistent symptoms in people with obsessive-compulsive
disorder (OCD), social anxiety disorder, and posttraumatic
stress disorder. It is less sedating, does not cause memory
loss, does not impair coordination or driving skills, does
not interact dangerously with alcohol, appears to have little risk for overdose, and has little danger of dependence.
However, because it has a slower onset of action than the
benzodiazepines, buspirone may take as long as a month
for persons to feel its full effects. Buspirone should never
be used in combination with an MAO inhibitor.

 Generic name: ALPRAZOLAM

 Available in generic form: Yes

Brand name: Xanax

 Drug class: Benzodiazepine

Prescribed for: Panic disorder, generalized anxiety
disorder, social anxiety disorder, specific phobia, adjustment disorder with anxiety. Alprazolam may be used
with antidepressants to treat agitated depression and posttraumatic stress disorder. It is sometimes used in women
premenstrually to treat agitation and associated anxiety.

General information: The use of alprazolam and
other benzodiazepines has diminished somewhat
with the development of newer antidepressants with fewer
side effects. Benzodiazepines work by binding to benzodiazepine receptors found in the brain. Those receptors, in
turn, stimulate a specific neurotransmitter called gamma-

aminobutyric acid (GABA), the principal inhibitory neuro-transmitter in the brain, which is believed to reduce anxiety. Alprazolam is rapidly absorbed into the central nervous system; hence, it may produce euphoria and may have more addiction potential than benzodiazepines that are more slowly absorbed, such as oxazepam (Serax) or clonazepam (Klonopin).

Dosing information: Alprazolam is available in 0.25-, 0.5-, 1-, and 2-mg. tablets. Alprazolam is usually prescribed in an initial dose of 0.25 mg. three to four times a day. Doses may be increased gradually up to a maximum of 6 to 8 mg. a day. The usual therapeutic dose is from 1 to 4 mg. a day. Individuals who will benefit from the drug will usually experience a reduction in anxiety within a few days to a week. Physicians carefully monitor the dose of alprazolam and prescribe the lowest dose possible so as to decrease the possibility of dependence.

Common side effects: The most common side effects of benzodiazepines are sedation, a "spacey" feeling, impaired concentration, memory disturbances, and poor coordination. Benzodiazepines may interfere with driving skills by reducing reflexes and impairing coordination. Older people are more susceptible to these effects and are also at increased risk of falling when taking benzodiazepines.

Precautions: Some people may develop "paradoxical" responses that, due to loss of inhibition, may lead to bizarre behavior, anger, irritability, and anxiety. These reactions are more likely to occur in the elderly, people with brain damage, those with a history of an impulse-control disorder, and those suffering from borderline personality disorder, which is characterized by impulsivity and instability in interpersonal relationships, mood, and self-image. Benzodiazepines may impair breathing in persons with chronic obstructive pulmonary disease (COPD) or emphysema.

Warnings: Individuals with acute narrow-angle glaucoma should not take benzodiazepines. People suffering from sleep apnea, a sleep disorder characterized by long pauses in respiration during the night, should also avoid benzodiazepines because they decrease the ability to begin breathing again after such pauses, a potentially fatal risk. A shorter-acting benzodiazepine like alprazolam should never be suddenly stopped because of the risk of severe withdrawal reactions, such as seizures, intense rebound anxiety, and severe agitation. If alprazolam has been taken for four or more weeks, it should be tapered off gradually over a period of two to eight weeks. The drug should be decreased each week at a rate of 10 percent of the total daily dose.

Alcohol: People should not drink alcohol when taking benzodiazepines. When taken together, benzodiazepines and alcohol intensify side effects such as sedation, memory disturbance, motor incoordination, euphoria, and impaired judgment, and can seriously impair driving ability.

Food and beverages: No restrictions.

Possible drug interactions: The antidepressants fluoxetine (Prozac) and nefazodone (Serzone) and the pain medication propoxyphene (Darvon) may increase blood levels of alprazolam. Other medications that may produce sedation, such as antihistamines and certain sedating antidepressants, should be used with caution. Alprazolam should not be taken with the antifungal agents ketoconazole (Nizoral) or itraconazole (Sporanox), since these agents can raise blood levels of alprazolam to dangerously high levels. Certain drugs that affect the ability of the liver to function may increase the blood levels of most benzodiazepines; these medications include birth-control pills, ulcer drugs such as cimetidine (Tagamet), the antihypertensive medication propanolol (Inderal), and disulfiram (Antabuse), which is used to treat alcoholism.

Use in pregnancy and breast-feeding:
Pregnancy Category D

Alprazolam has not been studied in pregnant women. In animals, benzodiazepines have been shown to produce cleft palate in the fetus. Some studies suggest that benzodiazepines, especially chlordiazepoxide (Librium) and diazepam (Valium), may increase the risk of cleft lip and heart deformities in human fetuses, especially when taken by women in the first trimester. In general, the use of benzodiazepines during pregnancy should almost always be avoided, especially during the first trimester. Alprazolam should be used in pregnant women only if the benefits to the mother greatly outweigh any potential risks to the fetus and if alternative agents have been unsuccessful. Women on alprazolam should not breast-feed, since the effects on the baby are unknown.

Use in children: This medication has not been systematically studied in individuals under eighteen years of age. However, benzodiazepines are sometimes prescribed for children for brief periods of time to treat anxiety. The usual dose range is from 0.5 to 1 mg., three to four times a day.

Use in seniors: Older people should not use alprazolam and other benzodiazepines because these drugs increase the risk of falls and of accidents when driving.

☠ **Overdosage:** Taken alone in overdose, alprazolam does not produce life-threatening consequences; however, when taken with other agents such as alcohol or barbiturates, the risk of serious complications or death increases considerably. People who overdose on alprazolam should be taken to the emergency room. Bring the bottle of medication to the emergency room, since the date the medication was prescribed and the number of pills remaining in the bottle can provide helpful information to the treating physician.

☞ **Special considerations:** In susceptible individuals (i.e., those with a personal or family history of substance abuse, alcohol dependence, or alcohol abuse), the potential for addiction is considerable. Consequently, these persons should avoid using alprazolam and other benzodiazepines. When a benzodiazepine is indicated, psychiatrists today generally prescribe clonazepam (Klonopin) in preference to alprazolam because this medication has a slightly longer half-life so may be taken less frequently during the day, is more slowly absorbed, and has a slightly lower potential for abuse. People who have been on alprazolam for longer than one month sometimes experience great difficulty in stopping the medication. Physicians may have to reduce the medication slowly (by 10 percent of the daily dose per week). For persons with panic disorder, which is a chronic condition similar to depression, psychiatrists usually prefer to use antidepressants, either newer drugs such as the SSRIs, nefazodone (Serzone), mirtazapine (Remeron), or the older tricyclic antidepressants. In some cases, both a benzodiazepine and an antidepressant may be prescribed. The benzodiazepine is gradually reduced after the antidepressant takes full effect, usually after four to six weeks.

Generic name: **BUSPIRONE**

 Available in generic form: Yes

 Brand name: BuSpar

 Drug class: azapirone

Prescribed for: Generalized anxiety disorder, social anxiety disorder, mild to moderate agitation (associated with anxiety, dementia, and other neurologic disorders), premenstrual anxiety and agitation, and with SSRIs for medication-induced or residual anxiety and for sexual dysfunction resulting from SSRIs. Buspirone is also used with SSRIs in treating obsessive-compulsive disorder.

General information: Buspirone, the only approved medication in a class of drugs called azapirones, relieves anxiety symptoms primarily by altering serotonin-receptor sensitivity at a specific serotonin subtype ($5\text{-}HT_{1A}$). Buspirone is an excellent choice for individuals with a personal or family history of substance abuse or dependence, since it does not intensify the effects of alcohol and does not increase the risk of relapse in people who have a history of alcoholism or substance abuse. In contrast to benzodiazepines, buspirone does not need to be tapered off but may be abruptly stopped without severe withdrawal symptoms. Another major advantage of buspirone is that it does not interfere with memory or cognitive skills and does not increase the risk of falls or loss of coordination, both important concerns for older persons. In contrast to the SSRI antidepressants, buspirone does not interfere with normal sexual functioning. Unlike the benzodiazepines, it does not produce sedation. As with benzodiazepines, an overdose of buspirone is not life-threatening.

Dosing information: Buspirone is available in 5- and 10-mg. tablets and in a 15-mg. and 30-mg. Dividose. The advantage of the Dividose is that individuals may increase the dose when advisable, say from 5 to 10 mg., without obtaining a new prescription by simply dividing the tablet. The 15-mg. tablet is scored so that dosages of 5, 7.5, and 10 mg. may be obtained by breaking the tablet into different sections. Correspondingly, the 30-mg. Dividose may be divided into 10-, 15-, and 20-mg. doses. The usual starting dose is 7.5 mg. twice a day, with an increase to 15 mg. twice a day after the first week. The usual therapeutic dose in healthy adults (including seniors) is 30 to 60 mg. a day. Physicians often suggest taking more of the medication at bedtime to minimize any side effects. Buspirone works in a manner similar to antidepressants in that initial effects may not be felt for two to three weeks, with maximum benefit after six to eight weeks of treatment.

If buspirone is used with an SSRI, the usual initial dose is 5 mg. in the evening, with 5-mg. increases every four days to a week. To treat residual anxiety symptoms in depressed persons taking an SSRI, a typical total daily dose is between 10 and 20 mg. To treat agitation in older individuals who may have mild to moderate dementia, buspirone is prescribed in dosages between 30 and 60 mg. Some people with particularly severe anxiety or agitation may require higher doses, above 60 mg. a day. Although this is the maximum recommended dose, physicians have prescribed higher doses, up to 90 mg. a day, to treat such agitation in both adults and seniors.

Common side effects: The most common side effects of buspirone are dizziness and light-headedness. Similar to other serotonin agents, buspirone may produce nausea and headache. In individuals who are particularly sensitive to medications or who metabolize them slowly, buspirone may produce nervousness or excitement. In contrast to the SSRIs, buspirone does not produce sexual dysfunction or weight gain.

Precautions: If buspirone is prescribed with nefazodone (Serzone), a serotonin 5-HT$_2$ antagonist-type antidepressant, it is begun at a dose of 5 mg. in the evening and increased slowly because both drugs are metabolized in a similar fashion.

Warnings: Buspirone (BuSpar) should be prescribed initially in lower doses with SSRIs, since it is a serotonin agent and may produce a potentially deadly condition called serotonin syndrome. Initial symptoms include lethargy, restlessness, confusion, flushing, sweating, tremor, and involuntary muscle jerks. Over time, a small percentage of persons may develop muscle disorders, hyperthermia, and rigor, which may lead to respiratory problems, increased platelet clotting, destruction of the red blood cells by the kidneys and their excretion in urine, and kidney failure. This syndrome requires emergency medical treatment. Buspirone should never be prescribed with MAO inhibitors, since the combination can cause a dangerous rise in blood pressure.

Alcohol: Buspirone, when taken with alcohol, will not intensify alcohol's side effects, such as sedation, memory disturbance, and impaired judgment. However, people taking buspirone should not drink alcohol, since alcohol may worsen anxiety and depressive symptoms.

Food and beverages: No restrictions. If taking buspirone on an empty stomach upsets your stomach, try it with food or immediately after eating.

Possible drug interactions: Buspirone should never be prescribed with an MAO inhibitor; the combination can cause a dangerous rise in blood pressure. If prescribed with nefazodone (Serzone) or an SSRI, buspirone should be started at a lower dose and increased more slowly (e.g., 5 mg. in the evening with 5-mg. increases every three to four days). The antidepressant nefazodone (Serzone), the antibiotic erythromycin, the anti-ulcer drug cimetidine (Tagamet), and the antifungal agent itraconazole (Sporanox) may increase buspirone levels in the blood. Buspirone may increase the blood levels of an active metabolite of diazepam (Valium).

Use in pregnancy and breast-feeding: Pregnancy Category B

Buspirone has not been systematically studied in pregnant women. Animal studies have shown no fetal abnormalities. However, women taking buspirone should always consult with their physician if they are contemplating pregnancy or become pregnant. Buspirone should be taken by pregnant women only if the benefits outweigh any potential adverse effects on the fetus. Women taking buspirone should not breast-feed, since the effects on the baby are unknown. Small amounts of the drug can pass into the breast milk and be absorbed into the baby's bloodstream, leading to possible sedation and other unknown effects on the child's developing nervous system.

Use in children: Preliminary results from controlled clinical studies have not shown buspirone (in the form of a patch that is applied daily) to be an effective treatment for attention deficit hyperactivity disorder (ADHD) in children. However, clinical reports in the literature suggest that the tablet form of buspirone may be effective for selected cases of ADHD. Buspirone has not been systematically studied in the treatment of generalized anxiety disorder in children, although case reports indicate that it is beneficial. Other anecdotal reports suggest that buspirone may be effective in children for treating mixed anxiety and depression, and for agitation and anxiety associated with mental retardation. Tentative dosing guidelines for children suggest beginning with 2.5 mg. or 5 mg. in a single dose, and gradually increasing the dose to three times a day. The usual maximum dose in children is 20 mg. a day, and in adolescents, 60 mg. a day, both in three equal doses.

Use in seniors: Buspirone is especially safe in elderly persons and should be prescribed instead of benzodiazepines to treat anxiety and agitation, especially in seniors with dementia or other neurological disorders. In contrast to the benzodiazepines, buspirone does not increase the risk for falls, does not cause motor incoordination, and does not interfere with memory or concentration.

Overdosage: Taken alone, buspirone does not produce life-threatening effects with overdose; however, when taken with other agents such as alcohol and barbiturates, the risk of serious complications increases. People who overdose on buspirone should be taken to the emergency room. Bring the bottle of medication to the emergency room with the person, since the date it was prescribed and the number of pills remaining in the bottle can provide helpful information to the treating physician.

Special considerations: Buspirone is a unique anti-anxiety agent, the only drug of its kind to treat generalized anxiety disorder. It is frequently prescribed by psychiatrists in combination with antidepressants, especially SSRIs, to treat major depression, refractory obsessive-compulsive disorder, residual anxiety symptoms, and sexual dysfunction resulting from SSRIs. Because of the possibility of serotonin syndrome with this combination, psychiatrists begin buspirone at a low dose (5 mg.) and increase it gradually (5 mg. every four days to a week). Most individuals can tolerate its side effects.

 Generic name: CHLORDIAZEPOXIDE

 Available in generic form: Yes

 Brand name: Librium

 Drug class: Benzodiazepine

Rx **Prescribed for:** Panic disorder, generalized anxiety disorder, social anxiety disorder, specific phobia, adjustment disorder with anxiety, alcohol withdrawal symptoms. Chlordiazepoxide may be used with antidepressants to treat agitated depression and posttraumatic stress disorder.

General information: Benzodiazepines work by binding to benzodiazepine receptors found in the brain. These receptors, in turn, stimulate a specific neurotransmitter called gamma-aminobutyric acid (GABA), the principal inhibitory neurotransmitter in the brain, which is believed to reduce anxiety.

The use of chlordiazepoxide for most of the conditions listed above has declined due to the development of newer benzodiazepines that have a shorter half-life and fewer drug interactions, as well as the nonbenzodiazepine buspirone. Chlordiazepoxide's principal use these days is to treat alcohol withdrawal symptoms. While all the benzodiazepines may be used to treat alcohol withdrawal, chlordiazepoxide is most commonly prescribed because of its long half-life.

Dosing information: Chlordiazepoxide is available in 5-, 10-, and 25-mg. tablets. It is usually prescribed in doses of 25 mg., two to three times a day, with an increase in dose to control symptoms up to a maximum of 300 mg. a day. In the treatment of alcohol withdrawal, the physician will increase the dose of the chlordiazepoxide to the amount necessary to stop any withdrawal symptoms, such as tremor, increased heart rate, elevated blood pressure, sweating, and other symptoms. Chlordiazepoxide is able to control these symptoms by producing the same effects on the body as alcohol. Chlordiazepoxide is then gradually tapered off over a period of three days to a week. Physicians carefully monitor the dose of chlordiazepoxide and prescribe the lowest dose possible to decrease the possibility of dependence.

Common side effects: The most common side effects of benzodiazepines are sedation, a "spacey" feeling, impaired concentration, memory disturbances, and poor coordination. Benzodiazepines may interfere with driving skills by reducing reflexes and impairing coordination. Older people are more susceptible to these effects and also are at increased risk of falling when taking benzodiazepines.

Precautions: Some people may develop "paradoxical" responses that, due to loss of inhibition, may lead to bizarre behavior, anger, irritability, and anxiety. These reactions are more likely to occur in the elderly, people with brain damage, those with a history of an impulse-control disorder, and those suffering from borderline personality disorder, which is characterized by impulsivity and instability in interpersonal relationships, mood, and self-image. Benzodiazepines may impair breathing in individuals with chronic obstructive pulmonary disorder (COPD) or emphysema.

≷⊘≷**Warnings:** Individuals with acute narrow-angle glaucoma should not take benzodiazepines. People suffering from sleep apnea, a sleep disorder characterized by long pauses in respiration during the night, should also avoid benzodiazepines because they decrease the ability to begin breathing again after such a pause—a potentially fatal risk. Chlordiazepoxide should not be stopped suddenly because of the risk of withdrawal reactions, such as rebound anxiety or agitation; however, such withdrawal symptoms are usually mild in comparison to alprazolam (Xanax) or lorazepam (Ativan).

Alcohol: People should not drink alcohol when taking benzodiazepines. When taken together, benzodiazepines and alcohol intensify side effects such as sedation, memory disturbance, motor incoordination, euphoria, and judgment problems and can seriously impair driving ability.

Food and beverages: No restrictions.

Possible drug interactions: Other medications that may produce sedation, such as antihistamines and certain sedating antidepressants, should be used with caution. Some drugs that affect the ability of the liver to function may increase blood levels of most benzodiazepines; these medications include birth-control pills, anti-ulcer drugs such as cimetidine (Tagamet), the antihypertensive medication propanolol (Inderal), and disulfiram (Antabuse), which is used to treat alcoholism.

Use in pregnancy and breast-feeding:
Pregnancy Category D
Chlordiazepoxide has not been studied in pregnant women. In animals, benzodiazepines have been shown to produce cleft palate in the fetus. Some studies suggest that

benzodiazepines, especially chlordiazepoxide and diazepam (Valium), may increase the risk of cleft lip and heart
deformities in human fetuses, especially when taken by
women in the first trimester. In general, the use of benzodiazepines during pregnancy should almost always be
avoided, especially in the first trimester. Chlordiazepoxide
should be used in pregnant women only if the benefits to
the mother greatly outweigh any potential risks to the fetus and if alternative agents have been unsuccessful.
Women on chlordiazepoxide should not breast-feed, since
the effects on the baby are unknown.

Use in children: Since clinical experience in children under six years of age is limited, the use of the
drug in this age group is not recommended. If used in children and adolescents between ages six and seventeen, a
typical starting dose would be 5 mg. two to four times a
day, with a usual therapeutic dose of 10 mg. two to three
times a day.

Use in seniors: Older people should not use chlordiazepoxide and other benzodiazepines because
these drugs increase the risk of falls and of accidents when
driving. In the elderly, the metabolism of chlordiazepoxide
may be quite prolonged, leading to additional adverse side
effects, such as excessive sedation and confusion.

Overdosage: Taken alone in overdose, chlordiazepoxide does not produce life-threatening consequences. However, when taken with other agents such as
alcohol or barbiturates, the risk of serious complications
or death increases considerably. People who overdose on
chlordiazepoxide should be taken to the emergency room.
Bring the bottle of medication to the emergency room with
the person, since the date it was prescribed and the number of pills remaining in the bottle can provide helpful information to the treating physician.

Special considerations: In susceptible individuals (i.e., those with a personal or family history of substance abuse, alcohol dependence, or alcohol abuse), the potential for addiction is considerable. Consequently, chlordiazepoxide and other benzodiazepines should be avoided.

Generic name: CLONAZEPAM

 Available in generic form: Yes

 Brand name: Klonopin

Drug class: Benzodiazepine

Prescribed for: Panic disorder, generalized anxiety disorder, social anxiety disorder, simple phobia, adjustment disorder with anxiety, alcohol withdrawal. Clonazepam may be used with antidepressants to treat agitated depression and posttraumatic stress disorder. It is sometimes used in women for premenstrual agitation and associated anxiety.

General information: The use of clonazepam and other benzodiazepines has declined with the development of newer antidepressants with fewer side effects. Benzodiazepines work by binding to benzodiazepine receptors found in the brain. These receptors, in turn, stimulate a specific neurotransmitter called GABA, the principal inhibitory neurotransmitter in the brain, which is believed to reduce anxiety.

Clonazepam is not absorbed as rapidly into the central nervous system as alprazolam (Xanax) or lorazepam (Ativan); hence it produces less euphoria and may have less addiction potential.

Dosing information: Clonazepam is available in 0.5-, 1-, and 2-mg. tablets. It is usually begun at doses of 0.5 mg. two or three times a day and increased gradually to a maximum dose of 6 to 8 mg. a day. The usual therapeutic dose is 1 to 4 mg. a day. Most people begin to feel the effects of the medication within the first several days to a week. When used to treat panic disorder, persons need to continue medication for six months or longer. In some cases, clonazepam is prescribed along with an antidepressant. It is then gradually reduced after the antidepressant takes full effect, usually after four to six weeks. Physicians carefully monitor the dose of clonazepam and prescribe the lowest dose possible to decrease the possibility of dependence.

Common side effects: The most common side effects of benzodiazepines are sedation, a "spacey" feeling, impaired concentration, memory disturbances, and poor coordination. Clonazepam may produce slightly more sedation than the other benzodiazepines. Benzodiazepines may interfere with driving skills by reducing reflexes and impairing coordination. Older people are more susceptible to these effects and are also at increased risk of falling when taking benzodiazepines.

Precautions: Some people may develop "paradoxical" responses that, due to loss of inhibition, may lead to bizarre behavior, anger, irritability, and anxiety. These reactions are more likely to occur in the elderly, people with brain damage, those with a history of an impulse-control disorder, and those suffering from borderline personality disorder, which is characterized by impulsivity and instability in interpersonal relationships, mood, and self-image. Benzodiazepines may impair breathing in individuals with chronic obstructive pulmonary disorder (COPD) or emphysema.

Warnings: Individuals with acute narrow-angle glaucoma should not take benzodiazepines. People with sleep apnea, a sleep disorder characterized by long pauses in respiration during the night, should also avoid benzodiazepines because they decrease the ability to begin breathing again after such pauses—a potentially fatal risk. Clonazepam should never be stopped abruptly because of the risk of severe withdrawal reactions, such as seizures, intense rebound anxiety, and extreme agitation. If clonazepam has been taken for four or more weeks, it should be tapered off gradually over a period of two to eight weeks. The drug should be decreased each week at a rate of 10 percent of the total daily dose.

Alcohol: People should not drink alcohol when taking benzodiazepines. When taken together, benzodiazepines and alcohol intensify side effects, such as sedation, memory disturbance, motor incoordination, euphoria, and impaired judgment, and can seriously impair driving ability.

Food and beverages: No restrictions.

Possible drug interactions: Other medications that produce sedation, such as antihistamines and certain sedating antidepressants, should be used with caution. Some drugs that affect the ability of the liver to function increase blood levels of benzodiazepines; these medications include birth-control pills, anti-ulcer drugs such as cimetidine (Tagamet), the antihypertensive medication propranolol (Inderal), and disulfiram (Antabuse), which is used to treat alcoholism.

Use in pregnancy and breast-feeding:
Pregnancy Category C
Clonazepam has not been studied in pregnant women. In

animals, benzodiazepines have been shown to produce cleft palate in the fetus. Some studies suggest that benzodiazepines may increase the risk of cleft lip and heart deformities in human fetuses, especially when taken by women in the first trimester. In general, the use of benzodiazepines during pregnancy should almost always be avoided, especially in the first trimester. Clonazepam should be used in pregnant women only if the benefits to the mother greatly outweigh any potential risks to the fetus and if alternative agents have been unsuccessful. Women taking clonazepam should not breast-feed, since the effects on the baby are unknown.

Use in children: This medication has not been systematically studied in children; however, recent studies suggest that it may be effective to treat panic disorder in adolescents. Its effectiveness in younger children has been questionable. Dosages used in children have ranged from 0.5 to 1 mg. one to three times a day, with a total maximum daily dose up to 3 mg.

Use in seniors: Older people should not use clonazepam and other benzodiazepines because these drugs increase the risk of falls and of accidents when driving.

Overdosage: Taken alone in overdose, clonazepam does not produce life-threatening consequences; however, when taken with other agents such as alcohol or barbiturates, the risk of serious complications or death increases considerably. People who overdose on clonazepam should be taken to the emergency room. Bring the bottle of medication to the emergency room with the person, since the date it was prescribed and the number of pills remaining in the bottle can provide helpful information to the treating physician.

Special considerations: In susceptible individuals (i.e., those with a personal or family history of substance abuse, alcohol dependence, or alcohol abuse) the potential for addiction is considerable. Consequently, these persons should avoid using clonazepam and other benzodiazepines. Psychiatrists frequently prefer clonazepam to alprazolam (Xanax) to treat panic disorder because clonazepam has a slightly longer half-life so may be taken less frequently during the day. In addition, there is less risk for developing physical dependence and tolerance, and individuals may be more readily withdrawn from it. However, clonazepam requires a gradual reduction in dose so the person does not experience rebound anxiety or severe withdrawal reactions. Because of its slightly greater capacity to produce sedation, clonazepam is often prescribed at bedtime to ease any sleep difficulties associated with panic disorder or other anxiety disorders.

Generic name: CLORAZEPATE

 Available in generic form: Yes

 Brand name: Tranxene, Tranxene-SD, Tranxene-SD Half Strength

 Drug class: Benzodiazepine

Prescribed for: Panic disorder, generalized anxiety disorder, social anxiety disorder, simple phobia, adjustment disorder with anxiety, alcohol withdrawal. Clorazepate may be used with antidepressants to treat agitated depression and posttraumatic stress disorder.

General information: The use of clorazepate and other benzodiazepines has declined with the development of newer antidepressants with fewer side effects.

Benzodiazepines work by binding at benzodiazepine receptors found in the brain. Those receptors, in turn, stimulate a specific neurotransmitter called GABA, the principal inhibitory neurotransmitter in the brain, which is believed to reduce anxiety.

Dosing information: Clorazepate is available in 3.75-, 7.5-, and 15-mg. tablets and capsules. Tranxene-SD is available in a 22.5-mg. tablet; Tranxene-SD Half Strength is available in an 11.25-mg. tablet, taken only once a day. The usual starting dose is 7.5 mg. two to three times a day, with increases to up to 90 mg. a day to control anxiety symptoms. After a person is stabilized on a dose of clorazepate taken two to three times a day, he or she may be switched to the Tranxene-SD formulation. For instance, someone responding well to clorazepate 7.5 mg. taken three times a day may be switched to the 22.5-mg. Tranxene-SD tablet. Physicians carefully monitor the dose of clorazepate and prescribe the lowest dose possible to decrease the possibility of dependence.

Common side effects: The most common side effects are sedation, a "spacey" feeling, impaired concentration, memory disturbances, and poor coordination. Benzodiazepines may interfere with driving skills by reducing reflexes and impairing coordination. Older people are more susceptible to these effects and are also at increased risk of falling when taking benzodiazepines.

Precautions: Some people may develop "paradoxical" responses that, due to loss of inhibition, may lead to bizarre behavior, anger, irritability, and anxiety. These reactions are more likely to occur in the elderly, people with brain damage, those with a history of an impulse-control disorder, and those suffering from borderline personality disorder, which is characterized by impulsivity and instability in interpersonal relationships, mood, and self-image. Benzodiazepines may impair breathing in individuals with chronic obstructive pulmonary disorder (COPD) or emphysema.

Warnings: Individuals with acute narrow-angle glaucoma should not take benzodiazepines. People suffering from sleep apnea, a sleep disorder characterized by long pauses in respiration during the night, should also avoid benzodiazepines because they decrease the ability to begin breathing again after such a pause—a potentially fatal risk. Clorazepate should not be stopped suddenly because of the risk of withdrawal reactions, such as intense rebound anxiety and extreme agitation; however, such withdrawal symptoms are usually mild in comparison with those of alprazolam (Xanax) or lorazepam (Ativan).

Alcohol: People should not drink alcohol when taking benzodiazepines. When taken together, benzodiazepines and alcohol intensify side effects such as sedation, memory disturbance, motor incoordination, euphoria, and judgment problems, and can seriously impair driving.

Food and beverages: No restrictions.

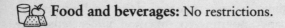

Possible drug interactions: Other medications that may produce sedation, such as antihistamines and certain sedating antidepressants, should be used with caution. Some drugs that affect the ability of the liver to function may increase blood levels of benzodiazepines; these medications include birth-control pills, anti-ulcer drugs such as cimetidine (Tagamet), the antihypertensive medication propanolol (Inderal), and disulfiram (Antabuse), which is used to treat alcoholism.

Use in pregnancy and breast-feeding: Pregnancy Category D

Clorazepate has not been studied in pregnant women. In animals, benzodiazepines have been shown to produce cleft palate in the fetus. Some studies suggest that benzodiazepines may increase the risk of cleft lip and heart deformities in human fetuses, especially when taken by women in the first trimester. In general, the use of benzodiazepines during pregnancy should almost always be avoided, particularly in the first trimester. Clorazepate should be used in pregnant women only if the benefits to the mother greatly outweigh any potential risks to the fetus and if alternative agents have been unsuccessful. Women taking clorazepate should not breast-feed, since the effects on the baby are unknown.

Use in children: This medication has not been systematically studied in children. It should not be used in children under the age of nine years. In children and adolescents, an initial dose should be in the 3.75- to 7.5-mg. range, taken once or twice a day as needed and as tolerated. The dosage should not be increased more than 7.5 mg a week. The usual maximum total daily dose in children is 60 mg.

Use in seniors: Older people should not use clorazepate and other benzodiazepines because these drugs increase the risk of falling and of accidents when driving. In the elderly, the metabolism of clorazepate may be quite prolonged, leading to more adverse side effects, such as excessive sedation and confusion.

Overdosage: Taken alone in overdose, clorazepate does not produce life-threatening consequences; however, when taken with other agents such as alcohol or barbiturates, the risk of serious complications or death

increases considerably. People who overdose on clorazepate should be taken to the emergency room. Bring the bottle of medication to the emergency room with the person, since the date it was prescribed and the number of pills remaining in the bottle can provide helpful information to the treating physician.

Special considerations: In susceptible individuals (i.e., those with a personal or family history of substance abuse, alcohol dependence, or alcohol abuse), the potential for addiction is considerable; consequently, clorazepate and other benzodiazepines should be avoided.

Generic name: DIAZEPAM

Available in generic form: Yes

Brand name: Valium

Drug class: Benzodiazepine

Prescribed for: Panic disorder, generalized anxiety disorder, social anxiety disorder, simple phobia, adjustment disorder with anxiety, alcohol withdrawal. Diazepam may be used with antidepressants to treat agitated depression and posttraumatic stress disorder.

General information: The use of diazepam and other benzodiazepines has diminished with the development of newer antidepressants with fewer side effects. Benzodiazepines work by binding at benzodiazepine receptors found in the brain. Those receptors, in turn, stimulate a specific neurotransmitter called GABA, the principal inhibitory neurotransmitter in the brain, which is believed to reduce anxiety.

Diazepam, together with chlordiazepoxide (Librium), is

one of the older benzodiazepines and was once one of the most widely prescribed medications. It is now used less frequently than the newer benzodiazepines. Its principal use now is to treat alcohol withdrawal symptoms. Diazepam is also available in an injectable form that may be administered intravenously or intramuscularly.

Dosing information: Diazepam is available in 2-, 5-, and 10-mg, tablets. The usual starting dose is 2 to 5 mg. two to three times a day, with increases up to 40 mg. a day to control anxiety symptoms. Physicians carefully monitor the dose of diazepam and prescribe the lowest dose possible to decrease the possibility of dependence.

Common side effects: The most common side effects are sedation, a "spacey" feeling, impaired concentration, memory disturbances, and poor coordination. Benzodiazepines may interfere with driving skills by reducing reflexes and impairing coordination. Older people are more susceptible to these effects and are also at increased risk of falling when taking benzodiazepines.

Precautions: Some people may develop "paradoxical" responses that, due to loss of inhibition, may lead to bizarre behavior, anger, irritability, and anxiety. These reactions are more likely to occur in the elderly, people with brain damage, those with a history of an impulse-control disorder, and those suffering from borderline personality disorder, which is characterized by impulsivity and instability of interpersonal relationships, mood, and self-image. Benzodiazepines may impair breathing in individuals with chronic obstructive pulmonary disorder (COPD) or emphysema.

Warnings: Individuals with acute narrow-angle glaucoma should not take benzodiazepines. People suffering from sleep apnea, a sleep disorder characterized by long pauses in respiration during the night, should also avoid benzodiazepines because they decrease the ability to begin breathing again after such a pause—a potentially fatal risk. Diazepam should not be stopped suddenly because of the risk of withdrawal reactions, such as intense rebound anxiety and extreme agitation; however, such withdrawal symptoms are usually mild in comparison to alprazolam (Xanax) or lorazepam (Ativan).

Alcohol: People should not drink alcohol when taking benzodiazepines. When taken together, benzodiazepines and alcohol intensify side effects such as sedation, memory disturbance, motor incoordination, euphoria, and judgment problems, and can seriously impair driving.

Food and beverages: No restrictions.

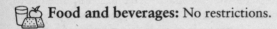

Possible drug interactions: Other medications that may produce sedation, such as antihistamines and certain sedating antidepressants, should be used with caution. Some drugs that affect the ability of the liver to function may increase blood levels of benzodiazepines; these medications include birth-control pills, anti-ulcer drugs such as cimetidine (Tagamet), the antihypertensive medication propanolol (Inderal), and disulfiram (Antabuse), which is used to treat alcoholism.

**Use in pregnancy and breast-feeding:
Pregnancy Category D**

Diazepam has not been studied in pregnant women. In animals, benzodiazepines have been shown to produce cleft palate in the fetus. Some studies suggest that benzodiazepines, especially diazepam and chlordiazepoxide (Librium), may increase the risk of cleft lip and heart deformities in human fetuses, especially when taken by women in the first trimester. In general, the use of benzodiazepines during pregnancy should almost always be avoided, particularly in the first trimester. Diazepam should be used in pregnant women only if the benefits to the mother greatly outweigh any potential risks to the fetus and if alternative agents have been unsuccessful. Women taking diazepam should not breast-feed, since the effects on the baby are unknown.

Use in children: This medication has not been systematically studied in children. It should not be used under the age of six months. In children and adolescents, an initial dose should be in the 1- to 2.5-mg. range, taken up to three to four times daily as needed and as tolerated. The usual maximum total daily dose is 10 mg.

Use in seniors: Older people should not use diazepam and other benzodiazepines because these drugs increase the risk of falling and of accidents when driving. In the elderly, the metabolism of diazepam may be quite prolonged, leading to more adverse side effects, such as excessive sedation and confusion.

Overdosage: Taken alone in overdose, diazepam does not produce life-threatening consequences; however, when taken with other agents such as alcohol or barbiturates, the risk of serious complications or death increases considerably. People who overdose on diazepam should be taken to the emergency room. Bring the bottle of medication to the emergency room with the person, since the date it was prescribed and the number of pills remaining in the bottle can provide helpful information to the treating physician.

Special considerations: In susceptible individuals (i.e., those with a personal or family history of substance abuse, alcohol dependence, or alcohol abuse), the potential for addiction is considerable; consequently, diazepam and other benzodiazepines should be avoided.

 Generic name: LORAZEPAM

 Available in generic form: Yes

 Brand name: Ativan

 Drug class: Benzodiazepine

Prescribed for: Panic disorder, generalized anxiety disorder, social anxiety disorder, simple phobia, adjustment disorder with anxiety. Lorazepam may be used with antidepressants to treat agitated depression and post-traumatic stress disorder. It is sometimes used in women for premenstrual agitation and anxiety.

General information: The use of lorazepam and other benzodiazepines has diminished with the development of newer antidepressants with fewer side effects. Benzodiazepines work by binding to benzodiazepine receptors found in the brain. These receptors, in turn, stimulate a specific neurotransmitter called GABA, the principal inhibitory neurotransmitter in the brain, which is believed to reduce anxiety. Lorazepam, similar to oxazepam (Serax) and unlike other benzodiazepines, has no active metabolites and can be used safely in people with liver disease or those taking other medications metabolized by the liver. Because lorazepam is rapidly absorbed into the central nervous system, it may produce euphoria and have more addiction potential than agents that are absorbed more slowly, such as oxazepam (Serax) or clonazepam (Klonopin).

Dosing information: Lorazepam is available in 0.5-, 1-, and 2-mg. tablets. The initial dose is usually 0.5 mg. three times a day, with increases up to a maximum of 6 to 8 mg. a day to control anxiety symptoms. Lorazepam is also available in an injectable form that may be given intramuscularly or intravenously. Physicians carefully monitor the dose of lorazepam and prescribe the lowest dose possible to decrease the possibility of dependence.

Common side effects: The most common side effects are sedation, a "spacey" feeling, impaired concentration, memory disturbances, and poor coordination. Benzodiazepines may interfere with driving skills by reducing reflexes and impairing coordination. Older people are more susceptible to these effects and are also at increased risk of falling when taking benzodiazepines.

Precautions: Some people may develop "paradoxical" responses that, due to loss of inhibition, may lead to bizarre behavior, anger, irritability, and anxiety. These reactions are more likely to occur in the elderly, people with brain damage, those with a history of an impulse-control disorder, and those suffering from borderline personality disorder, which is characterized by impulsivity and instability of interpersonal relationships, mood, and self-image. Benzodiazepines can impair breathing in persons with chronic obstructive pulmonary disorder (COPD) or emphysema.

Warnings: Benzodiazepines should not be used by anyone suffering from acute narrow-angle glaucoma. People suffering from sleep apnea, a sleep disorder characterized by long pauses in respiration during the night, should also avoid benzodiazepines because they decrease the ability to begin breathing again after such a pause—a potentially fatal risk. Lorazepam should never be stopped suddenly because of severe withdrawal reactions, such as seizures, intense rebound anxiety, and extreme agitation. If lorazepam has been taken for four or more weeks, it should be tapered off gradually over a period of two to eight weeks. The drug should be decreased each week at a rate of 10 percent of the total daily dose.

▽ **Alcohol:** People should not drink alcohol when taking benzodiazepines. When taken together, benzodiazepines and alcohol intensify side effects such as sedation, memory disturbance, motor incoordination, euphoria, and impaired judgment, and can seriously impair driving ability.

Food and beverages: No restrictions.

Possible drug interactions: Other medications that may produce sedation, such as antihistamines and certain sedating antidepressants, should be used with caution. Because lorazepam is metabolized differently from the other benzodiazepines, it may be taken by people with liver disease and other chronic medical illnesses or those taking multiple medications, since adverse drug interactions are less likely. For the most part, individuals taking birth-control pills, propanolol (Inderal), disulfiram (Antabuse), and cimetidine (Tagamet) or other anti-ulcer drugs do not have to worry about the effects of these medications on blood levels of lorazepam.

Use in pregnancy and breast-feeding: Pregnancy Category D

Lorazepam has not been studied in pregnant women. In animals, benzodiazepines have been shown to produce cleft palate in the fetus. Some studies suggest that benzodiazepines may increase the risk of cleft lip and heart deformities in human fetuses, especially when taken by women in the first trimester. In general, the use of benzodiazepines during pregnancy should almost always be avoided, particularly in the first trimester. Lorazepam should be used in pregnant women only if the benefits to the mother greatly outweigh any potential risks to the fetus and if alternative agents have been unsuccessful. Women on lorazepam should not breast-feed, since the effects on the baby are unknown.

Use in children: This medication has not been systematically studied in children. Its safety and effectiveness in children under the age of twelve has not been established. If used in children or adolescents, initial doses may be 0.25 to 0.5 mg. up to three times a day, with a total daily maximum dose of up to 6 mg.

Use in seniors: Older people should not use lorazepam and other benzodiazepines because these drugs increase the risk of falling and of accidents when driving.

Overdosage: Taken alone in overdose, lorazepam does not produce life-threatening consequences; however, when taken with other agents such as alcohol or barbiturates, the risk of serious complications or death increases. People who overdose on lorazepam should be taken to the emergency room. Bring the bottle of medication to the emergency room with the person, since the date it was prescribed and the number of pills remaining in the bottle can provide helpful information to the treating physician.

Special considerations: Lorazepam is frequently used by physicians to calm and relax people prior to surgery or medical procedures because of its relative safety in individuals taking multiple medications and those with liver disease.

Generic name: OXAZEPAM

 Available in generic form: Yes

 Brand name: Serax

 Drug class: Benzodiazepine

Prescribed for: Panic disorder, generalized anxiety disorder, social anxiety disorder, simple phobia, adjustment disorder with anxiety, alcohol withdrawal. Oxazepam may be used with antidepressants to treat agitated depression and posttraumatic stress disorder. It is sometimes used in women for premenstrual agitation and anxiety.

General information: The use of oxazepam and other benzodiazepines has diminished with the development of newer antidepressants with fewer side effects. Benzodiazepines work by binding to benzodiazepine receptors found in the brain. These receptors, in turn, stimulate a specific neurotransmitter called GABA, the principal inhibitory neurotransmitter in the brain, which is believed to reduce anxiety.

Oxazepam, similar to lorazepam (Ativan) and unlike other benzodiazepines, has no active metabolites and can be used safely in people with liver disease or those taking other medications metabolized by the liver. In addition, oxazepam is not absorbed as rapidly into the central nervous system as alprazolam or lorazepam; thus, it produces less euphoria and may have less addiction potential.

Dosing information: Oxazepam is available in 15-mg. tablets and 10-, 15-, and 30-mg. capsules. It is usually prescribed at a dose of 15 to 30 mg., taken three or four times a day. The maximum daily dose is usually 120 mg. Physicians carefully monitor the dose of oxazepam and prescribe the lowest dose possible to decrease the possibility of dependence.

Common side effects: The most common side effects are sedation, a "spacey" feeling, memory disturbances, impaired concentration, and poor coordination. Benzodiazepines may interfere with driving skills by reducing reflexes and impairing coordination. Older people are more susceptible to these effects and are also at increased risk of falling when taking benzodiazepines.

Precautions: Some people may develop "paradoxical" responses that, due to loss of inhibition, may lead to bizarre behavior, anger, irritability, and anxiety. These reactions are more likely to occur in the elderly, people with brain damage, those with a history of an impulse-control disorder, and those suffering from borderline personality disorder, which is characterized by impulsivity and instability of interpersonal relationships, mood, and self-image. Benzodiazepines can impair breathing in individuals with chronic obstructive pulmonary disorder (COPD) or emphysema.

Warnings: Benzodiazepines should not be used by anyone suffering from acute narrow-angle glaucoma. People suffering from sleep apnea, a sleep disorder characterized by long pauses in respiration during the night, should also avoid benzodiazepines because they decrease the ability to begin breathing again after such a pause—a potentially fatal risk. Oxazepam should never be stopped suddenly because of severe withdrawal reactions, such as intense rebound anxiety and extreme agitation. If oxazepam has been taken for four or more weeks, it should be tapered off gradually over a period of two to eight weeks. The drug should be decreased each week at a rate of 10 percent of the total daily dose.

⚗ **Alcohol:** People should not drink alcohol when taking benzodiazepines. When taken together, benzodiazepines and alcohol intensify side effects such as sedation, memory disturbance, motor incoordination, euphoria, and impaired judgment, and can seriously affect driving ability.

 Food and beverages: No restrictions.

Possible drug interactions: Be cautious about using other medications that may produce sedation, such as antihistamines and certain sedating antidepressants. Because oxazepam is metabolized slightly differently from the other benzodiazepines, it may be taken by people with liver disease and other chronic medical illnesses or those taking multiple medications, since adverse drug interactions are less likely. For the most part, individuals taking birth-control pills, propanolol (Inderal), disulfiram (Antabuse), and cimetidine (Tagamet) or other anti-ulcer drugs do not have to worry about the effects of these medications on blood levels of oxazepam.

Use in pregnancy and breast-feeding: Pregnancy Category D

Oxazepam has not been studied in pregnant women. In animals, benzodiazepines have been shown to produce cleft palate in the fetus. Some studies suggest that benzodiazepines may increase the risk of cleft lip and heart deformities in human fetuses, especially when taken by women during the first trimester. In general, the use of benzodiazepines during pregnancy should almost always be avoided, particularly in the first trimester. Oxazepam should be used in pregnant women only if the benefits to the mother greatly outweigh any potential risks to the fetus and if alternative agents have been unsuccessful. Women on oxazepam should not breast-feed, since the effects on the baby are unknown.

Use in children: This medication has not been systematically studied in children or adolescents. Its safety and effectiveness in children under six years of age have not been established. The absolute dosage for children between six and twelve years of age has not been established; if oxazepam is used in children, an initial dose would generally be 7.5 mg, up to two to three times a day, with a maximum total daily dose of 45 mg.

Use in seniors: Older people should not use oxazepam and other benzodiazepines because these drugs increase the risk of falling and of accidents when driving. However, oxazepam may be safer than other benzodiazepines because it has a relatively short half-life, no active metabolites, and is absorbed more slowly into the central nervous system.

Overdosage: Taken alone in overdose, oxazepam does not produce life-threatening consequences; however, when taken with other agents such as alcohol or barbiturates, the risk of serious complications or death increases. People who overdose on oxazepam should be taken to the emergency room. Bring the bottle of medication to the emergency room with the person, since the date it was prescribed and the number of pills remaining in the bottle can provide helpful information to the treating physician.

Special considerations: Because it has a relatively short half-life and no active metabolites, oxazepam may be a preferred benzodiazepine for use in elderly persons, individuals taking multiple medications, and those with liver disease and other chronic illnesses.

CHAPTER 4

Mood Stabilizers

To learn general information about this class of medications and the disorders they treat, read the first part of the chapter. To read about a specific mood-stabilizing medication, turn to the page indicated below.

BIPOLAR DISORDER

Bipolar illness (manic depression) takes people to extremes. Individuals with bipolar disorders describe themselves as having "higher highs" and "lower lows" than others. When they are "up," they are on top of the world, absolutely euphoric, endlessly energetic, convinced that they can do anything they set out to do—whether that means skiing the expert run without ever having taken a lesson or dropping out of business school to become a screenwriter. People with bipolar disorders can and do go over the edge, often becoming self-destructive and sometimes losing touch with reality. Their plunge downward from the exhilarating highs of mania into the depths of depression can be so wrenching that life seems unbearably painful.

The various types of bipolar illness—bipolar I, bipolar II, and cyclothymia—account for about 20 percent of all depressive disorders. They are among the most treatable mental illnesses if they are correctly diagnosed and treated. Unfortunately, affected individuals often are misdiagnosed or remain undiagnosed for years.

The cycles of despair and euphoria that are characteristic of bipolar illness can take various forms, but all involve episodes of hypomania (a mild form of mania) or mania, or mixed episodes (periods of at least one week of rapidly changing moods along with symptoms of mania and major depression). Hypomania usually imparts an intense sense of well-being, elation, and confidence and does not significantly impair functioning, although individuals may take dangerous risks or make impetuous decisions. Yet they also may become more productive, more passionate, or more charismatic than usual, all of which can be very appealing. In episodes of full-blown mania, impulsiveness and poor judgment become so extreme that they can destroy relationships, wreck careers, and wipe out personal finances. Some individuals develop psychotic symptoms, such as delusions and hallucinations, and require almost constant supervision to prevent physical harm. About 10 percent of people with a bipolar disorder experience only mania, without any depression. Mixed episodes seem to be more common among younger people and individuals over the age of sixty.

As shown in Table 4-1, bipolar disorder causes a wide range of symptoms. The following clusters of symptoms are common:

- *Changes in mood for a distinct period of time:* feeling happy, optimistic, euphoric, irritable

- *Changes in thinking:* thoughts speeding through one's brain, unrealistic self-confidence, difficulty concentrating, grandiose plans, delusions, hallucinations

- *Changes in behavior:* an increase in activity or socializing, immersion in plans and projects, talking very rapidly and much more than usual, excessive spending, impaired judgment, impulsive sexual involvement

- *Changes in physical condition:* less need for sleep, increased energy, fewer health complaints than usual

Table 4-1: Symptoms of a Manic Episode

A bipolar disorder is characterized by mood swings that include episodes of depression and of mania or hypomania (less severe mania). Common symptoms of mania are shown below. See Chapter 2, Table 2-1, for common symptoms of depression.

• Feel unusual excitement, enthusiasm, energy, or irritability

• Experience an uncharacteristic change in mood or functioning

• Develop a sense of supreme self-confidence and inflated ability

• Have grandiose thoughts and plans

• Sleep very little and feel no need for more rest

• Talk more than usual and feel a sense of pressure to keep talking

• Think and talk rapidly, jumping from one idea to another

• Be easily distracted by irrelevant or unimportant comments or events

• Be physically and mentally restless

• Noticeably increase usual social, sexual, or work-related activities

• Get involved in activities or pleasurable pursuits likely to lead to painful consequences (e.g., sexual indiscretions, poor business investments, buying sprees, potentially dangerous sports or adventures)

The 9 in 10 people with bipolar illness who experience episodes of depression as well as mania or hypomania may develop the depressive symptoms described in Chapter 2, including a depressed mood, loss of interest or pleasure in activities, feelings of worthlessness and hopelessness, lack of appetite, sleep difficulties, lack of energy, and thoughts of suicide.

Cycles

The cycle of mood swings can vary greatly. Initially, in many instances, the period between episodes of depression, mania, or hypomania becomes shorter, with episodes occurring more and more frequently. In time, as part of its natural course, the condition may stabilize, with the interval between emotional extremes growing longer.

Although most people with bipolar disorders have some periods of normal moods, 5 to 15 percent of those diagnosed with mood disorders (women more often than men) experience "rapid cycling"—four or more manic or major depressive episodes in a year, each lasting at least twenty-four hours and ending with a switch to the opposite psychological state, that is, from depression to mania or the reverse, or with a period of stability.

In ultra-rapid cycling, episodes of depression, mania, or hypomania may last only twenty-four hours. Some therapists have reported cases of ultra-ultra-rapid cycling, in which several or even many episodes occur daily. In continuous cycling, individuals swing from depression to mania or hypomania and back again without ever feeling normal for any sustained period of time.

Like unipolar depression, bipolar illnesses can follow a seasonal pattern, with individuals regularly sinking into depression at certain times of the year and then swinging into hypomania or mania a few months later. About half of those with bipolar disorder develop symptoms of psychosis (such as hallucinations and delusions), which may reflect their sense of power, knowledge, or inflated worth. More rarely, these symptoms involve completely different themes, such as a delusion of being controlled by others.

Types

Bipolar I disorder always includes at least one manic or mixed episode, often with one or more episodes of major depression. People in the depressive phase of bipolar I disorder feel worthless, helpless, and hopeless; derive no pleasure from life; cannot concentrate or remember clearly; eat and sleep more or less than usual; withdraw from friends and relatives; complain of insomnia, aches, pains, fatigue, and other physical problems; and may consider or attempt suicide.

Bipolar I disorder can begin with an episode of mania or of depression. In those who experience a depression first (which is more common in women), the interval from the first depression to the first manic episode is typically one to two years, although in some instances mania does not develop for ten years or more. When individuals initially diagnosed as having major depression develop mania, their diagnosis changes to bipolar I disorder. More than 90 percent of persons who experience a single manic episode go on to have additional ones.

Bipolar II disorder, a new diagnosis added to the *Diagnostic and Statistical Manual of Mental Disorders, Fourth Edition (DSM-IV)*, consists of one or more major depressive episodes along with at least one episode of hypomania. Individuals with this type of bipolar disorder never develop full-blown mania; their "highs" are less extreme than those with bipolar I disorder. Because hypomania is more muted and lower-keyed than mania, bipolar II disorder can be more difficult to recognize. In people who have been depressed for a long time, a period of normal happiness may seem like hypomania, or vice versa. An estimated 60 to 70 percent of hypomanic disorders occur immediately before or after a major depression.

How Common Are Bipolar Disorders?

Nearly 2 million American adults suffer from a bipolar disorder. According to the National Institute of Mental Health (NIMH), about 1 in 100 people will develop this illness. Bipolar disorders affect both sexes and all races equally, but are more common in upper socioeconomic and more highly educated groups.

Bipolar disorders usually begin in the late teens or early twenties. According to NIMH's epidemiological data, the median age for onset is eighteen years in men and twenty in women. In previous studies, the median age was somewhat older—in the mid-twenties—suggesting that, like major depression, bipolar illness is occurring earlier in life. If the illness is untreated, the average number of episodes of depression or mania over a ten-year period in bipolar I disorder is four; the number of episodes of depression and hypomania in bipolar II disorder tends to be higher.

What Causes Bipolar Disorders?

Like major depression, bipolar disorders may stem from a complex combination of many factors: genetic, chemical, hormonal, psychological, social, and developmental. However, most mental-health professionals now believe that bipolar illnesses are caused primarily by abnormal brain functioning.

Heredity plays an important role in susceptibility. Close relatives of people with bipolar illnesses are far more likely than others to develop either depression or a bipolar disorder themselves. The risks are highest if an individual's identical twin or both parents have bipolar disorder.

Researchers have theorized that bipolar illness stems from a defect in the brain's internal clock, or pacemaker, that controls daily and seasonal rhythms. Others feel that psychosocial stressors—a loved one's death, a serious accident, or other life traumas—may somehow sensitize the brain and make it more susceptible to mood swings. It is also possible that depression, mania, or hypomania alter brain chemistry in ways that create a predisposition to future episodes.

How Bipolar Disorder Feels

An episode of hypomania usually begins suddenly, with a pleasant sense of well-being or energy. Sometimes this mild mania—hypomania—persists for a long period without becoming more severe. In other cases, it intensifies day by day. As the intensity increases, mania takes on an edge. Affected individuals feel out of control of their emotions and behavior, so that normally amiable people may become increasingly impulsive, irritable, and angry. The euphoria of those in a manic state is so intense that not even a family tragedy or a terrible disaster can dispel their high; yet if their plans are frustrated, their boisterous sense of well-being may turn to irritation that quickly shifts into uncontrollable fury. Some people typically become hostile rather than exhilarated; a few become paranoid and violent and may assault others verbally or physically.

During a manic episode, individuals typically talk rapidly and incessantly, usually in a loud voice. They answer questions at great length, continue talking when others speak, and sometimes talk when no one is listening. Their speech may be riddled with jokes, puns, word plays, or amusing but irrelevant witticisms. They may act in extremely theatrical ways, as if they were playing the part of a character in a play—dressing up in strange outfits, wearing garish makeup, offering money or advice to passing strangers.

Persons in a manic state may not be able to sit still or sleep. Some go for days with little more than two or three hours of rest, yet do not feel tired. In addition to being more physically active than usual, they often become socially frenetic, throwing parties, going to bars, calling up friends in the middle of the night. Tossing aside normal inhibitions, some become sexually hyperactive or promiscuous. They may initiate sex with their regular partner far more often than usual or enter into sexual liaisons with casual acquaintances or strangers.

Because mania impairs judgment, individuals sometimes make decisions with harmful long-term consequences—spending too much money, committing themselves to unrealistic deadlines, quarreling with family members who interfere with their plans. Others may announce that they are writing a screenplay, marketing a brilliant invention, or starting a business. However, even when their plans are based in reality these individuals are too easily distracted or are involved in too many projects to follow through.

In severe mania, thinking is no longer logical. The manic person speaks in an uncontrollable rush, flitting from subject to subject, sometimes becoming incoherent. Thoughts seem to take shape too quickly to be put into words. As in psychotic disorders, these individuals cannot distinguish between what is real and what is not. Some develop grandiose delusions and see themselves as invincible, all-powerful, or specially favored by God; some may even "hear" Jesus Christ explaining the need for a special crusade. Others become paranoid and so angry and frightened that they feel, as one person put it, trapped in "the bleakest caves of the mind—caves you never knew were there." Some individuals with extremely severe mania may become catatonic, not speaking, barely moving, or assuming and maintaining weird postures.

Seeking Help

Bipolar disorders often strike people of great personal charm, creativity, and charisma. Initially it may be impossible for them—and difficult for those close to them—to understand or admit that anything is wrong. Often it is only when their behavior becomes outrageous, when they run up thousands of dollars on their credit cards or get into a brawl, that friends or family members realize that something is seriously wrong.

The primary medications used to treat bipolar disorders are mood stabilizers (lithium and anticonvulsants) and antidepressants. They are also used for milder forms of bipolar disorder, such as cyclothymia, which is characterized by less severe episodes of mania and depression. Lithium carbonate, a naturally occurring salt, and the anticonvulsants carbamazepine (Tegretol) and divalproex (Depakote) are first-line treatments, regardless of whether an individual has symptoms of mania or depression. They treat manic and depressive episodes and largely prevent recurrences of both. Because antidepressants can push bipolar depressed individuals into a manic phase or speed up their cycling from depression to mania, psychiatrists usually first prescribe lithium, carbamazepine (Tegretol), or divalproex (Depakote), and add an antidepressant later only if needed. Symptoms usually diminish within seven to fourteen days.

When individuals do not improve on one mood stabilizer, they may be given another one as well. Other drugs being used experimentally to treat mania in bipolar illness include clonazepam (Klonopin), a benzodiazepine (see Chapter 3, page 178); verapamil (Isoptin or Calan), a treatment for arrhythmias (irregular heartbeats) and high blood pressure; and, more recently, the anti-seizure medications gabapentin (Neurontin) and lamotrigine (Lamictal).

LITHIUM CARBONATE

Some researchers theorize that lithium regulates the movement of calcium in and out of nerve cells; others suggest that it controls the sensitivity of various receptors on the nerve cells. Whatever its mechanism of action, lithium successfully reduces both the number and the intensity of manic episodes for as many as 70 percent of those with bipolar illness. About 20 percent become completely free of symptoms.

Individuals with less severe bipolar disorders, such as bipolar type II disorder (in which major depressions alternate with hypomanic—less than full-blown manic—episodes) or cyclothymia (minor depressions and hypomania) also benefit from lithium. Those with rapid cycling disorder (four or more mood-disorder episodes a year), concurrent mania and depression (called "mixed" bipolar disorder), mania involving irritability rather than euphoria, or a problem with drugs or alcohol may not respond as well to lithium.

Lithium may work by itself or in combination with other medications. If administered early in a hypomanic episode, lithium can produce benefits in a few days. If not given until full-blown mania develops, lithium alone may not be a sufficient therapy. In such cases, both benzodiazepines and neuroleptics (antipsychotics) have proven helpful and often are necessary for extremely agitated and psychotic patients. Although antipsychotic drugs, such as haloperidol (Haldol) (see page 310), have been more widely used, recent Treatment Guidelines published by the American Psychiatric Association recommend benzodiazepines—most often clonazepam (Klonopin) (see page 178) and lorazepam (Ativan) (see page 190)—as alternatives to treat agitation in the absence of psychosis. These agents are frequently as effective as neuroleptics in treating acute mania prior to the onset of action of the mood stabilizer and do not pose a risk of tardive dyskinesia (see Glossary, page 457, and Chapter 6, page 292).

Side Effects

As many as 75 percent of individuals treated with lithium experience some side effects. Most are minor and can be reduced or eliminated by lowering the dose or changing the timing of the medication. The most common side effects of lithium include hand tremor, fatigue, weight gain, nausea, diarrhea, and skin rashes.

Some side effects of lithium necessitate day-to-day adjustments in lifestyle or additional medications for relief of these effects. About 60 percent of those taking lithium experience increased thirst and frequent urination. They should drink ten to twelve glasses of water a day to replace fluids and prevent dehydration. A single daily dose of lithium at bedtime (rather than divided doses) or a lower dose may help to relieve these problems. The thyroid function of some lithium users, most often women or individuals with existing thyroid abnormalities, may be impaired. This condition (hypothyroidism) tends to appear after six to eighteen months of lithium treatment and may sometimes require thyroid hormone replacement treatment. Other users may experience changes in parathyroid gland function, which can increase blood levels of calcium and parathyroid hormones, and may require medication to lower calcium levels in their blood. About 5 percent develop psychological symptoms (mood changes, anxiety, delirium, aggressiveness, sleep disturbances, apathy, or confusion).

Half of those taking lithium develop a hand tremor. This often becomes less noticeable after several weeks on the drug; if it does not, the beta-blocker propranolol (Inderal) can be used to treat the tremor. Other possible side effects include an increase in white blood cells, impaired memory and concentration (particularly in those with neurological disorders), changes in heart rhythm (usually harmless), hair thinning or straightening, and, less commonly, changes in kidney structure, which usually do not affect the kidneys' ability to function.

Precautions

The gap between the therapeutic and the toxic level of lithium is very narrow. Adequate fluid intake is essential to prevent harmful effects, and persons should take care to drink ample amounts of fluid and make sure their salt and water intake is sufficient during hot weather and exercise. Using careful trial-and-error testing, doctors usually prescribe the lowest possible dose that will prevent episodes of mania and depression.

Lithium requires conscientious monitoring by a psychiatrist or a physician experienced in the use of psychiatric drugs. Regular tests of the level of lithium in the blood and assessments of kidney and thyroid-gland function are essential. Monitoring for potential toxic effects, particularly those involving the central nervous system, such as slurred speech, dizziness, vertigo, incontinence, somnolence, restlessness, confusion, stupor, and seizures, is also important.

Warnings

Taking lithium at the time of conception or during the first trimester of pregnancy has been linked to heart defects in the fetus, although data now suggest that this risk may be less than had been thought in the past. Nonetheless, electroconvulsive therapy—ECT—is a safer treatment alternative for women with bipolar disorder who are pregnant or who want to have a child. Those who are taking lithium are advised to wait until they have used it for at least two years without any episodes of mania or depression before discontinuing the drug and attempting to conceive. In the event of a serious relapse, lithium or certain antidepressants can be used after the first trimester. The dose of lithium often needs to be higher during pregnancy, but it must be stopped or the dose reduced two weeks before delivery. Women taking lithium should not breast-feed their babies.

Overdose

Because of the narrow gap between therapeutic and toxic levels of lithium, there is a high risk of accidental overdose. Symptoms include confusion, lethargy, seizures, and

ANTIDEPRESSANTS

150 mg 100 mg	20 mg	10 mg
150 mg	40 mg	20 mg
bupropion sustained-release (Wellbutrin-SR) bupropion sustained-release (Zyban-SR) PAGE 61	citalopram (Celexa) PAGE 66	fluoxetine (Prozac) PAGE 85
		50 mg 100 mg
50 mg	30 mg	150 mg 200 mg
100 mg	15 mg	250 mg
fluvoxamine (Luvox) PAGE 91	mirtazapine (Remeron) PAGE 102	nefazodone (Serzone) PAGE 106

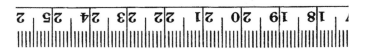

ANTIDEPRESSANTS (cont.)

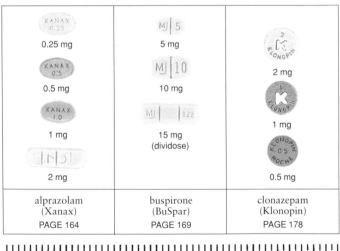

10 mg		
20 mg	25 mg	150 mg
30 mg	50 mg	75 mg
40 mg	100 mg	37.5 mg
paroxetine (Paxil)	sertraline (Zoloft)	venlafaxine extended-release (Effexor-XR)
PAGE 115	PAGE 126	PAGE 141

ANTIANXIETY MEDICATIONS

0.25 mg	5 mg	2 mg
0.5 mg	10 mg	1 mg
1 mg	15 mg (dividose)	0.5 mg
2 mg		
alprazolam (Xanax)	buspirone (BuSpar)	clonazepam (Klonopin)
PAGE 164	PAGE 169	PAGE 178

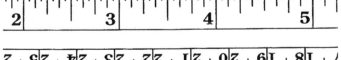

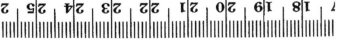

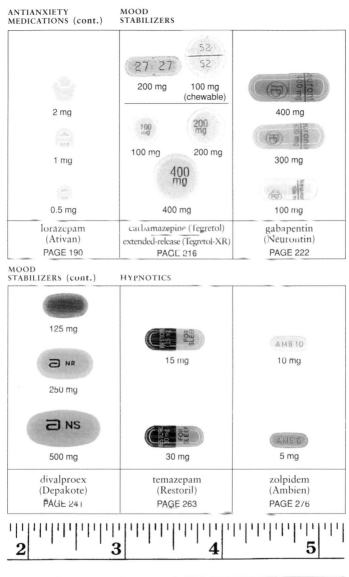

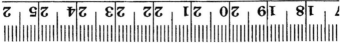

ANTIPSYCHOTICS

25 mg	LILLY 4112 — 2.5 mg	LILLY 4115 — 5 mg	R | 1 — 1 mg
100 mg	LILLY 4116 — 7.5 mg	LILLY 4117 — 10 mg	R 2 — 2 mg
			R 3 — 3 mg
			R 4 — 4 mg
clozapine (Clozaril) PAGE 316	olanzapine (Zyprexa) PAGE 322	risperidone (Risperdal) PAGE 332

AD / AH MEDICATIONS   COGNITIVE ENHANCERS

CIBA — 5 mg CIBA — 10 mg	TH — 18.75 mg TI — 37.5 mg	5 — 5 mg
CIBA — 20 mg		
CIBA 16 — 20 mg	TK — 37.5 mg (chewable) TJ — 75 mg	10 — 10 mg
methylphenidate (Ritalin Hydrochloride) methylphenidate sustained-release (Ritalin-SR) PAGE 364	pemoline (Cylert) PAGE 360	donepezil (Aricept) PAGE 375

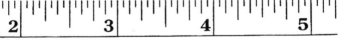

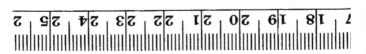

coma. Without immediate treatment, a lithium overdose can be fatal.

ANTICONVULSANT MEDICATIONS

Carbamazepine (Tegretol) and divalproex (Depakote) are anticonvulsants—drugs created to control or prevent seizures—that are also used both to treat and prevent manic behavior. They have proved as effective as lithium and often help individuals who do not respond to lithium. Anticonvulsants, which have varied effects on the central nervous system, may help in the treatment of bipolar illness by controlling "kindling," a term used to describe repeated electrical stimulation of the brain. Sometimes triggered by psychological stresses, kindling produces activity in pathways of the nervous system that sets off a cascade of events leading to seizures and manic behavior.

The anticonvulsants are effective in treating mania, although other medications may be needed if the person becomes depressed. In some cases, an anticonvulsant may be added to an antidepressant for depression that is resistant to treatment. An anticonvulsant can be used in combination with lithium for individuals who do not improve on lithium alone or as a single medication for those who develop serious side effects while taking lithium. Anticonvulsants may also be the first choice for those who experience four or more episodes of mania per year (rapid cycling), have concurrent mania and depression, a drug or alcohol problem, or mania involving irritability rather than euphoria.

Side Effects

Carbamazepine (Tegretol) may cause blurred vision, constipation, dry mouth, dizziness, drowsiness, rash, and difficulty in awakening. As with many other drugs, these side effects tend to be more common and more severe during the early phases of treatment and diminish as therapy progresses. This drug also can cause severe allergic reactions. The most common of these is dermatitis (skin rash), which often goes away when carbamazepine is stopped and then restarted. If periodic tests indicate the development of liver abnormalities, the drug cannot be continued or used again.

The side effects of valproic acid (Depakene) include indigestion, heartburn, and nausea, which may be alleviated by taking the medication with food or taking the coated form (which produces less stomach upset), divalproex (Depakote). About 18 percent of individuals, particularly women, experience some weight gain. Other possible side effects include tremor, drowsiness, hair loss, and diarrhea.

Warnings

Persons taking carbamazepine (Tegretol) must undergo regular blood tests because of its most serious adverse effect, aplastic anemia. This condition, in which the bone marrow stops making blood cells, is rare, occurring in only one of 125,000 individuals taking this drug, but it can be fatal. A somewhat more common risk is leukopenia, a drop in total white blood cells, which occurs in about 10 percent of persons. Unexplained fatigue, flu-like symptoms, or fever may signify either of these problems. All individuals taking anticonvulsants should undergo liver-function tests before treatment because these drugs can damage the liver, and preexisting liver disease may preclude their use. Divalproex (Depakote), in particular, has been reported to produce liver failure, usually in the first six months of treatment. Consequently, liver-function tests are recommended at regular intervals, especially during the first six months of treatment.

Both carbamazepine (Tegretol) and divalproex (Depakote) have been linked to spina bifida and other neural-tube defects in the babies of women who took these drugs during pregnancy. For this reason, women should avoid these drugs if they think they might be pregnant or are contemplating pregnancy. Women who take these agents after delivery should not breast-feed their babies.

Overdose

The first symptoms of an overdose may appear one to three hours after taking too much of an anticonvulsant. These include difficulty in breathing, muscle twitching, drowsiness, dizziness, tachycardia (rapid heartbeat), and coma, and require immediate emergency treatment.

New Treatments for Bipolar Disorders

Three relatively new anticonvulsant medications are effective alternatives in treating bipolar disorders. Gabapentin (Neurontin), released in the United States in 1994, is approved by the FDA to treat seizure disorders. This medication is generally well tolerated; common side effects are tiredness, dizziness, and digestive problems. Unlike lithium, carbamazepine (Tegretol), and divalproex (Depakote), blood levels of gabapentin (Neurontin) do not have to be tested periodically, and this drug is safer during pregnancy. Its disadvantages are relatively high cost and lack of a standard dosing range. It may be used in combination with another mood stabilizer.

Another recent medication is lamotrigine (Lamictal), approved in 1995, which some psychiatrists believe may be effective in treating both the manic and depressive phases of bipolar disorder. Generally well tolerated, it has not been associated with liver damage, weight gain, or severe drowsiness, and also is safer during pregnancy.

A major side effect of lamotrigine (Lamictal) is the development of a severe skin rash, which occurs in approximately 10 percent of users. One in 1,000 patients may develop Stevens-Johnson syndrome, a potentially life-threatening condition characterized by painful, weeping skin lesions. To lessen this risk, lamotrigine (Lamictal) is slowly increased to its therapeutic level over a four-week period. Other reported side effects are headache, dizziness, digestive problems, and visual disturbances, such as double or blurred vision.

Lastly, oxcarbazepine (Trileptal) was approved by the FDA in early 2000 to treat seizure disorders. It is chemically similar to carbamazepine but has a number of advantages: fewer side effects, fewer drug-drug interactions, a lower incidence of rash than carbamazepine, and a relative lack of adverse effects upon the liver.

Generic name: **CARBAMAZEPINE**

 Available in generic form: Yes

 Brand name: Tegretol, Tegretol-XR, Tegretol chewable tablets, and Tegretol suspension

 Drug class: Mood stabilizer; anticonvulsant

 Prescribed for: Seizure disorders, bipolar disorder, borderline personality disorder, agitation (especially in people with dementia), schizoaffective disorder.

General information: Carbamazepine was originally approved for the treatment of seizure disorders, especially those affecting the brain's temporal lobes, and for severe facial pain (trigeminal neuralgia). In the early 1980s researchers found that this drug is also an effective treatment for acute mania and for prevention of recurrences of mania and depression in bipolar individuals. It is believed to control "kindling," repeated electrical stimulation of the brain. Sometimes triggered by psychological stresses, kindling produces activity in pathways of the nervous system that sets off a cascade of events leading to seizures and manic behavior. Although the FDA has not approved the drug for bipolar disorders, substantial clinical and research evidence supports its use.

Carbamazepine can be used alone or in combination with lithium in the treatment of bipolar disorder. When combined with lithium, carbamazepine is usually prescribed for those persons who have not responded completely to lithium and still experience symptoms such as irritability or elevated mood. Carbamazepine is also especially effective in treating people who are "rapid cyclers" (those who have four episodes of mania per year). It may also be useful in treating mania accompanied by irritability rather than euphoria. It is less effective in treating acute depression than acute mania.

Dosing information: Carbamazepine is available in an oral suspension at a dose of 100 mg. per 5 cc. of liquid, in 100-mg. chewable tablets, and in 200-mg. tablets. It is usually begun at a dose of 200 mg. twice a day, with 200-mg.-a-day increases every three to five days. The usual therapeutic dosages are based on achieving the desired blood levels, but frequently are between 400 and 1,200 mg. a day, although higher doses are not uncommon. Carbamazepine blood levels need to be periodically monitored, with the usual therapeutic levels between 4 and 12 micrograms per milliliter. The higher the blood levels, the more frequently side effects occur. For this reason, physicians attempt to treat persons at the lower therapeutic range.

With use, carbamazepine speeds up its own metabolism. This means that after a month or so, blood levels of the drug may drop substantially, often by a third or more, and the dose must be increased. Blood levels are usually measured once a week during the first two weeks, approximately twelve hours after the last dose. Whenever possible, physicians prescribe the medication in a single dose at bedtime to decrease the frequency of side effects, especially sedation, during the day.

Common side effects: The most common side effects of carbamazepine are sedation, fatigue, nausea, and dizziness. When the dose is increased, people may complain of visual disturbances such as double vision and jerky eye movements (nystagmus). These symptoms are usually temporary. Some motor incoordination or clumsiness may occur at higher levels.

Precautions: Dizziness, drowsiness, and problems in walking (ataxia) may occur with normal therapeutic levels of carbamazepine. Reducing the dose decreases these symptoms. Approximately 5 to 15 percent of people taking carbamazepine may develop a rash and usually must stop taking this drug because of the risk of a more severe disorder called Stevens-Johnson syndrome, a potentially fatal rash characterized by painful, weeping skin lesions.

Warnings: Very rare but serious adverse drug reactions to carbamazepine include leukopenia, an absolute decrease in the white-blood-cell count, and aplastic anemia, a condition where the bone marrow stops making all blood cells. Consequently, people at risk for such conditions should not take this drug. (Mild anemia, which is a decrease in red blood cells, may occur in approximately 5 percent of people and is usually not serious.) It is estimated that the rate of aplastic anemia is approximately 1 in 125,000 persons. Approximately 10 percent of people taking the drug will experience a decrease in their white-blood-cell count (leukopenia) to a count of less than 3,000 cells per cubic millimeter. (The normal count is usually between 7,000 and 10,000 cells per cubic millimeter.) Approximately 2 percent of people will experience both a persistent decrease in their white-blood-cell count and a decrease in their platelet count, which leads to bleeding abnormalities. If you take carbamazepine and develop a fever, sore throat, infection, weakness, or bruises, contact your physician immediately.

Carbamazepine occasionally has adverse effects on the liver, including elevation of selected liver enzymes, as well as increases in bilirubin, a bile pigment, which leads to a yellow skin pallor, especially noticeable in the whites of the eyes. Consequently, people with liver disease should not take this medication. If periodic blood levels assessing liver function show an increase in the liver enzymes SGOT, SGPT, or GGT to three times normal, carbamazepine must be stopped.

Individuals may also experience a syndrome called inappropriate antidiuretic hormone, a syndrome that produces a decrease in serum sodium. Individuals who are alcoholic are at greater risk. If serum sodium levels are lowered, fluid restriction usually corrects the condition. If a person taking carbamazepine experiences confusion or disorientation, the physician will measure the serum sodium level to rule out a more severe decrease in sodium levels.

♈ **Alcohol:** People should not drink alcohol if they are taking carbamazepine, since alcohol may increase its rate of metabolism and lower blood levels. Since the most common side effect of carbamazepine is sedation, the additional sedating effects of alcohol may produce significant daytime drowsiness and fatigue. Also, because alcohol acts as a depression-producing agent, it may decrease a person's response to carbamazepine's antidepressant effects. People who consume large quantities of alcohol may increase their risk of a condition called syndrome of inappropriate antidiuretic hormone (SIADH), which causes a reduction in blood sodium levels and, if pronounced, may lead to confusion, seizures, and coma.

Food and beverages: No restrictions.

Possible drug interactions: Carbamazepine stimulates the liver to metabolize medications (including itself) more rapidly. This may result in lower blood levels of many other drugs, including birth-control pills. Contraceptive failure is of special concern because carbamazepine can produce fetal abnormalities. Carbamazepine may also reduce the blood levels of phenytoin (Dilantin), an antiseizure medication, the anticoagulant warfarin (Coumadin), tricyclic antidepressants, neuroleptics (antipsychotic medications), methadone, benzodiazepines, over-the-counter theophylline-containing preparations used for cold or flu symptoms, and the antibiotic doxycycline, and decrease their effectiveness. Phenobarbital, an older medication used in treating anxiety, may decrease blood levels of carbamazepine.

Other drugs may increase carbamazepine blood levels. These include the anti-ulcer medication cimetidine (Tagamet), the antihypertensive agent diltiazem (Cardizem), the antidepressants fluoxetine (Prozac) and fluvoxamine (Luvox), the antibiotics doxycycline and erythromycin, the antifungal agent ketoconazole (Nizoral), and the mood stabilizer and anti-seizure medication divalproex (Depakote).

Use in pregnancy and breast-feeding: Pregnancy Category D

Carbamazepine has been reported to produce birth defects, including craniofacial abnormalities, developmental delays, spinal-cord or neural-tube defects, and decreased size or absence of fingernails. Consequently, carbamazepine should not be used during pregnancy, especially in the first trimester. If it is necessary to use carbamazepine during pregnancy, the woman should start taking 1 mg. a day of folate early in the pregnancy; this may reduce the risk of some fetal abnormalities.

Whenever possible, carbamazepine's use should be restricted to the second and third trimesters. If it is used during the first trimester, an ultrasound and an alpha-fetoprotein blood test to assess spinal-cord defects should be performed at weeks eighteen to twenty. If a mood stabilizer is required during pregnancy, it should preferably be prescribed after the first trimester. Lithium is preferred over carbamazepine and divalproex (Depakote) during the second or third trimesters, since lithium's risk of fetal malformation is greatest during the first trimester, when the baby's heart is developing and lithium has been reported to produce heart abnormalities. Women taking carbamazepine should avoid breast-feeding, since small amounts will pass into the breast milk and be absorbed into the baby's bloodstream. This can lead to possible sedation and unknown effects on the child's developing nervous system.

Use in children: Carbamazepine has been used to treat severe aggression and temporal lobe seizures in children. It has not been studied in children or adolescents with bipolar disorder. If used in children over the age of six, the initial dose is usually 100 mg. a day with food, with 100-mg. increases weekly. The usual total daily dose in children between six and twelve is 400 to 800 mg. in two or three doses, and for children over twelve years of age the dose is between 400 and 1,200 mg. a day in two or three doses.

Use in seniors: In general, lower doses are prescribed for seniors. Because carbamazepine speeds up the metabolism of other drugs, older people taking multiple medications should have their blood levels of both carbamazepine and other drugs carefully monitored. Because it produces significant sedation and higher doses may lead to dizziness on rising and an unsteady gait, carbamazepine requires special caution in older people to decrease the likelihood of falls.

Overdosage: Carbamazepine is potentially fatal in overdose. It will produce neuromuscular symptoms such as jerky eye movements (nystagmus), muscle jerks (myoclonus), and increased reflexes (hyperreflexia). Other symptoms include severe nausea and vomiting. With even higher doses, seizures, cardiac arrhythmias, and coma may ensue. Persons who overdose with carbamazepine should be taken to the emergency room at once. They are almost always hospitalized because of the high risk of death and the need to monitor blood pressure, respirations, and cardiac and kidney functioning. If an overdose is suspected, bring the bottle of medication to the emergency room with the person, since the date it was prescribed and the number of pills remaining in the bottle can provide helpful information to the treating physician.

Special considerations: Carbamazepine may be prescribed for people with bipolar disorder who fail to respond to lithium or who cannot tolerate its side effects. As with lithium, frequent blood tests are necessary. Despite these limitations and with careful monitoring, carbamazepine is a reasonable alternative to lithium, and its benefits usually outweigh its risks in treating bipolar disorder.

 Generic name: **GABAPENTIN**

 Available in generic form: No

 Brand name: Neurontin

 Drug class: Anti-seizure medication and mood stabilizer

℞ **Prescribed for:** Seizure disorders, bipolar disorder, pain disorders.

🦉 **General information:** The FDA approved gabapentin as a treatment for complex partial seizures in 1994. Since 1996, it has also been used to treat persons with bipolar disorder who do not improve with lithium or with the more standard mood stabilizers, divalproex (Depakote) or carbamazepine (Tegretol). Gabapentin may be especially effective in the treatment of the depressive phase of bipolar disorder. It is believed to control "kindling," repeated electrical stimulation of the brain. Sometimes triggered by psychological stresses, kindling produces activity in pathways of the nervous system that sets off a cascade of events leading to seizures and manic behavior.

Gabapentin can be used alone or in combination with lithium in the treatment of bipolar disorder. When combined with lithium, gabapentin is usually prescribed for those persons who have not responded completely to lithium and still experience symptoms such as irritability or elevated mood. Gabapentin may be especially effective in treating people who are "rapid cyclers" (those who have four episodes of mania per year). It may also be useful in treating mania accompanied by irritability rather than euphoria, and in individuals with prominent anxiety symptoms.

🔲 **Dosing information:** Gabapentin is available in 100-, 300-, and 400-mg. capsules. It is usually started at a dose of 300 mg. two or three times a day, with increases of 300 mg. every four to five days, to a usual maximal daily dose of 1,800 to 2,400 mg.

🫀 **Common side effects:** Gabapentin may produce tiredness, dizziness, and gastrointestinal symptoms. Other side effects reported in clinical trials are problems with walking (ataxia), tremor, jerky eye movements (nystagmus) and double vision.

Precautions: Gabapentin is not metabolized by humans but is excreted unchanged by the kidney. Consequently, although it may be used safely in people with liver disease, for those with kidney disease, including renal insufficiency, or those in hemodialysis, the dosage of the medication needs to be reduced.

Warnings: Gabapentin has fewer serious side effects than older medications, such as lithium, divalproex (Depakote), and carbamazepine (Tegretol), and it does not require routine blood-level monitoring.

Alcohol: People should not drink alcohol if they are taking gabapentin, since the most common side effect of gabapentin is sedation and the additional sedating effects of alcohol may produce significant daytime drowsiness and tiredness. Also, alcohol acts as a depression-producing agent and may decrease a person's response to gabapentin's antidepressant effects. People who consume large quantities of alcohol may increase their risk of a condition called syndrome of inappropriate antidiuretic hormone (SIADH), which causes a reduction in blood sodium levels and, if pronounced, may lead to confusion, seizures, and coma.

Food and beverages: No restrictions.

Possible drug interactions: If taken with another mood stabilizer, such as carbamazepine (Tegretol) or divalproex (Depakote), gabapentin may increase tiredness, dizziness, problems with walking (ataxia), visual jerkiness (nystagmus), and double vision. If prescribed with carbamazepine (Tegretol), blood levels of gabapentin may be lowered. Antacids may reduce absorption of gabapentin into the bloodstream.

Use in pregnancy and breast-feeding: Pregnancy Category C

Gabapentin is safer than lithium, carbamazepine (Tegretol), and divalproex (Depakote) in pregnancy, but there have been no large, well-controlled studies. Gabapentin is not recommended during pregnancy, especially during the first trimester, because it is not known whether it increases birth defects or spontaneous miscarriages. Some women who have been taking gabapentin may experience a recurrence of mania if they discontinue it in pregnancy. In these circumstances, the physician should discuss the need to restart gabapentin or seek an alternative medication or treatment. Women taking gabapentin should not breast-feed, since small amounts will pass into the breast milk and be absorbed into the baby's bloodstream. This could lead to possible sedation and other unknown effects on the child's developing nervous system.

Use in children: The effectiveness of gabapentin in children under the age of twelve has not been established. It may be used for children over the age of twelve whose bipolar disorder does not improve with conventional medications. However, there are few data as to its effectiveness in this age group.

Use in seniors: No systematic clinical studies have been conducted in seniors. However, persons over age sixty-five treated with gabapentin have not reported more or different side effects than younger individuals. Older people who take gabapentin may develop dizziness and problems with walking (ataxia), which may increase the risk for falls; consequently, the drug is usually prescribed in lower doses for seniors.

Overdosage: Significant overdoses can cause double vision, slurred speech, drowsiness, tiredness, diarrhea, breathing abnormalities, and seizures. People who overdose with gabapentin require hospitalization because of the potential for serious side effects and the need for supportive hospital care. If overdose is suspected, bring the bottle of medication to the emergency room with the person, since the date it was prescribed and the number of pills remaining in the bottle can provide helpful information to the treating physician.

 Special considerations: Gabapentin is a relatively new anti-seizure medication that may be prescribed in combination with other mood stabilizers like lithium, carbamazepine (Tegretol), and divalproex (Depakote) for bipolar individuals who do not completely improve on these drugs. For people who cannot tolerate the side effects or who do not improve on lithium, carbamazepine (Tegretol), or divalproex (Depakote), gabapentin may be prescribed as an alternative drug. People generally tolerate this medication extremely well, and many prefer it to the other mood stabilizers. Its major limitation is its high cost.

 Generic name: LAMOTRIGINE

 Available in generic form: No

 Brand name: Lamictal

Drug class: Anti-seizure medication and mood stabilizer

Prescribed for: Seizure disorders and bipolar disorder

General information: The FDA approved lamotrigine to treat seizures in 1995; it has been used for many years in Europe. According to recent reports in the psychiatric literature, lamotrigine is effective not only in treating both the manic and depressive phases of bipolar disorder, but it may also be especially effective in treating major depression. Of the mood stabilizers, it is least likely to cause weight gain, and it appears more effective for bipolar depression than the others.

Lamotrigine can be used alone or in combination with lithium in the treatment of bipolar disorder. When combined with lithium, lamotrigine is usually prescribed for those persons who have not responded completely to lithium and still experience symptoms such as irritability or elevated mood. Lamotrigine may be especially effective in treating people who are "rapid cyclers" (those who have four episodes of mania per year). It may also be useful in treating mania accompanied by irritability rather than euphoria.

Dosing information: Lamotrigine is available in 25-, 100-, 150-, and 200-mg. tablets. Treatment is usually begun at a dose of 25 mg. a day and increased in weekly increments of 25 mg. The usual therapeutic dosage range is between 100 and 300 mg. a day. Blood-level monitoring is not required with this medication.

Common side effects: Approximately 10 percent of persons develop a rash. Other common side effects are gastrointestinal symptoms (nausea, diarrhea, and cramping), difficulty with walking (ataxia), dizziness, sedation, headache, double vision, and blurred vision.

Precautions: Because it is not possible to predict which rashes may become life-threatening (see below), lamotrigine should be discontinued at the first sign of a rash and the physician informed. In most cases, life-threatening rashes develop within the first two to eight weeks of treatment, although some cases have been reported after six months of treatment.

⧉⊘⧉ **Warnings:** One in 1,000 adults taking lamotrigine and 1 in 50 to 100 children develop severe and potentially life-threatening rashes, including Stevens-Johnson syndrome, which is characterized by painful, weeping skin lesions and can be fatal. Lamotrigine is not approved for persons under age sixteen. Other than age, there are no known risk factors that predict the occurrence or the severity of a rash associated with lamotrigine, although the risk may increase if lamotrigine is combined with divalproex (Depakote) or if the recommended initial dose or dose escalation is exceeded. An initial dose of 25 mg. a day, with an increase in 25-mg. increments every week, minimizes the risk of rash. Persons who are also taking divalproex (Depakote) should take a reduced dosage of lamotrigine, beginning with a dose of 25 mg. every other day for two weeks, followed by 25 mg. once a day for two weeks, with a very gradual dose increase thereafter at the rate of 25 mg. every two weeks. The usual maximum daily dose of lamotrigine is 150–200 mg. Persons who are also taking carbamazepine (Tegretol) can increase the dose in normal increments. Then the usual maximum daily dose of lamotrigine is 400–500 mg.

▽ **Alcohol:** People taking lamotrigine should not drink alcohol because alcohol may increase its rate of metabolism and lower blood levels of the drug. Since a common side effect of lamotrigine is sedation, the additional sedating effects of alcohol may produce significant daytime drowsiness and tiredness. Also, alcohol acts as a depression-producing agent and may obscure a person's response to lamotrigine's antidepressant effects.

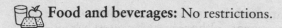 **Food and beverages:** No restrictions.

Possible drug interactions: Those taking divalproex (Depakote) should begin lamotrigine at a lower dose of 25 mg. every other day for two weeks and increase by 25 mg. every two weeks. This slower dose increase is necessary because divalproex decreases lamotrigine's elimination from the bloodstream by half. When used with carbamazepine (Tegretol), higher doses of lamotrigine may be necessary because carbamazepine increases lamotrigine's removal from the bloodstream, substantially reducing its blood levels.

Use in pregnancy and breast-feeding: Pregnancy Category C

Lamotrigine is safer than lithium, carbamazepine (Tegretol), and divalproex (Depakote) in pregnancy, but there have been no large, well-controlled studies of this drug. Lamotrigine decreases fetal folate concentration in rats, an effect that may indicate increased risk of fetal abnormalities in humans. If it is necessary to use lamotrigine during pregnancy, the woman should start taking 1 mg. a day of folate early in the pregnancy, since folate may reduce the risk of some fetal abnormalities.

Lamotrigine should be used during pregnancy only if the potential benefits justify the possible risks to the fetus. Some pregnant women who had been taking lamotrigine may experience a recurrence of mania if they discontinue it. In these circumstances, the physician should discuss the need to restart lamotrigine or seek an alternative medication or treatment. Women taking lamotrigine should not breast-feed, since small amounts will pass into the breast milk and be absorbed into the baby's bloodstream, affecting the child's developing nervous system.

Use in children: Lamotrigine should not be used in children under age sixteen because of a high rate of serious, potentially life-threatening rashes.

Use in seniors: Lower doses of lamotrigine may be prescribed in seniors, although its use in older people has not been systematically studied.

Overdosage: People who overdose with lamotrigine are nearly always hospitalized because of potential life-threatening effects of severe rash. The most common effects of overdose are dizziness, headaches, extreme tiredness, and coma. Persons overdosing on this medication are generally closely monitored in the emergency room or in a hospital setting. If an overdose is suspected, bring the bottle of medication to the emergency room with the person, since the date it was prescribed and the number of pills remaining in the bottle can provide helpful information to the treating physician.

Special considerations: Lamotrigine may be an effective alternative to more standard mood-stabilizing agents. However, because of the risk of life-threatening rashes, this medication should be used with caution, especially by people who are also taking divalproex (Depakote), which raises blood levels considerably and thereby increases the risk for adverse side effects, especially a serious rash.

 Generic name: LITHIUM CARBONATE LITHIUM CITRATE

 Available in generic form: Yes

Brand name: Eskalith, Lithane, Lithotabs, Eskalith CR (sustained release), Lithobid (sustained release), Cibalith-S (suspension)

Drug class: Mood stabilizer

Prescribed for: Bipolar disorder (both mania and depression), agitation (especially in persons with dementia), augmentation of the antidepressant effect of antidepressant medications, schizoaffective disorder, schizophrenia, borderline personality disorder.

General information: When used to treat mania, the full effects of lithium usually take one to two weeks to appear. Because of this, physicians also commonly prescribe an antipsychotic medication to treat psychosis. In the past, the drug of choice was haloperidol (Haldol), but now an atypical antipsychotic agent, such as risperidone (Risperdal), is often preferred. In addition to, or instead of, an antipsychotic agent, physicians frequently prescribe a sedating benzodiazepine such as clonazepam (Klonopin) to calm individuals and to treat their agitation until lithium becomes fully effective. After a few days or a week, the antipsychotic and the benzodiazepine are tapered off and stopped. Because lithium may affect electrical conduction in the heart, people over the age of forty and those with cardiac disease should have a baseline electrocardiogram (EKG) prior to beginning lithium treatment.

Lithium's primary limitations are its side effects, in particular weight gain and mental sluggishness, which many people find bothersome or troubling. More than half of people treated with lithium eventually stop taking it for these reasons.

Dosing information: Lithium is available in 300-mg. tablets and capsules and 300- and 450-mg. tablets of the sustained-release form (Eskalith CR and Lithobid). It is also available in a liquid form, lithium citrate (Cibalith-S), at a dose of 8 meq. (milliequivalents) per 5 cc. Many different dosing regimens may be used. A generally accepted strategy is to begin with a lithium dose of 300 mg. twice a day, with a 300-mg. daily increase every three to five days. Lithium levels must be obtained through a weekly blood test approximately twelve hours after the last dose, until manic symptoms subside or until the lithium level is stabilized between 0.9 meq. and 1.2 meq. per liter. Some physicians will then change the timing of doses to all at bedtime, which may decrease side effects during the day. People usually respond to lithium doses of between 900 and 1,800 mg. a day, although there is wide variability. Once a person has responded to lithium, lithium levels are generally tested once a month for the first three months and every three months thereafter.

Common side effects: The most common side effect is frequent urination because lithium decreases the kidneys' ability to concentrate urine. This effect usually stops when lithium is discontinued, though in some cases it may persist for months. People who experience frequent urination should drink ten to twelve glasses of water a day to replace fluids and prevent dehydration.

One-fourth of persons taking lithium complain of memory difficulties. Another frequent side effect is weight gain, which may be considerable. Approximately some 7 percent of persons develop a rash, and may develop acne and psoriasis. These reactions are usually time-limited. Gastrointestinal side effects, especially nausea and diarrhea, frequently occur early in lithium treatment and may be alleviated by increasing the dose gradually or initially using divided doses. Common neurological side effects of lithium include tremor or other involuntary movements of the upper extremities and blurred vision. Some people also experience dizziness, an unstable gait, slurred speech, and jerky eye movements (nystagmus).

Precautions: Lithium may affect the thyroid gland and produce hypothyroidism, a disorder characterized by lethargy, tiredness, depression, and weight gain. All persons need to undergo laboratory tests prior to beginning lithium, including blood tests to evaluate thyroid function, electrolytes, kidney function, and blood counts. A urine sample is necessary to determine the kidneys' ability to concentrate urine, since lithium can affect this process. These tests are usually repeated every six months to a year, and sooner if the person experiences symptoms.

Warnings: Lithium affects the electrical rhythm of the heart, and individuals who have certain heart irregularities should not take this medication. In particular, persons with cardiac conduction abnormalities (called heart block) should not use lithium.

Lithium is usually not prescribed for people who have kidney problems. Long-term use of lithium may damage the kidneys. Lithium must be used with caution by anyone with a history of thyroid disease, in particular hypothyroidism, because it may produce or worsen this condition.

Alcohol: Many people with bipolar disorder abuse alcohol and other illicit drugs in an effort to treat the manic phase of their illness. Although the sedating effects of alcohol may seem beneficial in the short term, continued use increases the frequency and severity of depressive episodes. People taking lithium should not drink alcohol, which acts as a depression-producing agent and may obscure their response to lithium. Because alcohol can cause significant dehydration, it may also cause lithium levels to soar, leading to side effects and/or toxicity.

Food and beverages: There are no restrictions. If you experience side effects such as nausea, diarrhea, or stomach cramps, take lithium during or within an hour following a meal. The longer-acting (sustained-release) forms of the drug usually decrease the severity and frequency of gastrointestinal side effects.

Possible drug interactions: Lithium has a very narrow therapeutic range, meaning that the gap between the therapeutic and the toxic blood level is very small. Those who are taking a diuretic medication, such as furosemide (Lasix), to treat hypertension need to take lithium cautiously. Diuretics decrease the kidneys' ability to remove lithium from the blood, resulting in much higher lithium blood levels and potentially serious side effects, including severe gastrointestinal symptoms, cardiac arrhythmias, stupor, and coma. Lithium may be used safely with antipsychotic medications, benzodiazepines, and antidepressants. The antibiotic tetracycline may increase lithium blood levels. Over-the-counter theophylline-containing compounds, often used for cold or flu symptoms, may decrease lithium blood levels. Nonsteroidal anti-inflammatory drugs (NSAIDs), such as ibuprofen (Motrin, Nuprin, Advil, and Midol) and indomethacin (Indocin), may decrease the kidneys' ability to clear lithium from the blood, leading to higher lithium levels.

Use in pregnancy and breast-feeding: Pregnancy Category D

Lithium taken in pregnancy has been reported to increase cardiac abnormalities in newborns. The risk of serious cardiac abnormalities in children whose mothers have taken lithium is approximately twenty times greater than that in the general population and is highest when lithium is taken during the first trimester. Because the risk of any major birth defect appears to be two to three times greater in women who are taking lithium, its use in pregnancy should be avoided whenever possible, especially in the first trimester. If used after the first trimester, the dose may need to be 50 to 100 percent more than usual because of the body's increased water volume, but it should be reduced to a normal level one to two weeks before delivery. Women taking lithium should avoid breast-feeding, since small amounts will pass into the breast milk and be absorbed into the baby's bloodstream. This can lead to possible sedation and other unknown effects on the child's developing nervous system.

Use in children: Lithium has not been studied in children under the age of twelve. Adolescents with bipolar disorder have been successfully treated with lithium.

Use in seniors: Lower doses of lithium are generally prescribed for seniors. For older persons who also have dementia, the adverse effects on memory can be especially troubling. In addition, those who have a tremor due to Parkinson's disease will experience a significant worsening in their tremor. Since many older people take cardiac medications, lithium must be used cautiously because of the risk of side effects on the heart.

Overdosage: Lithium can be extremely toxic in overdose. In severe cases, individuals experience seizures, kidney failure, and eventually death. At slightly less toxic levels, there may be intense nausea and diarrhea, abnormal arm movements, confusion, circulatory failure, and coma. Individuals who overdose with lithium should be taken to the emergency room; they are nearly always hospitalized because of potentially fatal side effects. If an overdose is suspected, bring the bottle of medication to the emergency room with the person, since the date it was prescribed and the number of pills remaining in the bottle can provide helpful information to the treating physician.

 Special considerations: Because of the frequent side effects people experience when taking lithium (memory disturbance, weight gain, frequent urination, thirst, tremor, nausea, diarrhea, acne, and rash), a majority of people placed on lithium eventually stop taking it. The newer mood-stabilizing medications—divalproex (Depakote), gabapentin (Neurontin), and lamotrigine (Lamictal)—are usually better tolerated and are currently prescribed more often. Persons taking lithium must have periodic monitoring of their blood lithium levels as well as other blood and urine tests.

Generic name: OXCARBAZEPINE

 Available in generic form: No

 Brand name: Trileptal

Drug class: Mood stabilizer; anticonvulsant

Prescribed for: Seizure disorders, bipolar disorder, borderline personality disorder, agitation (especially in people with dementia), schizoaffective disorder, atypical panic disorder.

General information: The FDA approved oxcarbazepine in January 2000 for the treatment of seizure disorders, especially those affecting the brain's temporal lobes. Oxcarbazepine is chemically similar to carbamazepine (Tegretol); it was developed to have efficacy similar to carbamazepine (Tegretol), while improving that drug's side-effect profile.

Oxcarbazepine shares similar pharmacologic properties with carbamazepine (Tegretol) in the treatment of acute mania and for prevention of recurrences of mania and depression in bipolar individuals. Like carbamazepine (Tegretol), the FDA has not approved the use of oxcarbazepine for bipolar disorders, but there is substantial clinical and research evidence to support this use.

Dosing information: Oxcarbazepine is available in 150-, 300-, and 600-mg. tablets. Like carbamazepine, oxcarbazepine may be used alone or in combination with another mood stabilizer (e.g., lithium, valproate [Depakote]) in the treatment of bipolar disorders. When used alone, oxcarbazepine is begun at a dose of 300 mg. twice a day, with 300-mg.-a-day increases every third day until a dose of 1,200 mg. a day is reached. The usual therapeutic dosages range from 1,200 mg. a day to 2,400 mg. a day. If clinically indicated, the dose may be increased by a maximum of 600 mg. a day at weekly intervals. When oxcarbazepine is used in conjunction with another mood stabilizer, the starting dose is also 300 mg. twice a day; however, the dosage of the other mood stabilizer may need to be lowered if indicated. When a second mood stabilizer is used, the recommended daily dose of oxcarbazepine is 1,200 mg. a day, in divided doses of 600 mg. twice a day.

Unlike carbamazepine (Tegretol), oxcarbazepine does not speed up its own metabolism, so dosage readjustments are not necessary. A laboratory test to measure serum levels of oxcarbazepine or its metabolite is not currently available.

Common side effects: The most common side effects of oxcarbazepine include headaches, sedation, dizziness, tiredness, and nausea. When the dose is increased, the most frequent complaints are visual disturbances, such as double vision and jerky eye movements (nystagmus), problems in walking, nausea, and vomiting.

Precautions: Oxcarbazepine may affect mental alertness, making it difficult to concentrate. Drowsiness, dizziness, and problems in walking (ataxia) are generally more common at the beginning of therapy and subside over time. Therefore, people should exercise caution when driving a motor vehicle or operating machinery, especially during the beginning phase of therapy.

Unlike carbamazepine (Tegretol), oxcarbazepine is associated with a very low incidence of rash. This probably results from a safer metabolite formed from oxcarbazepine. The metabolite from carbamazepine (Tegretol) is associated with a higher incidence of toxicity.

Warnings: In rare cases, oxcarbazepine may lower serum sodium levels (hyponatremia), which return to normal when the drug is reduced or discontinued. In general, oxcarbazepine-induced hyponatremia occurs during the first three months of treatment, and requires close monitoring of sodium levels.

Oxcarbazepine does not appear to induce the adverse drug reactions of leukopenia and aplastic anemia, conditions that occur on rare occasions with carbamazepine (Tegretol). This is probably attributable to the differing metabolites of the two drugs.

In addition, oxcarbazepine does not appear to have adverse effects on the liver, obviating the need for periodic blood tests to assess liver function. According to the manufacturer, even in persons with mild to moderate liver problems, the liver's ability to handle oxcarbazepine or its metabolite is not significantly altered, so dosage adjustment is not required. Because over 95 percent of oxcarbazepine's metabolite is excreted by the kidneys, patients with kidney disease may require a lower dosage.

Alcohol: Since a common side effect of oxcarbazepine is sedation, the additional sedating effects of alcohol can produce significant daytime drowsiness and tiredness. Also, alcohol acts as a depression-producing agent, so may obscure a person's response to oxcarbazepine's antidepressant effects.

Food and Beverages: No restrictions.

Possible drug interactions: For the most part, oxcarbazepine exhibits fewer drug interactions than its counterpart, carbamazepine (Tegretol). However, while it does not stimulate the liver to speed up its own metabolism like carbamazepine, it does stimulate certain liver enzymes to metabolize certain medications more rapidly. This may result in lower blood levels of those drugs, including combination birth control pills that contain ethinyl estradiol (Estinyl) and levonorgestrel (Alesse). Contraception may fail because of lower blood levels of these hormones.

Oxcarbazepine inhibits the liver enzyme that metabolizes other drugs, including phenytoin (Dilantin), an anticonvulsant. When phenytoin is given with oxcarbazepine, its blood levels may increase as much as 40 percent, potentially leading to phenytoin toxicity. Similarly, when phenobarbital's metabolism is inhibited by oxcarbazepine, increased phenobarbital levels may lead to toxic levels.

In addition, some drugs stimulate the liver enzymes that metabolize oxcarbazepine, thereby decreasing the blood levels of oxcarbazepine and its metabolite. Examples include divalproex (Depakote), verapamil (Calan), carbamazepine (Tegretol), as well as phenobarbital and phenytoin.

Use in pregnancy and breast-feeding: Pregnancy Category C

Because the chemical structures of oxcarbazepine and carbamazepine (Tegretol) are closely related, and carbamazepine (Tegretol) is known to produce birth defects, it is likely that oxcarbazepine may also have harmful effects on the fetus. While there are insufficient data at this time to be certain, use during pregnancy should be avoided if at all possible. The drug should be considered only if the potential benefit justifies the risk to the fetus.

Oxcarbazepine and its metabolite are excreted in human breast milk. Because of the potential for adverse reactions in the infant, it is recommended that the mother discontinue the drug while breast-feeding or avoid breast-feeding.

Use in children: Oxcarbazepine is indicated for use as an anticonvulsant in children. The pediatric dosage is 5 to 15 mg. of oxcarbazepine per kilogram of body weight. Its use in children has been limited to the treatment of seizures. Its use as a mood stabilizer in children is probably comparable to carbamazepine; however, the available data are insufficient to confirm this.

Use in seniors: In general, lower doses of oxcarbazepine are prescribed for seniors. Customary doses have resulted in higher blood levels than in younger people, because of age-related reductions in kidney function; over 95 percent of oxcarbazepine's metabolite is excreted by the kidneys.

Overdosage: The manufacturer cites isolated cases of overdose, with all patients recovering after treatment of symptoms. While there is no specific antidote, the drug may be removed by gastric lavage or its absorption limited by administering activated charcoal. Persons who overdose with oxcarbazepine should be taken to the emergency room at once for treatment. Bring the bottle of medication to the emergency room with the person, since the date it was prescribed and the number of pills remaining in the bottle can provide helpful information to the treating physician.

Special considerations: Oxcarbazepine was designed to provide a compound chemically similar to carbamazepine (Tegretol) and with similar clinical efficacy, but with an improved side-effect profile. Clinical experience with oxcarbazepine as a mood stabilizer thus far indicates that it compares favorably with carbamazepine (Tegretol), although further experience is needed. The side effects associated with oxcarbazepine and its metabolite, however, are fewer than with carbamazepine and its metabolite.

The current disadvantage of oxcarbazepine is cost. Unlike carbamazepine (Tegretol), it is not available in generic form, so its cost is considerably higher than carbamazepine (Tegretol). There is also a clinical disadvantage in using oxcarbazepine because laboratories currently do not offer tests of the drug's serum levels, which can help physicians gauge dosing.

 Generic name: **VALPROIC ACID, DIVALPROEX**

 Available in generic form: Yes

 Brand name: Depakene (valproic acid), Depakote (divalproex)

Drug class: Anti-seizure medication and mood stabilizer

 Prescribed for: Seizure disorders, bipolar disorder (both mania and depression), schizophrenia, schizoaffective disorder, borderline personality disorder, agitation, especially in association with dementia.

General information: There are two forms of this medication: the valproic acid formulation (Depakene), and divalproex, a compound that contains both valproic acid and sodium divalproex (Depakote). Most persons tolerate divalproex better. Divalproex has been found to be as effective as lithium both in treating acute mania and in preventing its recurrence. Divalproex is especially useful in treating persons with rapid-cycling mania (frequent recurrences of mania), dysphoric or mixed mania (characterized by symptoms of both mania and depression), irritable mania, and mania associated with a drug or alcohol problem. It is unclear whether divalproex is effective in treating acute depression in bipolar individuals. It is believed to be effective in bipolar disorder by controlling "kindling," repeated electrical stimulation of the brain. Sometimes triggered by psychological stresses, kindling produces activity in pathways of the nervous system that sets off a cascade of events leading to seizures and manic behavior. Persons generally tolerate divalproex better than lithium for the prevention and treatment of acute mania.

Dosing information: Valproic acid is available in 250-mg. capsules and in a syrup in a concentration of 250 mg. per 5 cc. Divalproex comes in an enteric-coated tablet available in 125-, 250-, and 500-mg. sizes and in a 125-mg. sprinkled capsule that can be pulled apart and mixed with food, such as applesauce. The usual starting dose of divalproex is 250 mg. twice a day, with increases of 250 mg. every three to four days. The usual required dose is between 1,000 and 3,000 mg. a day; the dose is increased until the drug's blood-plasma level reaches between 50 and 125 micrograms per milliliter. Divalproex levels are monitored weekly until a stable dose is achieved, then monthly for three months, then every three months. Blood-plasma levels are usually measured twelve hours after the last dose.

In contrast to carbamazepine (Tegretol), divalproex does not speed up its own metabolism; consequently, the dose does not have to be increased after one or more months of treatment. Physicians often prescribe divalproex once a day at bedtime to reduce daytime sedation, although it is sometimes taken twice a day, with a larger dose at bedtime and a smaller dose in the morning.

Common side effects: Divalproex produces sedation, tremor, and problems with walking (ataxia). People also frequently complain of weight gain, nausea, diarrhea, and other gastrointestinal side effects. The enteric-coated form of divalproex produces fewer digestive problems. People frequently experience a mild tremor and hair loss (alopecia), probably resulting from the drug's interference with zinc and selenium absorption. To prevent hair loss, physicians recommend multivitamins that contain zinc and selenium (e.g., Centrum Silver).

Precautions: Divalproex may cause a considerable weight gain. Because excessive weight is associated with an increased risk of diabetes, hypertension, heart disease, and premature death, persons who gain excessive weight should participate in a medically supervised program to reduce this weight gain (diet, exercise, and medication).

Warnings: The most severe adverse drug reaction associated with divalproex is liver toxicity or liver failure, which occurs in approximately 1 of every 500,000 individuals over age ten. Since it is impossible to predict when liver toxicity will occur, liver-function tests are recommended before treatment and every six months thereafter. Divalproex has been reported to reduce the platelet count, resulting in bleeding and coagulation (blood-clotting) problems, but this is a relatively rare side effect.

Alcohol: People should not drink alcohol if they are taking divalproex, since alcohol may increase the rate of metabolism of divalproex and lower its blood levels. Since a common side effect of divalproex is sedation, the additional sedating effects of alcohol may produce significant daytime drowsiness and tiredness. Also, alcohol acts as a depression-producing agent and may decrease a person's response to divalproex's antidepressant effects.

Food and beverages: No restrictions. If gastrointestinal side effects are troubling, take divalproex with food.

Possible drug interactions: Unlike carbamazepine (Tegretol), which stimulates liver metabolism, divalproex may inhibit various liver enzymes and reduce the metabolism of other drugs, leading to increases in their blood levels. Certain drugs may decrease divalproex blood levels; these include phenobarbital, carbamazepine (Tegretol), and two medications used to treat tuberculosis, rifampin and ethosuximide. Drugs that may increase blood levels of divalproex include the antidepressants fluoxetine (Prozac) and fluvoxamine (Luvox), phenothiazine-type antipsychotic medications such as chlorpromazine (Thorazine), thioridazine (Mellaril), and others, nonsteroidal anti-inflammatory agents (NSAIDS) such as aspirin and ibuprofen (Motrin), the antibiotic erythromycin, and the anti-ulcer drug cimetidine (Tagamet).

Use in pregnancy and breast-feeding: Pregnancy Category D

Divalproex has been reported to produce birth defects, including spinal-cord or neural-tube defects such as spina bifida and failure of the brain to develop. To avoid this risk, divalproex always should be discontinued before an anticipated pregnancy. If divalproex must be continued during pregnancy, the woman should take 1 mg. a day of folate as early in the pregnancy as possible, since folate has been shown to reduce the risk of some fetal abnormalities. Use of divalproex should be restricted whenever possible to the second and third trimesters. If divalproex is used during the first trimester, an ultrasound and an alpha-fetoprotein blood test to assess spinal-cord defects should be performed at weeks eighteen to twenty. If the woman remains on divalproex throughout her pregnancy, she should take vitamin K during the last months to decrease the risk of excessive bleeding prior to delivery or during delivery. If a mood stabilizer is required during pregnancy, it should preferably be prescribed after the first trimester. Lithium is preferred over carbamazepine (Tegretol) and divalproex during the second or third trimesters, since lithium's risk of fetal malformation is greatest during the first trimester when the fetus's heart is developing, and lithium has been reported to produce heart abnormalities. Women taking divalproex should not breast-feed, since small amounts of divalproex will pass into the breast milk and be absorbed into the baby's bloodstream. This can lead to possible sedation and other unknown effects on the child's developing nervous system.

Use in children: Divalproex should be avoided whenever possible as a treatment for seizure disorders in children younger than two years of age, who have the highest risk of liver damage. Divalproex has not been systematically studied in children with mood disorders or bipolar illness, but it is believed to be well tolerated and effective in treating mania in adolescents. Blood tests of liver function and red-blood-cell counts are recommended prior to using divalproex, then weekly for the first month, every month thereafter for children under age ten and every four to six months in children over ten and adolescents.

Use in seniors: Lower doses are generally prescribed in seniors, often at bedtime. Divalproex's possible sedating effects may be more troubling in older persons.

Overdosage: In overdose, divalproex produces significant sedation and confusion, progressing to coma. People may also experience seizures, cardiac arrhythmias, and decreased breathing, requiring placement on a ventilator. Individuals who overdose with divalproex are nearly always hospitalized because of the risk of death and the need for ICU monitoring. If an overdose is suspected, bring the bottle of medication to the emergency room with the person, since the date it was prescribed and the number of pills remaining in the bottle can provide helpful information to the treating physician.

Special considerations: Divalproex is a first-line treatment to prevent mania and depression in bipolar persons. The main disadvantages are its side effects, which include significant sedation, weight gain, and hair loss. Doctors may add divalproex to lithium in persons who have not shown a full response to lithium alone. There are no significant adverse drug interactions between lithium and divalproex. Divalproex may be an especially good drug for agitation in individuals with dementia or bipolar disorder and for those with manic irritability or euphoria. While it is not clear whether divalproex is as effective in treating acute depression in bipolar persons, it may help prevent recurrence of depression.

CHAPTER 5

Medications Used to Treat Insomnia

To learn general information about this class of medications and the disorders they treat, read the first part of the chapter. To read about a specific drug used to treat insomnia, turn to the page indicated below.

ON ANY GIVEN NIGHT, 1 IN 3 PEOPLE HAS A PROBLEM falling or staying asleep. According to the National Commission on Sleep Disorders Research, 40 million men, women, and children have chronic sleep problems; another 20 to 30 million occasionally have difficulty getting the rest they need. Mental-health professionals define sleep disorders as persistent disturbances in the quantity or quality of sleep for a month or more that interfere with an individual's ability to function normally. There are four primary types of sleep disorders:

- *Insomnia:* a problem in falling asleep, staying asleep, or feeling rested after sleep

- *Hypersomnia:* a problem involving too much sleep or extreme daytime sleepiness

- *Circadian rhythm sleep disorders:* problems in falling asleep or staying awake at appropriate times

- *Parasomnias:* problems that occur during sleep

Each year, an estimated 15 to 30 percent of American adults seek professional help for insomnia. About 30 percent of them have a chronic sleep problem. Insomnia can begin at any age, but the likelihood increases with age. Younger people are more likely to have problems falling asleep. Since sleep patterns change with aging, older people complain more of difficulty staying asleep or of waking too early.

Insomnia is frequently a symptom of something else that is wrong: stress, physical pain, discomfort or illness, another type of sleep disorder, lifestyle habits, such as irregular work hours, or worry about a particular event or problem. Sometimes temporary sleep difficulties turn into chronic ones. Although most people who are apprehensive or upset about a life crisis eventually return to normal sleep patterns after a night or two of poor sleep, some continue to have sleep difficulties even after the stressful situation has eased. Increasingly anxious and exhausted, they try harder and harder to get more sleep, but end up frustrated. Each night of poor sleep reinforces their anxiety about not sleeping, and their sleep problems may persist for weeks, months, or even years.

About one-third of those with insomnia have an underlying mental disorder, usually depression or an anxiety disorder. Depressed individuals have characteristic changes in their sleep patterns, including a shorter than usual time from sleep onset to dream or rapid eye movement (REM) sleep. Insomnia may also occur in individuals with anxiety disorders, such as posttraumatic stress disorder (PTSD), obsessive-compulsive disorder, and psychiatric disorders such as Alzheimer's disease and schizophrenia.

Many substances, including alcohol, drugs of abuse, and prescription medications, can disrupt sleep. Sleeping pills, called hypnotics, themselves may also be a culprit. An estimated 20 percent of all cases of insomnia are complicated by withdrawal reactions from sleeping pills. People who have taken them for more than two to four weeks and then stop typically find it hard to sleep well without them. This condition, called rebound insomnia, often produces very vivid and frightening dreams; sleep usually returns to normal within several weeks. To avoid this problem, sleeping pills or other medications to treat insomnia should generally be taken for only a short period of time.

Physicians may prescribe a sedating antidepressant such as trazodone (Desyrel) or a hypnotic agent such as temazepam (Restoril) for persons who are depressed, together with an antidepressant, for the first two to four weeks of therapy. The reason is that certain antidepressants, such as fluoxetine (Prozac), venlafaxine (Effexor), and bupropion (Wellbutrin or Zyban), may worsen sleep patterns during the first month or two of treatment. Other antidepressants—nefazodone (Serzone), mirtazapine (Remeron), trazodone (Desyrel), and some of the older tricyclic antidepressants—improve sleep.

It is important to remember that there is no perfect sleeping pill. Good sleep hygiene is usually the best long-term solution to sleep difficulties (see Table 5-1).

Table 5-1: How to Sleep Like a Baby

• Keep regular hours for going to bed and getting up in the morning. Stay as close as possible to this schedule on weekends as well as weekdays.

• Develop a sleep ritual—such as stretching, meditation, yoga, prayer, or reading a not-too-exciting novel—to ease the transition from wakefulness to sleep.

• Don't drink coffee late in the day. The effects of caffeine can linger for up to eight hours.

• Don't smoke. Nicotine is an even more powerful stimulant—and sleep saboteur—than caffeine.

• Don't rely on alcohol to get to sleep. Alcohol disrupts normal sleep stages, so you won't sleep as deeply or as restfully as you normally would.

• Don't nap during the day if you're having problems sleeping through the night.

BENZODIAZEPINES

With the exception of zolpidem (Ambien) and Zaleplon (Sonata), the sleeping pills most often used today are benzodiazepines, which are safer than older medications like barbiturates. They decrease the amount of time it takes to fall asleep and increase total sleep time. Physicians often choose one drug over another on the basis of its half-life—the length of time it remains in the body—and the residual effects individuals may feel the next day.

Side Effects

Sleeping pills with long half-lives remain in the body for a longer period and may affect alertness and cause drowsiness and confusion. Some pills with short half-lives have been linked to other problems, including amnesia and agitation. For individuals with insomnia who also suffer from depression, psychiatrists may prescribe a sedating antidepressant in low doses, either alone or with another antidepressant, to improve sleep (see Table 5-2).

Precautions

Individuals who take benzodiazepine sleeping pills for more than two weeks may develop dependence and addiction. Since these drugs lose their effectiveness as sleep inducers with continued use, people sometimes increase the doses in an attempt to replicate the initial effect. Those who stop taking benzodiazepines after prolonged use typically develop rebound insomnia, and their sleep is even more disturbed than before they used the drugs. Careful tapering off of dosages over the course of a few nights can prevent this problem.

The elderly metabolize sleeping medications more slowly. This means that the drugs remain in their bodies longer, and they become more prone to the side effects

Table 5-2: Drugs Commonly Used for Insomnia

CLASS AND MEDICATION	TRADE NAME
Short half-life benzodiazepines[a]	
estazolam	ProSom
temazepam	Restoril
triazolam	Halcion
Short half-life non-benzodiazepine[b]	
zaleplon	Sonata
zolpidem	Ambien
Long half-life benzodiazepine[c]	
flurazepam	Dalmane

[a]Half-life 3–16 hours
[b]Half-life 1–3 hours
[c]Half-life 30–100 hours

noted below and to an increased risk of falling. A National Institutes of Health (NIH) consensus conference on treating sleep problems in the elderly recommended that clinicians consider sleeping pills only after a thorough assessment of the possible causes of the insomnia, improvements in sleep hygiene, and behavioral treatments. If all these prove unsuccessful, sleeping pills are prescribed, but only in low doses and for short periods of time.

Although it is difficult to overdose on benzodiazepines alone, combining them with alcohol, barbiturates, or narcotics can be fatal. Immediate emergency treatment is essential.

Warnings

The benzodiazepines may interfere with breathing, especially in people with chronic respiratory problems. The long-acting hypnotic benzodiazepines, especially flurazepam (Dalmane), may impair daytime coordination, memory, driving skills, and thinking and may disrupt normal sleep stages. Confusion, hallucinations, and other psychiatric disturbances may occur, especially in the elderly. Benzodiazepines should not be used in pregnancy to treat insomnia because of the risk of birth defects in the fetus.

The non-benzodiazepines zolpidem (Ambien) and zaleplon (Sonata) have rapid onsets of action; people taking them fall asleep within fifteen to thirty minutes. They have a short half-life of approximately one to three hours, so individuals who experience early-morning awakening and can't fall back to sleep may respond better to a longer-acting agent such as temazepam (Restoril). In contrast to the benzodiazepine-type hypnotic agents, zolpidem and zaleplon may not lead to tolerance in individuals taking the medication for longer than two weeks; that is, they may not need higher doses to achieve the same benefit.

ANTIDEPRESSANTS

Three antidepressants—amitriptyline (Elavil), doxepin (Sinequan), and trazodone (Desyrel)—are frequently used to treat insomnia. Both amitriptyline (Elavil) and doxepin (Sinequan) are older tricyclic antidepressants that produce sedation when taken at bedtime. For sleep, physicians frequently will prescribe amitriptyline (Elavil) and doxepin (Sinequan) in doses ranging from 25 to 100 mg. The major problem with these medications is their side effects—dry mouth, blurred vision or difficulty focusing at close range, constipation, problems in urinating—which are caused by decreased stimulation of the nerves that affect the muscles controlling these functions. Other common side effects are orthostatic hypotension (a drop in blood pressure when going from lying down to sitting or from a sitting to a standing position), drowsiness during the day, and confusion. A profile of amitriptyline (Elavil) is found in Chapter 2, pages 50–56, and of doxepin (Sinequan) on pages 81–85.

The atypical antidepressant trazodone (Desyrel) is often prescribed for insomnia. Trazodone affects serotonin receptors, but unlike the selective serotonin reuptake inhibitors (SSRIs), it is one of the most sedating antidepressants. A typical dose for individuals with insomnia is 50 to 100 mg. at bedtime. In addition, trazodone is often prescribed with SSRI-type antidepressants, especially fluoxetine (Prozac), to treat sleep disturbance produced by these medications.

One problem with trazodone is orthostatic hypotension. Older people taking this drug should be very cautious and get out of bed slowly so they don't become dizzy and fall. A small number of men taking this drug (about 1 in 6,000) develop prolonged and painful erections (priapism), a condition that may require emergency surgery and lead to permanent impotence. A profile of trazodone is found in Chapter 2, pages 137–141.

 Generic name: ESTAZOLAM

 Available in generic form: No

 Brand name: ProSom

Drug class: Hypnotic benzodiazepine

 Prescribed for: Primary insomnia or insomnia secondary to depression, anxiety disorders, or a medical illness.

General information: Estazolam is one of the newer benzodiazepines approved for treating insomnia. Its half-life of approximately sixteen hours may lead to daytime sedation. Temazepam is generally preferred over estazolam because its metabolism is not affected in individuals with liver disease or reduced liver function, and it has no active metabolites. Nonetheless, estazolam is considered an effective medication for sleep.

Dosing information: Estazolam is available in 1- and 2-mg. tablets. The usual dose in healthy adults is either 1 or 2 mg. taken shortly before bedtime. Both the 1- and 2-mg. tablets are scored, so individuals can increase their doses by .5 mg. of the 1-mg. tablet or 1 mg. of the 2-mg. tablet, up to a dose of 4 mg. a day, if required.

Common side effects: The most common side effects are sedation, fatigue, tiredness, nausea, and dizziness. At higher levels, people may complain of visual disturbances, such as double vision and jerky eye movements (nystagmus), and impaired coordination while walking (ataxia).

Precautions: People who have an alcohol or substance use disorder should not take estazolam, since it can lead to addiction and contribute to a relapse in those who are recovering alcoholics.

Individuals who take benzodiazepine sleeping pills for more than two weeks may develop dependence and addiction. Since these drugs lose their effectiveness as sleep inducers with continued use, people may increase the doses in an attempt to replicate the initial effect. Those who stop taking benzodiazepines after prolonged use typically develop rebound insomnia, and their sleep is even more disturbed than before they used the drugs. Careful tapering off of dosages over the course of a few nights can prevent this problem.

Warnings: Individuals with narrow-angle glaucoma should not take benzodiazepines. People with chronic obstructive pulmonary disease (COPD) should not take estazolam or other benzodiazepines because they may decrease their ability to breathe, which can be fatal. Those with sleep apnea, a disorder characterized by long pauses in respiration during sleep, should not take benzodiazepines such as estazolam. These drugs decrease the ability to begin breathing again after such a pause—a potentially fatal effect. People with liver disease should not take estazolam because it is metabolized by the liver; the drug's effect on the body will be magnified, producing greater sedation, memory disturbance, and incoordination.

☒ **Alcohol:** People should not drink alcohol when taking benzodiazepines. When taken together, benzodiazepines and alcohol intensify side effects such as sedation, memory disturbance, motor incoordination, euphoria, and impaired judgment, and can seriously affect driving ability. In addition, alcohol frequently disrupts sleep and leads to early morning awakening.

☒ **Food and beverages:** There are no restrictions. Avoid caffeine-containing beverages, such as coffee, tea, cocoa, and colas, since caffeine is a frequent contributor to sleep problems. The nicotine contained in cigarettes also interferes with sleep.

☒ **Possible drug interactions:** Alcohol and narcotics— meperidine (Demerol), hydrocodone (Vicodin), oxycodone (Percodan), and others—may increase estazolam's sedative effects and can be fatal. *Do not drink alcohol* or take narcotic agents if you are taking sleeping medications. Also, do not combine estazolam with other sleep medications, especially the older barbiturates, such as phenobarbital, secobarbital (Seconal), and others, since this combination is potentially fatal. Propranolol (Inderal), a medication used to treat hypertension, birth-control pills, anti-ulcer drugs such as cimetidine (Tagamet), and disulfiram

(Antabuse) may increase the amount of estazolam in the body.

🐾 Use in pregnancy and breast-feeding: Pregnancy Category X

Pregnant women should not take estazolam because benzodiazepines may increase the risk of birth defects, such as cleft palate and heart deformities, especially when taken in the first trimester. In general, the use of benzodiazepines during pregnancy should almost always be avoided. If taken immediately prior to delivery, estazolam may decrease a newborn's breathing. Women who are breast-feeding should not take estazolam because it will pass into breast milk and be absorbed by the baby, leading to potential breathing problems and possible unknown effects on the child's developing nervous system.

👤 Use in children: Estazolam has not been studied and is not recommended in children.

🏠 Use in seniors: The dose of estazolam in seniors is usually 1 mg. The elderly metabolize sleeping medications more slowly. This means that the drugs remain in their bodies longer, and they become more prone to the side effects noted above and to an increased risk of falling. A National Institutes of Health (NIH) consensus conference on treating sleep problems in the elderly recommended that clinicians consider sleeping pills only after a thorough assessment of the possible causes of the insomnia, improvements in sleep hygiene, and behavioral treatments. If all these prove unsuccessful, sleeping pills are prescribed, but only in low doses and for short periods of time.

☠️ Overdosage: The most common symptoms of overdose are excessive sleepiness, problems with walking (ataxia), slurred speech, confusion, and daytime

drowsiness. Large doses of estazolam are usually not fatal. However, combining it with alcohol, barbiturates, or certain other medications considerably increases the risk of death. People who take an overdose should always be brought to a hospital emergency room. Bring the bottle of medication to the emergency room with the person, since the date it was prescribed and the number of pills remaining in the bottle can provide helpful information to the treating physician.

 Special considerations: Estazolam is a good medication for insomnia, but because of its sixteen-hour half-life, it may produce daytime sedation.

Generic name: FLURAZEPAM

 Available in generic form: Yes

 Brand name: Dalmane

Drug class: Hypnotic benzodiazepine

Prescribed for: Primary insomnia or insomnia secondary to depression, anxiety disorders, or a medical illness.

General information: If flurazepam were formulated today, it would probably not be approved as a treatment for insomnia because it has a long half-life of between two and four days. With daily use, individuals frequently sleep better after the second and third night of treatment than on the first night, because the blood level of the medication builds up in the body. However, with continued use, the amount of flurazepam in the body continues to increase and may lead to daytime drowsiness, lack of coordination, and memory disturbance. Physicians who may not be knowledgeable about newer medications sometimes prescribe flurazepam. However, its use is strongly discouraged because of the likelihood of daytime sedation and problems with concentration, memory, and coordination.

Dosing information: Flurazepam is available in 15- and 30-mg. capsules. The usual daily dose is 30 mg. in adults and 15 mg. in older people, taken at bedtime. It should be prescribed for only a brief period of time (two weeks or less).

Common side effects: The most common side effects are memory disturbance, daytime drowsiness, and loss of motor coordination. Even a single nighttime dose of flurazepam impairs a person's driving ability the next day because a significant amount of the drug remains in the body. Other side effects include problems with walking (ataxia), slurred speech, and nausea.

Precautions: People who have an alcohol or substance use disorder should not take flurazepam, since it can lead to dependence, withdrawal symptoms, and addiction, and can contribute to a relapse in those who are recovering alcoholics.

Individuals who take benzodiazepine sleeping pills for more than two weeks may develop dependence and addiction. Since these drugs lose their effectiveness as sleep inducers with continued use, people may increase the doses in an attempt to replicate the initial effect. Those who stop taking benzodiazepines after prolonged use typically develop rebound insomnia, and their sleep is even more disturbed than before they used the drugs. Careful tapering off of dosages over the course of a few nights can prevent this problem.

⅏**Warnings:** Individuals with acute narrow-angle glaucoma should not take benzodiazepines. People with chronic obstructive pulmonary disease (COPD) should not take flurazepam or other benzodiazepines because they may decrease their ability to breathe, which can be fatal. Those with sleep apnea, a disorder characterized by long pauses in respiration during sleep, also should not take benzodiazepines such as flurazepam because these drugs decrease the ability to begin breathing again after such a pause—a potentially fatal effect. People with liver disease should not take flurazepam, since it is metabolized by the liver; the drug's effect on the body will be magnified, producing greater sedation, memory disturbance, and incoordination.

𝜑 **Alcohol:** People should not drink alcohol when taking benzodiazepines. When taken together, benzodiazepines and alcohol intensify side effects such as sedation, memory disturbance, motor incoordination, euphoria, and impaired judgment, and can seriously affect driving ability. In addition, alcohol frequently disrupts sleep and leads to early-morning awakening.

▦ **Food and beverages:** There are no restrictions. Avoid caffeine-containing beverages, such as coffee, tea, cocoa, and colas, since caffeine is a frequent contributor to sleep problems. Nicotine in cigarettes also interferes with sleep.

▨ **Possible drug interactions:** Alcohol and narcotic drugs—meperidine (Demerol), hydrocodone (Vicodin), oxycodone (Percodan), and others—may increase flurazepam's sedative effects and potentially could be fatal. *Do not drink alcohol* or take narcotic agents if you are taking sleeping medications. Also, do not combine flurazepam with other sleep medications, especially the older barbiturates, such as phenobarbital, secobarbital (Seconal), and others, since this combination is potentially fatal. Propranolol (Inderal), a medication used to treat hypertension, birth-control pills, anti-ulcer drugs such as cimetidine (Tagamet), and disulfiram (Antabuse) increase the amount of flurazepam in the body, heightening the effects resulting from its longer half-life.

Use in pregnancy and breast-feeding: Pregnancy Category D

Pregnant women should not take flurazepam because benzodiazepines may increase the risk of birth defects, such as cleft palate and heart deformities, especially when taken in the first trimester. In general, the use of benzodiazepines during pregnancy should almost always be avoided. If taken immediately prior to delivery, flurazepam may decrease the newborn's breathing. Women who are breast-feeding should not take flurazepam because it will pass into the breast milk and be absorbed by the baby, leading to potential breathing problems and possible unknown effects on the child's developing nervous system.

Use in children: Flurazepam has not been studied and is not recommended for use in children.

Use in seniors: Because of its long half-life, flurazepam is not recommended for older people. If it is prescribed, the usual dose is 15 mg. The elderly metabolize sleeping medications more slowly. This means that the drugs remain in their bodies longer, and they become more prone to the side effects noted above and to an increased risk of falling. A National Institutes of Health (NIH) consensus conference on treating sleep problems in the elderly recommended that clinicians consider sleeping pills only after a thorough assessment of the possible causes of the insomnia, improvements in sleep hygiene, and behavioral treatments. If all these prove unsuccessful, sleeping pills are prescribed, but only in low doses and for short periods of time.

 Overdosage: The most common symptoms of overdose are excessive sleepiness, problems with walking (ataxia), slurred speech, confusion, and daytime drowsiness. Large doses of flurazepam are usually not fatal, but when combined with alcohol, barbiturates, or certain other medications, the risk of death is considerably increased. People who take an overdose should always be brought to a hospital emergency room. Bring the bottle of medication to the emergency room with the person, since the date it was prescribed and the number of pills remaining in the bottle can provide helpful information to the treating physician.

 Special considerations: In general, flurazepam should not be prescribed as a medication to treat insomnia. The benzodiazepine temazepam (Restoril) has a shorter half-life and is better tolerated. The newer benzodiazepine estazolam (ProSom) and the non-benzodiazepine zolpidem (Ambien) are other preferred alternatives.

 Generic name: TEMAZEPAM

 Available in generic form: Yes

Brand name: Restoril

Drug class: Hypnotic benzodiazepine

Prescribed for: Primary insomnia or secondary insomnia caused by depression, anxiety disorders, or a medical illness.

General information: Temazepam, which has a half-life of approximately eight to twelve hours with no active metabolites, is the preferred benzodiazepine to treat insomnia. Its metabolism is not affected by liver disease or reduced liver function. People with early-morning awakening benefit, since its ideal half-life enables them to get a full night's sleep. For individuals who desire to sleep during very long airplane flights, temazepam is a good option. Because it is absorbed more slowly than flurazepam (Dalmane) or triazolam (Halcion), it should be taken approximately an hour before going to sleep.

Dosing information: Temazepam is available in 7.5-, 15-, and 30-mg. capsules. The usual dose in adults is 30 mg. taken an hour before bedtime.

Common side effects: The most common side effects are daytime sedation, fatigue, occasional nausea, and dizziness. At higher doses, people may complain of visual disturbances, such as double vision and jerky eye movements (nystagmus), and impaired coordination while walking (ataxia) or clumsiness.

Precautions: People who have an alcohol or substance use disorder should not take temazepam, since it can lead to dependence or addiction and contribute to a relapse for those who are recovering alcoholics.

Individuals who take benzodiazepine sleeping pills for more than two weeks may develop dependence and addiction. Since these drugs lose their effectiveness as sleep inducers with continued use, people may increase the doses in an attempt to replicate the initial effect. Those who stop taking benzodiazepines after prolonged use typically develop rebound insomnia, and their sleep is even more disturbed than before they used the drugs. Careful tapering off of dosages over the course of a few nights can prevent this problem.

꧁ Warnings: Individuals with narrow-angle glaucoma should not take benzodiazepines. People with chronic obstructive pulmonary disease (COPD) should not take temazepam or other benzodiazepines because they can decrease their ability to breathe, which can be fatal. Those with sleep apnea, a disorder characterized by long pauses in respiration during sleep, should not take benzodiazepines such as temazepam because these drugs decrease the ability to begin breathing again after such a pause—a potentially fatal effect. Since temazepam is metabolized differently from the other hypnotic benzodiazepines, it may be safely used by people with liver disease or diminished liver function.

꧂ Alcohol: People should not drink alcohol when taking benzodiazepines. When taken together, benzodiazepines and alcohol intensify side effects such as sedation, memory disturbance, motor incoordination, euphoria, and impaired judgment, and can seriously affect driving ability. In addition, alcohol frequently disrupts sleep and leads to early-morning awakening.

꧃ Food and beverages: There are no restrictions. Avoid caffeine-containing beverages, such as coffee, tea, cocoa, and colas, since caffeine is a frequent contributor to sleep problems. The nicotine contained in cigarettes also interferes with sleep.

꧄ Possible drug interactions: Alcohol and narcotics—meperidine (Demerol), hydrocodone (Vicodin), oxycodone (Percodan), and others—may increase temazepam's sedative effects and can be fatal. *Do not drink alcohol* or take narcotic agents if you are taking sleeping medications. Also, do not combine temazepam with other sleep medications, especially the older barbiturates, such as phenobarbital, secobarbital (Seconal), and others, since this combination is potentially fatal. Propranolol (Inderal), a medication used to treat hypertension, birth-control pills, and anti-ulcer drugs such as cimetidine (Tagamet) may increase the amount of temazepam in the body.

Use in pregnancy and breast-feeding: Pregnancy Category X

Pregnant women should not take temazepam because benzodiazepines may increase the risk of birth defects, such as cleft palate and heart deformities, especially when taken in the first trimester. In general, the use of benzodiazepines during pregnancy should almost always be avoided. Although this has not been systematically studied, it is thought that temazepam may pass into the fetus's bloodstream through the placenta. If taken immediately prior to delivery, temazepam may decrease the newborn's breathing. Women who are breast-feeding should not take temazepam because it will pass into the breast milk and be absorbed into the baby's bloodstream, leading to potential breathing problems and possible unknown effects on the child's developing nervous system.

Use in children: Temazepam has not been studied and is not recommended for use in children.

Use in seniors: The usual dose in seniors is 7.5 or 15 mg. The elderly metabolize sleeping medications more slowly. This means that the drugs remain in their bodies longer, and they become more prone to the side effects noted above and to an increased risk of falling. A National Institutes of Health (NIH) consensus conference on treating sleep problems in the elderly recommended that clinicians consider sleeping pills only after a thorough assessment of the possible causes of the insomnia, improvements in sleep hygiene, and behavioral treatments. If all these prove unsuccessful, sleeping pills are prescribed, but only in low doses and for short periods of time.

Overdosage: The most common symptoms of overdose are excessive sleepiness, problems with walking (ataxia), slurred speech, confusion, and daytime drowsiness. Large doses of temazepam are usually not fatal. However, combining it with alcohol, barbiturates, or certain other medications considerably increases the risk of death. People who take an overdose should always be brought to a hospital emergency room. Bring the bottle of medication to the emergency room with the person, since the date it was prescribed and the number of pills remaining in the bottle can provide helpful information to the treating physician.

Special considerations: Temazepam is an excellent benzodiazepine for insomnia. Because of its intermediate half-life of approximately eight to twelve hours and lack of active metabolites, it generally leads to a good night's sleep. It is also a good medication to take on very long airplane flights if you want to sleep for eight or more hours. Because temazepam is absorbed slowly, it is less likely to cause amnesia than the short-acting and rapidly absorbed triazolam (Halcion).

Generic name: TRIAZOLAM

 Available in generic form: Yes

 Brand name: Halcion

Drug class: Hypnotic benzodiazepine

 Prescribed for: Primary insomnia or insomnia secondary to depression, anxiety disorders, or a medical illness.

General information: Triazolam has a short half-life of approximately three to four hours. It can produce memory loss, especially at higher doses of 0.5 mg. or more. Transatlantic or transpacific airline passengers who have taken triazolam have reported that they don't remember arriving at their destination, especially if they also drank alcohol on the plane. Memory problems like these, along with reports of agitation, paranoia, depression, and hallucinations, led to triazolam's removal from the market in Great Britain. Many psychiatrists in the United States prefer not to prescribe triazolam because of the risk of amnesia, memory disturbance, and rebound insomnia.

Dosing information: Triazolam is available in 0.125-, 0.25-, and 0.5-mg. tablets. The usual dose in healthy adults is either 0.125 mg. or 0.25 mg. If at all possible, avoid taking the 0.5-mg. tablet or two 0.5-mg. tablets because of reports of violent behavior, paranoia, and amnesia at these dosage levels.

Common side effects: The most common side effects are memory disturbance, daytime drowsiness, and impaired motor coordination, although these risks are less than with longer-acting hypnotic benzodiazepines such as flurazepam (Dalmane). Even a single nighttime dose of triazolam may potentially impair a person's driving ability the next day because some of the drug may remain in the bloodstream, especially in older people or those with liver disease or diminished liver function. Other side effects are problems with walking (ataxia), slurred speech, and nausea.

Precautions: People who have an alcohol or substance use disorder should not take triazolam, since it can lead to dependence, addiction, and contribute to a relapse in those who are recovering alcoholics. At high doses, such as 0.5 mg., paranoia, worsening of depression, and amnesia may occur. These effects are less frequent at the 0.125- and 0.25-mg. dosages. Drinking when taking this medication heightens such effects.

Individuals who take benzodiazepine sleeping pills for more than two weeks may develop dependence and addiction. Since these drugs lose their effectiveness as sleep inducers with continued use, people may increase the doses in an attempt to replicate the initial effect. Those who stop taking benzodiazepines after prolonged use typically develop rebound insomnia, and their sleep is even more disturbed than before they used the drugs. Careful tapering off of dosages over the course of a few nights can prevent this problem.

≷⊘≷**Warnings:** Individuals with narrow-angle glaucoma should not take benzodiazepines. People with chronic obstructive pulmonary disease (COPD) should not take triazolam or other benzodiazepines because they may decrease the ability to breathe, which can be fatal. Those with sleep apnea, a condition characterized by long pauses in respiration during sleep, also should not take benzodiazepines such as triazolam because these drugs decrease the ability to begin breathing again after such a pause—a potentially fatal effect. People with liver disease should not take triazolam, since it is metabolized by the liver and its effects on the body will be magnified, producing greater sedation, memory disturbance, and incoordination.

▽ **Alcohol:** People should not drink alcohol when taking benzodiazepines. When taken together, benzodiazepines and alcohol intensify side effects such as sedation, memory disturbance, motor incoordination, euphoria, and impaired judgment, and can seriously affect driving ability. In addition, alcohol frequently disrupts sleep and leads to early-morning awakening.

Food and beverages: There are no restrictions. Avoid caffeine-containing beverages, such as coffee, tea, cocoa, and colas, since caffeine is a frequent contributor to sleep problems. The nicotine contained in cigarettes also interferes with sleep.

Possible drug interactions: Alcohol and narcotic drugs—meperidine (Demerol), hydrocodone (Vicodin), oxycodone (Percodan), and others—may increase triazolam's sedative effects and potentially could be fatal. *Do not drink alcohol* or take narcotic agents if you are taking sleeping medications. Also, do not combine triazolam with other sleep medications, especially the older barbiturates, such as phenobarbital, secobarbital (Seconal), and others, since this combination may potentially be fatal. Propranolol (Inderal), a medication used to treat hypertension, birth-control pills, anti-ulcer drugs such as cimetidine (Tagamet), and disulfiram (Antabuse) may increase the amount of triazolam in the body. The antidepressants nefazodone (Serzone) and fluvoxamine (Luvox) inhibit the metabolism of triazolam, leading to higher blood levels and an increased risk for amnesia, daytime sedation, and impaired motor coordination. If you are taking triazolam (Halcion) for sleep and your physician prescribes nefazodone (Serzone) or fluvoxamine (Luvox), your dose of triazolam should be reduced.

**Use in pregnancy and breast-feeding:
Pregnancy Category X**

Pregnant women should not take triazolam because benzodiazepines may increase the risk of birth defects such as cleft palate and heart deformities, especially when taken in the first trimester. In general, the use of benzodiazepines during pregnancy should almost always be avoided. If taken immediately prior to delivery, triazolam may decrease the newborn's breathing. Women who are breast-feeding should not take triazolam because it will pass into the breast milk and be absorbed by the baby, leading to potential breathing problems and possible unknown effects on the child's developing nervous system.

Use in children: Triazolam has not been studied in children and is not recommended for use in children.

Use in seniors: The usual dose in seniors is 0.125 mg. Because triazolam produces a higher rate of amnesia and confusion than other benzodiazepine sleeping pills, physicians may avoid using it in older people.

Overdosage: In overdose, triazolam produces significant sedation and confusion, leading to coma. People may experience seizures, decrease in breathing (requiring placement on a ventilator), and cardiac arrhythmias. Persons who overdose on triazolam may be hospitalized because of the risk of death and the need for monitoring in an ICU. Combining triazolam with alcohol, barbiturates, or certain other medications increases the risk of death. If an overdose is suspected, bring the bottle of medication to the emergency room with the person, since the date it was prescribed and the number of pills remaining in the bottle can provide helpful information to the treating physician.

Special considerations: Triazolam is used less frequently than in the past because it can produce amnesia. However, a dose of 0.125 or 0.25 mg. at bedtime generally does not cause this problem. If you do not drink alcohol or take other medications such as barbiturates or narcotics, the risk of daytime sedation and other side effects, such as amnesia, paranoia, or agitation, is lessened.

Generic name: **ZALEPLON**

 Available in generic form: No

 Brand name: Sonata

 Drug class: Non-benzodiazepine hypnotic

Prescribed for: Primary insomnia or insomnia secondary to depression, anxiety disorders, or a medical illness.

General Information: Zaleplon is one of the newer nonbenzodiazepine hypnotic agents. Its chemical structure is unrelated to benzodiazepines, barbiturates or antihistamines. The drug is rapidly absorbed following oral administration, producing peak blood levels in about one hour. Its half-life is approximately one hour, which is significantly shorter than zolpidem (Ambien), with a half-life of about two hours. Zaleplon is effective for rapid sleep induction, and its short duration of action offers the advantage of being able to take it later in the night without excess residual effects in the morning.

Dosing information: Zaleplon is available in 5- and 10-mg. capsules. The recommended dose of zaleplon for a non-elderly healthy adult of average weight is 10 mg. For elderly and low-weight individuals, the manufacturer recommends using a 5-mg. dose. The maximum recommended dose is 20 mg.

Interestingly, Japanese people experienced higher blood levels following a standard dose than did people of other races. This may be attributed to differences in body weight or differences in metabolism of the drug in this population. Therefore, for Japanese people, and perhaps for other Asian people, a lower dose of 5 mg. may be all that is needed.

To minimize daytime drowsiness and other related side effects, zaleplon should be taken shortly before going to bed, allowing four hours or more of sleep time.

Common side effects: The reported side effects of zaleplon are dose-related; that is, more people experienced these side effects when taking higher doses. The most frequent complaints are headaches, dizziness, lightheadedness, and difficulty with coordination (ataxia). At higher doses (20 mg.), people have complained of memory loss, nausea, confusion, loss of personal identity (depersonalization), and daytime drowsiness.

Precautions: The use of hypnotics, including zaleplon, is recommended for the short-term treatment of insomnia. Generally, treatment should be limited to no longer than seven to ten days. Long-term use may induce tolerance to the effects of hypnotics. (Although development of tolerance to zaleplon was not noted over a four-week period, the drug was not studied for longer than four weeks.)

People who have a history of alcohol or substance abuse should not take zaleplon. Zaleplon has been reported to cause dependence, especially when used regularly for long periods or at high doses. When taken for periods of more than a few weeks, zaleplon should not be abruptly discontinued, because withdrawal symptoms (e.g., rebound insomnia, nervousness) may occur.

Warnings: Zaleplon is metabolized by the liver and excreted by the kidneys. People with liver disease should not take zaleplon. In people with mild-to-moderate kidney disease, dosage adjustment was not required, but those with severe kidney disease should not take zaleplon.

Some people have experienced unusual changes after

taking zaleplon, especially at higher doses, including aggressiveness, memory loss, nausea, confusion, loss of identity (depersonalization), and agitation.

Alcohol: People should not drink alcohol when taking zaleplon. When taken together, zaleplon and alcohol intensify side effects such as sedation, memory disturbance, incoordination, euphoria, and impaired judgment, and can seriously affect driving ability. In addition, alcohol seriously disrupts sleep and leads to early-morning awakening.

Food and beverages: Taking zaleplon shortly after a heavy, high-fat meal may delay the absorption of the drug, and hence its effectiveness in inducing sleep. Avoid caffeine-containing beverages, such as coffee, tea, cocoa, and colas, since caffeine is a frequent contributor to sleep problems. The nicotine contained in cigarettes also interferes with sleep.

Possible drug interactions: Cimetidine (Tagamet), an anti-ulcer drug, inhibits the metabolism of zaleplon, resulting in higher blood levels. People taking cimetidine (Tagamet) should use a lower 5-mg. dose of zaleplon, and should separate the dose time by at least two to three hours.

Medications such as narcotic analgesics that affect the central nervous system may increase zaleplon's sedative effect, as well as cause other CNS side effects. Do not combine zaleplon with other sleep medications, especially barbiturates, such as phenobarbital, secobarbital (Seconal) and others, because this combination may potentially be fatal.

Use in pregnancy and breast-feeding: Pregnancy Category C

The use of zaleplon in pregnant women has not been studied, and the drug is not recommended for use during pregnancy.

Zaleplon is excreted in human breast milk, reaching peak levels one hour after taking the drug. Women who are breast-feeding should not take zaleplon.

Use in children: Zaleplon has not been studied in children and is not recommended for use in children.

Use in seniors: Seniors may be more sensitive to zaleplon. Because of its fast onset of action and short half-life, zaleplon may induce amnesia in some older individuals. Therefore, the usual dose should not exceed 5 mg. The elderly metabolize sleeping medications more slowly. This means that these drugs remain in their bodies longer, and they become more prone to the side effects noted above, and to an increased risk of falling. A National Institutes of Health (NIH) consensus conference on treating sleep problems in the elderly recommended that clinicians consider sleeping pills only after a thorough assessment of the possible causes of the insomnia, improvements in sleep hygiene, and behavioral treatments. If all these measures prove unsuccessful, sleeping pills are prescribed, but only in low doses and for short periods of time.

Overdosage: There are limited data on the treatment of zaleplon overdose. The most common signs and symptoms are central nervous system (CNS) depression, including drowsiness, confusion, problems with walking (ataxia), and slurred speech. Even in more serious cases, zaleplon overdose is seldom fatal. However, when the drug is combined with alcohol, barbiturates, or certain other medications, the risk of death is significantly increased. Bring the bottle of medication to the hospital emergency room with the patient, since the date it was prescribed and the number of pills remaining in the bottle can provide helpful information to the treating physician.

 Special considerations: Zaleplon is a fast-acting, nonbenzodiazepine hypnotic with a short half-life. The clinical advantage of zaleplon in the short-term management of insomnia is its relatively rapid onset of action and clearance of the drug from the body, so that it does not cause daytime drowsiness and hangover.

As with other sedative-hypnotics, there is a potential risk for abuse and dependence, although this is far less likely than with the benzodiazepines and barbiturates. Moreover, in overdosage, zaleplon and newer hypnotics like zolpidem (Ambien) are far safer than are the older sedative-hypnotics.

 Generic name: ZOLPIDEM

 Available in generic form: No

 Brand name: Ambien

Drug class: Non-benzodiazepine hypnotic

Prescribed for: Primary insomnia or insomnia secondary to depression, anxiety disorders, or a medical illness.

General information: Zolpidem is a short-acting hypnotic agent that induces and maintains sleep. Unlike the benzodiazepines, it is not effective in treating anxiety disorders and does not serve as a muscle relaxant. Persons who use zolpidem for several weeks or more do not develop rebound insomnia or tolerance to the medication, as they may with benzodiazepines. As a result, higher doses are not necessary to continue the same desired effect. Zolpidem preserves normal sleep stages, with only minor effects on REM. Zolpidem's primary limitation is its short half-life of just three to four hours. Because of this, people who experience early-morning awakening may not benefit from its use.

Dosing information: Zolpidem is available in 5- and 10-mg. tablets. The usual recommended dose for healthy adults is 10 mg. a day. Because of its short half-life, few people experience daytime drowsiness or sedation. In addition, because of its rapid absorption, people experience its sedative effects within a short period of time, usually in fifteen to thirty minutes. For this reason, the medication should be taken immediately before bedtime.

Common side effects: The most common side effects are drowsiness, fatigue, diarrhea, nausea, and dizziness. At higher levels, people may complain of visual disturbances, such as double vision and jerky eye movements (nystagmus), and impaired coordination.

Precautions: People who have an alcohol or substance use disorder should not take zolpidem, since it may lead to dependence or addiction and may contribute to a relapse in those who are recovering alcoholics.

Warnings: People with chronic obstructive pulmonary disease (COPD) should not take zolpidem because it may decrease the ability to breathe, which can be fatal. Those with sleep apnea, a condition characterized by long pauses in respiration during sleep, should not take zolpidem because this drug decreases the ability to begin breathing again after such a pause—a potentially fatal effect. People with liver disease or decreased liver function should not take zolpidem because it is metabolized by the liver, and its effects on the body will be magnified, producing greater sedation, memory disturbance, and incoordination.

▽ **Alcohol:** People should not drink alcohol when taking zolpidem. When taken together, zolpidem and alcohol intensify side effects such as sedation, memory disturbance, motor incoordination, euphoria, and impaired judgment, and can seriously affect driving ability. In addition, alcohol frequently disrupts sleep and leads to early-morning awakening.

Food and beverages: Because food reduces its absorption, zolpidem should not be taken with food or immediately after a meal. Avoid caffeine-containing beverages, such as coffee, tea, cocoa, and colas, since caffeine is a frequent contributor to sleep problems. The nicotine contained in cigarettes also interferes with sleep.

Possible drug interactions: Alcohol and narcotic drugs—meperidine (Demerol), hydrocodone (Vicodin), oxycodone (Percodan), and others—may increase zolpidem's sedative effects and potentially be fatal. *Do not drink alcohol* or take narcotic agents if you are taking zolpidem. Do not combine zolpidem with other sleep medications, especially the older barbiturates, such as phenobarbital, secobarbital (Seconal), and others; this combination may potentially be fatal.

Use in pregnancy and breast-feeding: Pregnancy Category B

Although zolpidem has not been systemically studied in pregnant women, they should not take zolpidem because it may increase the risk of birth defects. Women who are pregnant or who are contemplating pregnancy should not use zolpidem unless its possible benefits to the mother outweigh any potential unknown risks to the fetus and unless alternative treatments have been unsuccessful. Women who are breast-feeding should not take zolpidem because it will pass into the breast milk and be absorbed into the baby's bloodstream, leading to potential breathing problems and possible unknown effects on the child's developing nervous system.

Use in children: Zolpidem has not been studied in children and is not recommended for use in children.

Use in seniors: The usual dose in seniors is 5 mg. Because of its fast onset of action and short half-life, zolpidem may produce amnesia in some older individuals. The elderly metabolize sleeping medications more slowly. This means that the drugs remain in their bodies longer, and they become more prone to the side effects noted above and to an increased risk of falling. A National Institutes of Health (NIH) consensus conference on treating sleep problems in the elderly recommended that clinicians consider sleeping pills only after a thorough assessment of the possible causes of the insomnia, improvements in sleep hygiene, and behavioral treatments. If all these prove unsuccessful, sleeping pills are prescribed, but only in low doses and for short periods of time.

Overdosage: The most common symptoms of overdose are excessive sleepiness, problems with walking (ataxia), slurred speech, confusion, and daytime drowsiness. Large doses of zolpidem are usually not fatal. However, combining it with alcohol, barbiturates, or certain other medications increases the risk of death considerably. People who take an overdose should always be brought to a hospital emergency room. Bring the bottle of medication to the emergency room with the person, since the date it was prescribed and the number of pills remaining in the bottle can provide helpful information to the treating physician.

Special considerations: Zolpidem is an excellent medication to treat insomnia. It may have special usefulness for treatment of jet lag. Because of its short half-life and fast onset of action, people taking the medication fall asleep rapidly and usually do not experience amnesia when they wake up or have daytime drowsiness.

CHAPTER 6

Antipsychotic Medications

To learn general information about this class of medications and the disorders they treat, read the first part of the chapter. To read about a specific antipsychotic medication, turn to the page indicated below.

PSYCHOTIC DISORDERS

Psychosis is a condition in which individuals are unable to distinguish between what is real and what is not. The most common psychotic symptoms are *hallucinations,* sensations involving any of the senses that a person experiences as real even though there is no evidence that they exist; *delusions,* fixed beliefs that a person clings to despite evidence that they are false; and *thought disorders,* disturbances in a person's capacity to reason or think logically.

Many factors, including mental disorders such as major depression and bipolar illness, physical illnesses such as brain tumors or infections, and reactions to drugs or toxic substances, can impair an individual's perceptions, thoughts, and emotional responses. Some psychotic episodes are acute and interfere only briefly with a person's ability to distinguish between the real and the unreal. If such episodes are induced by illness, injury, or substance use, appropriate treatment of the underlying cause can lead to a quick and full recovery. Other forms of psychosis, such as schizophrenia, can be chronic, with symptoms flaring up or persisting for decades.

For those affected and their loved ones, psychosis can be extremely frightening. Psychotic symptoms always require prompt professional evaluation.

Schizophrenia

Schizophrenia, one of the most debilitating mental disorders, profoundly impairs an individual's sense of reality. As the National Institute of Mental Health (NIMH) puts it, schizophrenia, which is characterized by abnormalities in brain structure and chemistry, destroys "the inner unity of the mind" and weakens "the will and drive that constitute our essential character." It affects every aspect of psychological functioning, including the ways people think, feel, view themselves, and relate to others.

Individuals with schizophrenia may hear, see, or feel things that do not exist—a voice telling them to jump from a bridge, a statue crying tears of blood, a spaceship beaming a light upon them. Frightened and vulnerable, they may devote all their energy to warding off the demons within. Unable to take care of themselves, they may look messy and disheveled. They often move in unusual ways, such as rocking or pacing, or repeat certain gestures again and again. They may believe that someone or something, such as the devil, is putting thoughts into their heads or controlling their actions. Some think they are reincarnations of Christ or Napoleon. About a third attempt to take their own lives, often in response to a command they hear inside their heads. The symptoms of schizophrenia are summarized in Table 6-1.

Schizophrenia is most likely to occur between the ages of seventeen and twenty-four. One-half to 1 percent of the world population—about 1 in every 150 people—suffers from this disorder. According to NIMH's epidemiological data, the total lifetime prevalence for schizophrenia in the United States ranges from 1 to 1.9 percent. This means that between 2.5 million and 4.75 million Americans may have schizophrenia at any one time.

Schizophrenia typically consists of several stages. During the prodromal phase, a period ranging from months to years, individuals withdraw from social interactions, pay

Table 6-1: The Symptoms of Schizophrenia

CHARACTERISTIC SYMPTOMS OF SCHIZOPHRENIA

• Hallucinations

• Delusions

• Inability to think in a logical manner

• Talking in rambling or incoherent ways

• Making odd or purposeless movements or not moving at all

• Repeating others' words or mimicking their gestures

• Showing few, if any, feelings; responding with inappropriate emotions

• Lacking will or motivation to complete a task or accomplish something

• Functioning at a much lower level than in the past at work, in interpersonal relations, or in taking care of oneself

less attention to keeping clean and dressing appropriately, or act in peculiar ways. In the acute, or active, phase, individuals develop "positive symptoms." They may experience delusions and become convinced that space aliens have taken control of their bodies or hallucinate and hear voices mocking them. Some talk nonstop, rambling on without making any clear point; others repeatedly shake their heads, tap their feet, or assume odd postures or positions. After positive symptoms subside, individuals enter the residual phase, which is characterized by "negative" symptoms, such as apathy, flattened emotions, or inappropriate emotional reactions (for example, laughing when someone is hurt).

For centuries, the quest for a cure for this frightening and often tragic disease led to desperate methods, including spraying a strong stream of water at a patient's spine, injecting horse serum, and administering huge doses of vitamins. While they do not cure schizophrenia and other psychotic disorders, for the vast majority of individuals with schizophrenia, antipsychotic drugs are the foundation of treatment today. They make most people with schizophrenia feel more comfortable and in control of themselves, help organize chaotic thinking, and reduce or eliminate delusions or hallucinations, allowing fuller participation in normal activities. Even those who do not improve significantly on medication almost invariably do still worse without it.

Because tranquilization, or sedation, is a common side effect, antipsychotic drugs used to be called "major tranquilizers." They are now referred to as "antipsychotics" or "neuroleptics" (because their side effects mimic neurological diseases like Parkinsonism).

Most of these drugs have a similar mode of action. While some may act more quickly than others, almost all are equally effective. But they can have problematic side effects, including uncontrollable facial tics, tongue tremors, and jaw movements known as tardive dyskinesia, which may be irreversible. In most cases, "positive" symptoms, such as hallucinations and delusions, decrease in intensity after one or two weeks of treatment with an antipsychotic medication. However, almost one-third of those given conventional antipsychotics continue to have residual or "negative" symptoms, such as apathy and lack of motivation. In the past, little, if anything, could be done to relieve these negative symptoms. A relatively new medication, the atypical antipsychotic drug clozapine (Clozaril), can help to relieve both positive and negative symptoms in individuals who do not improve with conventional antipsychotic medications or who develop intolerable side effects. Other recently released atypical antipsychotic medications, risperidone (Risperdal), olanzapine (Zyprexa), and quetiapine (Seroquel), have also shown promise in treating negative symptoms like apathy and withdrawal. While some individuals with schizophrenia recover completely, many thousands—perhaps as many as 200,000—live on the street or in homeless shelters.

Although neuroscientists do not completely understand how antipsychotic drugs work, many believe that psychotic symptoms result in part from an excess of the neurotransmitter dopamine, increased sensitivity of the dopamine receptors, or altered activity in specific dopamine pathways within the brain. Antipsychotic drugs may work, at least to some extent, by preventing dopamine from binding to dopamine receptor sites in the brain. More recently, serotonin has also been implicated as a possible neurochemical contributor to schizophrenia. The new "atypical" antipsychotic agents have proven beneficial because they also act on serotonin receptors.

Conventional Antipsychotic Drugs

Over the last thirty years, many studies have confirmed the efficacy of antipsychotic medications in treating psychotic symptoms, such as delusions, hallucinations, and disorganized speech and thinking, in individuals with schizophrenia, major depression, bipolar illness, and brain disorders such as Huntington's disease or traumatic brain injury. Antipsychotic drugs may also be used in the treatment of borderline or schizotypal personality disorders, somatization disorder, severe obsessive-compulsive disorder, and a neurological disorder known as Tourette's syndrome, which is characterized by vocal and motor tics. These drugs have also proven valuable in treating individuals who become aggressive or intensely agitated, but they should not be used as a treatment for chronic aggression or agitation if an individual does not have psychotic symptoms.

Antipsychotic drugs are categorized both by their chemical similarities and by their potency (low, intermediate, or high), a classification based on the dosage required to achieve a desired effect. Thus, haloperidol (Haldol) is called a high-potency conventional neuroleptic because less of it is needed to reduce psychotic symptoms. Chlorpromazine

(Thorazine) is a low-potency conventional neuroleptic because more of the drug is required to achieve a similar benefit. Perphenazine (Trilafon) is an intermediate-potency conventional agent. The dose equivalents of the antipsychotic medications are based on their relative potencies as compared with 100 mg. of chlorpromazine (Thorazine). For instance, a 2-mg. dose of haloperidol (Haldol) and a 10-mg. dose of perphenazine (Trilafon) achieve approximately the same effect as 100 mg. of chlorpromazine (Thorazine) (see Table 6-2).

Table 6-2: Antipsychotic Medication Drug Potencies

GENERIC NAME	BRAND NAME	EQUIVALENT DOSE TO 100 MG. OF CHLORPROMAZINE (THORAZINE)
chlorpromazine	Thorazine	100 mg.
clozapine	Clozaril	50 mg.
fluphenazine	Prolixin	2 mg.
haloperidol	Haldol	2 mg.
loxapine	Loxitane	10 mg.
mesoridazine	Serentil	50 mg.
molindone	Moban	10 mg.
olanzapine	Zyprexa	2.5 mg.
perphenazine	Trilafon	1.0 mg.
pimozide	Orap	1.5 mg.
quetiapine	Seroquel	100 mg.
risperidone	Risperdal	0.5 mg.
thioridazine	Mellaril	100 mg.
thiothixene	Navane	5 mg.
trifluoperazine	Stelazine	5 mg.
ziprasidone	Geodon	20 mg.

The reversal of psychotic symptoms is often gradual, occurring over a period of several weeks to several months. Without continued treatment after the remission of acute psychotic symptoms, the relapse rate for individuals with schizophrenia can be as high as 15 percent per month. By comparison, those who continue to take antipsychotic medications have a relapse rate of 1.5 to 3 percent per month. Individuals who have chronic, relapsing schizophrenia may continue to take the lowest possible dose of medication for years.

Although some antipsychotic medications act more rapidly than others, most are equally effective, differing only in dosages, side effects, and cost. Nonetheless, for unknown reasons, different individuals often tend to respond better to one drug than another. The only way to determine which drug and which dose will help a person most and cause the fewest side effects is by trial and error, a process that, although necessary, can be time-consuming and sometimes distressing.

Side Effects

Antipsychotic drugs differ in the side effects they produce (see Table 6-3).

Low-potency conventional antipsychotics tend to be very sedating and often lower blood pressure, especially when the person moves from a sitting to standing position (orthostatic hypotension). High-potency conventional medications can cause abnormal movements such as Parkinson-like trembling and involuntary movements (called extrapyramidal symptoms), but are less sedating and less likely to lower blood pressure. Intermediate-potency conventional antipsychotics are mildly sedating and have some blood-pressure-lowering effects, though far fewer than the low-potency agents. Also, the intermediate-potency conventional antipsychotics produce fewer extrapyramidal symptoms than the high-potency agents. Regardless of potency, side

Table 6-3: Major Side Effects of Conventional Antipsychotic Agents Based on Their Potencies

	Sedation and Fatigue	Postural Hypotension	Anticholinergic Effects[1]	Extrapyramidal Symptoms[2]
Low-potency	+ + +	+ + +	+ + +	+
Intermediate-potency	+ +	+ +	+ +	+ +
High-potency	+	+	+	+ + +

+   mild effects
+ +   moderate effects
+ + +   severe effects

[1] Dry mouth, blurred vision, constipation, confusion
[2] Tremor, muscle stiffness and spasms, stooped posture, lack of facial expression (mask-like face)

effects such as dry mouth, blurred vision, constipation, difficulty in urinating, dizziness on sitting or standing (orthostatic hypotension), and drowsiness are most likely to occur during the first few weeks of therapy. These usually disappear, or the individual adjusts to them, after a few weeks. Other side effects include increased heart rate; rash; sensitivity to sunlight or heat; weight gain; muscle spasms in the head or neck; slowing and stiffening of muscle activity in the face, body, arms, and legs; drooling; hand tremor; and seizures in seizure-prone individuals. Some of these effects are obviously uncomfortable or distressing, but they do not cause lasting impairment. In some cases additional medications can prevent or relieve troubling side effects. For example, beta-blockers can relieve *akathisia,* a condition where individuals become so restless that they are unable to sit still and constantly need to move.

Some persons develop what is called an acute dystonic reaction during the first hours or days of treatment. They may experience tightening of the face and neck and spasms of the muscles of the head and/or back. Sometimes the eye muscles are affected, causing the eyes to roll upward and "lock" in this position. This problem can be rapidly alleviated by the intramuscular injection of an anticholinergic drug such as diphenhydramine (Benadryl) or benztropine (Cogentin).

Antipsychotic drugs affect many hormones in the body, especially the sex-related hormones. Unfortunately, these side effects often last as long as the person remains on the medication. Both men and women may develop enlargement of the breasts and occasional fluid discharge from the nipples. The medication amantadine (Symmetrel) can sometimes decrease the severity of these effects. Antipsychotics can also affect sexual desire and performance. Some men may have difficulty achieving or maintaining an erection, may experience retrograde ejaculation, or may develop priapism. Both men and women may have trouble achieving orgasm. Again, these effects usually remain as long as the person is on the medication.

After several weeks of drug therapy, some individuals may talk and gesture less, seem apathetic, and have difficulty initiating spontaneous gestures, such as moving the arms when talking. This condition, called *akinesia,* is sometimes mistaken for depression. On occasion, long-term drug treatment can lead to rabbit syndrome, which consists of lip movements that mimic the chewing of a rabbit. It can be treated effectively with anticholinergic drugs such as diphenhydramine (Benadryl).

Warnings

The most disabling and difficult-to-treat side effect of the traditional antipsychotic medications is *tardive dyskinesia,* a neurological disorder marked by involuntary movements that can affect any muscle group in the body, most often the face. According to the American Psychiatric Association Task Force on Tardive Dyskinesia, 15 to 20 percent of individuals undergoing long-term treatment with traditional antipsychotics show some signs of this problem. The most significant risk factors are increasing age and duration of treatment. The incidence among young adults who are taking typical antipsychotic agents is about 5 percent per year of treatment and rises with age. The newer "atypical" antipsychotic agents (see page 295) are associated with a much lower risk of tardive dyskinesia, and clozapine is believed not to produce it. In older persons, the rate may be as high as 20 to 25 percent after one year of treatment with further increases up to 60 percent after five years of treatment.

Individuals with tardive dyskinesia may, without meaning or wanting to, frown, blink, grimace, smile, pout, pucker, smack their lips, bite, clench, chew, or stick out their tongues. Others may rock, twist, squirm, tap their fingers, or shrug their shoulders. This condition does not affect mental function but can be so severe that walking, eating, and even breathing become difficult. There is no known cure, and some cases are irreversible, although scientists are studying various medications that may alleviate the condition.

Because of the risk of tardive dyskinesia, some states, among them California and New Jersey, require that patients give their informed consent specifically for the possibility of this condition before antipsychotic drugs can be prescribed. If it is not possible to obtain consent because an individual is acutely psychotic, psychiatrists must educate family members about the risk and obtain their consent. The patient is then informed of the risk after symptoms ease.

Regular examinations every six months can check for early signs of tardive dyskinesia, such as small wormlike movements under the surface of the tongue. Some individuals with this disorder who are switched from a traditional antipsychotic to clozapine (Clozaril) or risperidone (Risperdal) show improvement. In other cases, it becomes necessary to weigh the therapeutic benefits of the antipsychotic medication against the risk for tardive dyskinesia and decide which course to pursue on the basis of this risk/benefit assessment.

All antipsychotic agents may produce agranulocytosis, a rare, potentially fatal condition where there is a significant reduction in infection-fighting white blood cells.

A rare but life-threatening side effect of any antipsychotic medication is *neuroleptic malignant syndrome* (NMS), where there is an elevation of body temperature, severe muscle stiffness, rigidity, paralysis of the eye muscles, and a significant increase in heart rate, blood pressure, and sweating. The atypical antipsychotics may not produce muscle rigidity but can cause NMS. Increases in white-blood-cell counts and blood chemistry abnormalities are also frequent. The person may also become delirious, leading to coma. NMS is a medical emergency, requiring immediate hospitalization and treatment in an intensive-care unit. NMS may be more common with high-potency, conventional agents, such as haloperidol (Haldol).

General Precautions

Individuals taking any antipsychotic medication should be careful about using other medications and should avoid alcohol, which not only makes psychotic symptoms worse but can also be dangerously sedating. The question of continued use during pregnancy must always be decided on a case-by-case basis by the woman, her psychiatrist, and her obstetrician.

Low-Potency Conventional Antipsychotic Drugs

These medications include chlorpromazine (Thorazine), mesoridazine (Serentil), and thioridazine (Mellaril). All the low-potency medications require higher doses to achieve a therapeutic response similar to those of other antipsychotics. They are often used in the early treatment of an otherwise healthy young person who becomes psychotic and agitated because they can help control physical activity that might harm the individual or others. In addition to sedation, side effects include low blood pressure, photosensitivity, sexual dysfunction, constipation, and blurred vision.

Intermediate-Potency Conventional Antipsychotic Drugs

These medications include loxapine (Loxitane), molindone (Moban), and perphenazine (Trilafon). They are less sedating than the low-potency drugs and cause fewer movement abnormalities than high-potency antipsychotics. Some must be used with caution in seizure-prone individuals. Molindone (Moban) is the only antipsychotic agent that does not cause weight gain, and it may also pose less risk of seizures.

High-Potency Conventional Antipsychotic Drugs

These medications include fluphenazine (Prolixin), haloperidol (Haldol), pimozide (Orap), thiothixene (Navane), and trifluoperazine (Stelazine). High-potency antipsychotics are less sedating and less likely to lower blood pressure. However, they can cause extrapyramidal symptoms and agitated restlessness. Psychiatrists often prescribe an additional medication—usually an anticholinergic drug, such as benztropine (Cogentin) or trihexyphenidyl (Artane)—to reduce these side effects.

Pimozide (Orap) has proved helpful for delusional disorders, such as erotomania, and for involuntary tics, and has shown promise for treatment of both negative and positive symptoms in schizophrenia.

Atypical Antipsychotic Drugs

As noted above, almost one-third of individuals given conventional antipsychotics continue to experience residual symptoms, such as apathy and social withdrawal. In the past, little, if anything, could be done to relieve these negative symptoms. A major breakthrough in treatment came with the development of a different type of antipsychotic medication, called "atypical."

The atypical antipsychotic agent clozapine (Clozaril), which was the first of these agents available in the United States, can help with both positive and negative symptoms, such as lack of motivation and withdrawal, for individuals who do not improve with conventional medications or who develop intolerable side effects. In one study, 30 percent of those with so-called refractory schizophrenia who were not helped by other antipsychotics improved with clozapine. It may also be useful in refractory cases of schizoaffective disorder and psychotic depression.

Clozapine, which is believed to act on receptors for subtypes of dopamine and serotonin, is less likely than many other antipsychotics to cause chronic neurological side effects such as tardive dyskinesia. Its side effects include heavy salivation, sedation, increased heart rate, low blood pressure, and seizures.

Although clozapine is highly effective and helps reduce the length of hospital stays, it has one serious drawback: About 1 percent of those who use it may develop agranulocytosis. For this reason, individuals taking this drug must have their blood checked prior to treatment, weekly for the first six months of continuous treatment, and every other week thereafter. Individuals must discontinue

clozapine if their white-blood-cell counts drop dangerously low (less than 3,000 white blood cells per mm^3).
Fortunately, once the drug is stopped, the white-blood-cell
counts usually return to normal. The need for frequent
monitoring makes use of this drug very costly, an estimated $5,300 to $9,000 annually. Mental-health advo-
cates argue that only a fraction of those who might benefit
from clozapine have been able to afford it.

Other Atypical Antipsychotic Drugs

Newer atypical medications, risperidone (Risperdal), olanzapine (Zyprexa), quetiapine (Seroquel), and ziprasidone
(Geodon), which block receptors for subtypes of serotonin
as well as dopamine, became available in the United States
in the 1990s and early 2000s. In clinical trials, these medications, unrelated chemically to other antipsychotic drugs,
have produced fewer neurological side effects, such as
acute dystonic reactions (muscle spasms), tremors, and
akathisia (a subjective sense of motor restlessness). They
may cause neuroleptic malignant syndrome and produce
tardive dyskinesia with long-term use, but at a rate much
lower than conventional agents. Side effects include agitation, anxiety, and insomnia.

Although less is known about the use of risperidone
(Risperdal), olanzapine (Zyprexa), quetiapine (Seroquel),
and ziprasidone (Geodon) over time than about older, conventional antipsychotics, they have shown promise in significantly reducing both positive and negative symptoms
of schizophrenia. They produce fewer side effects than
clozapine (Clozaril) and the conventional antipsychotics
and do not require intensive—and expensive—blood monitoring. According to manufacturers' estimates, the cost of
a year's dose ranges between one-half and two-thirds the
cost of clozapine (Clozaril). Zaprasidone (Geodon), the
newest of the atypical antipsychotics, may prove beneficial
in treating depressive symptoms in schizophrenic patients

because of its effects in blocking the reuptake of both serotonin and norepinephrine.

LOW-POTENCY CONVENTIONAL ANTIPSYCHOTIC MEDICATIONS

GENERIC NAME	BRAND NAME	DRUG CLASS
chlorpromazine	Thorazine	Phenothiazine
mesoridazine	Serentil	Phenothiazine
thioridazine	Mellaril	Phenothiazine

 Generic name: CHLORPROMAZINE MESORIDAZINE THIORIDAZINE

 Brand name: Thorazine, Serentil, Mellaril

 Drug class: Phenothiazine

 Available in generic form: Yes

Prescribed for: Schizophrenia, schizoaffective disorder, acute mania, psychotic depression, severe obsessive-compulsive disorder, agitation in persons with dementia.

 General information: The low-potency antipsychotic drugs of the phenothiazine class have been available for many years. These drugs are called low-potency medications because the amount of medication needed to achieve a similar therapeutic response is higher than with the other antipsychotic medications. These drugs, the oldest antipsychotics, also have some of the most problematic side effects.

As indicated in the introduction to this chapter, many neuroscientists believe that the psychotic symptoms of schizophrenia result in part from an excess of the neurotransmitter dopamine, increased sensitivity of the dopamine receptors, or altered activity in specific dopamine pathways within the brain. Conventional antipsychotic medications are believed to work by blocking dopamine receptor sites in the hypothalamus. The blocking of dopamine receptors also produces troublesome side effects such as Parkinson-like symptoms. Because of the numerous side effects and problems with these medications, newer atypical antipsychotic medications are used more frequently.

Dosing information: Chlorpromazine (Thorazine) is available in tablets, extended-release spansules, suppositories, syrup, concentrate, and ampules for intramuscular injection. Mesoridazine (Serentil) is available in tablets, concentrates, and ampules for injection. Thioridazine (Mellaril) does not have an injectable form but is available in tablets, concentrate, and suspension. Most persons who are acutely psychotic respond to doses of chlorpromazine between 400 and 1,000 mg. a day, doses of thioridazine between 400 and 800 mg. a day, and doses of mesoridazine between 200 and 500 mg. a day. Unfortunately, higher doses than these are often used. According to current belief, higher doses are not necessary because persons will respond to these medications at lower doses if sufficient time is allowed for them to work. Thioridazine has an upper-limit dose restriction of 800 mg.; doses above this have been reported to produce retinal pigmentation, which may lead to significant visual problems. Mesoridazine, a metabolite of thioridazine, does not produce this condition, nor does chlorpromazine.

Common side effects: Sedation is the most common problem with the low-potency conventional antipsychotic medications. Other common side effects are sexual dysfunction (especially with thioridazine (Mellaril), in the form of retrograde ejaculation in males), orthostatic hypotension, and significant anticholinergic effects (see Glossary), including dry mouth, blurred vision, constipation, and confusion. Since all conventional antipsychotics block dopamine receptors in the hypothalamus, they may increase blood prolactin levels, leading to breast enlargement and milk secretion in both women and men. Weight gain is often quite significant. All the conventional antipsychotic medications may produce rashes and photosensitivity (an increased susceptibility to sunburn), but chlorpromazine is especially likely to do so. Anyone taking chlorpromazine and other conventional antipsychotics should apply sunscreen before going outdoors.

Precautions: All antipsychotic medications may lower the seizure threshold; this may occur more often with chlorpromazine. Men with enlarged prostates who take low-potency antipsychotics may experience difficulty in urinating and urinary retention. Individuals with narrow-angle glaucoma may have dangerous increases in the internal eye pressure, leading to visual disturbances and even blindness. Because of the effects of antipsychotic medications on the hypothalamus, individuals become very sensitive to extreme heat and must be cautious about avoiding high temperatures.

All antipsychotic medications have the potential to produce neurologic side effects. Although these are more likely to occur with the high-potency agents, the low-potency conventional antipsychotics may produce dystonia (muscle spasms in the tongue, jaw, and neck); pseudo-Parkinsonism, characterized by a pill-rolling tremor, muscle stiffness, stooped posture, mask-like face, drooling, akinesia (a decrease in voluntary motor movements so the person walks stiffly); and akathisia (an inner sense of motor restlessness that causes people to become agitated, pace constantly, and wring their hands). Doctors sometimes confuse akathisia with psychotic depression. A decrease in antipsychotic medication may improve symptoms in cases of akathisia. If the problem is psychotic depression, an increase in antipsychotic medication may be required.

The low-potency conventional antipsychotic agents produce excessive weight gain more frequently than high-potency agents do. Since excessive weight is associated with an increased risk of diabetes, hypertension, heart disease, and premature death, people who gain excessive weight should participate in medically supervised programs to reduce this weight gain (diet, exercise, and medication) or should be switched to a high-potency conventional antipsychotic (haloperidol) or an atypical antipsychotic (risperidone) that produces less weight gain. Also, periodic weight checks are encouraged while on the medication.

§∅§**Warnings:** Both chlorpromazine (Thorazine) and thioridazine (Mellaril) have been reported to produce agranulocytosis, a potentially fatal condition in which the bone marrow stops producing white blood cells, at rates of 1 in 5,000 to 1 in 10,000. Patients who have agranulocytosis or a lesser condition called leukopenia (a decrease in white blood cells) are more prone to infections. Chlorpromazine may infrequently produce a rare allergic form of hepatitis, but this condition, similar to agranulocytosis and leukopenia, is usually reversible when the medication is stopped.

Low-potency antipsychotics can lead to a potentially life-threatening condition, neuroleptic malignant syndrome (NMS), where there is an elevation of body temperature, severe muscle stiffness, rigidity, paralysis of the eye muscles, and a significant increase in heart rate, blood pressure, and sweating. Increases in white-blood-cell counts and blood-chemistry abnormalities also frequently occur. The person may also become delirious, leading to coma. NMS is a medical emergency requiring immediate hospitalization and treatment in an intensive-care unit. NMS can occur with any conventional antipsychotic drug but may be more common with high-potency agents such as haloperidol (Haldol).

People who take antipsychotic medication for a prolonged period of time may develop a condition called tardive dyskinesia, marked by involuntary movements of the tongue, fingers, and upper extremities, jaw movements, facial grimacing, smacking of the lips, twisting of the upper extremities and body, grunting while breathing, and various abnormal movements of the lower extremities. The condition does not affect mental function, but can be so severe that walking, eating, and even breathing become difficult. The risk of developing tardive dyskinesia appears to be related to the cumulative dose and length of treatment with antipsychotic medication. Individuals who are in state mental hospitals have rates in the range of 20 to 40 percent. The incidence rises with age, and women are at greater risk. Unfortunately, there is no known treatment for tardive dyskinesia, and it may be irreversible. Tapering off of the antipsychotic medication is recommended, but the condition may worsen in the short term.

▽ **Alcohol:** Individuals who are taking antipsychotic medications should not drink alcohol, since alcohol leads to even greater sedation, a significant side effect of low-potency conventional antipsychotic medications.

Food and beverages: There are no restrictions. Individuals should be discouraged from smoking, since nicotine lowers the blood levels of antipsychotic medications.

Possible drug interactions: Certain antacids may decrease absorption of antipsychotic drugs. Antihypertensive medications such as propranolol (Inderal), clonidine (Catapres), or guanethidine (Ismelin) should be closely monitored when taken with low-potency conventional antipsychotic medications (especially chlorpromazine [Thorazine]) because the antipsychotic drugs also lower blood pressure. Other medications that produce sedation, such as benzodiazepines, antihistamines, and narcotic-type pain medications like meperidine (Demerol), hydrocodone (Vicodin), and others, should be avoided because these drugs may interfere with an individual's breathing when combined with antipsychotics.

Use in pregnancy and breast-feeding: Pregnancy Category C

Women who are contemplating becoming pregnant or who are pregnant should not, whenever possible, take antipsychotic agents. Women who breast-feed should not take an antipsychotic medication because it passes into the breast milk and is absorbed into the baby's bloodstream, leading to potential adverse effects upon the child's developing nervous system.

Use in children: These medications have been used in children over the age of six months, but they should be prescribed cautiously by a child psychiatrist with special expertise in treating childhood schizophrenia, a relatively rare condition. The newer atypical antipsychotic medications are a recommended alternative.

Use in seniors: Seniors should avoid low-potency conventional antipsychotics because of their significant anticholinergic side effects, including sedation, dry mouth, constipation, difficulty in urinating, and confusion. The low-potency agents also cause orthostatic hypotension, which increases the risk of falls, an especially dangerous problem for seniors.

☠ **Overdosage:** The most common effects of over-dosage are excessive tiredness, a decrease in blood pressure, confusion, irregular heartbeats (arrhythmias), seizures, and significant muscle rigidity or spasms. People who take an overdose should always be brought to a hospital emergency room. Bring the bottle of medication to the emergency room with the person, since the date the medication was prescribed and the number of pills remaining in the bottle can provide helpful information to the treating physician.

Special considerations: The intermediate- and higher-potency conventional antipsychotic medications, such as perphenazine (Trilafon) and haloperidol (Haldol), or the newer atypical antipsychotic medications, such as risperidone (Risperdal) or olanzapine (Zyprexa), are frequently preferred over low-potency antipsychotics. While the cost of the newer medications is much higher, they have a much lower risk of tardive dyskinesia, acute dystonic reactions (see page 291), Parkinsonian side effects, and allergic reactions. However, in situations where significant sedation is required for an agitated, psychotic individual, the low-potency agents are still extremely useful.

INTERMEDIATE-POTENCY CONVENTIONAL ANTIPSYCHOTIC MEDICATIONS

GENERIC NAME	BRAND NAME	DRUG CLASS
loxapine	Loxitane	Dibenzoxazepine
molindone	Moban	Dihydroindolone
perphenazine	Trilafon	Phenothiazine

 Generic name: **LOXAPINE**
MOLINDONE
PERPHENAZINE

 Available in generic form: Yes

 Brand name: Loxitane, Moban, Trilafon

Drug class: Dibenzoxazepine, dihydroindolone, phenothiazine

Prescribed for: Schizophrenia, schizoaffective disorder, acute mania, psychotic depression, severe obsessive-compulsive disorder, agitation in persons with dementia.

General information: The three intermediate-potency conventional antipsychotic drugs represent three different chemical classes of medications. They are generally less sedating than low-potency antipsychotic drugs and cause fewer movement abnormalities, especially dystonia (see page 291), akinesia (decreased motor activity), and akathisia (internal sense of physical restlessness) than the high-potency antipsychotics. The intermediate-potency agents are just as effective therapeutically as the low-potency agents.

In general, an intermediate-potency conventional antipsychotic medication may be prescribed if those taking a low-potency conventional antipsychotic medication complain significantly of sedation or if those taking a high-potency agent develop troublesome extrapyramidal symptoms, such as muscle rigidity and akathisia.

As indicated in the introduction to this chapter, many neuroscientists believe that the psychotic symptoms of schizophrenia result in part from an excess of the neurotransmitter dopamine, increased sensitivity of the dopamine receptors, or altered activity in specific dopamine pathways within the brain. Conventional antipsychotic medications are believed to work by blocking dopamine receptor sites in the brain. The blocking of dopamine receptors also produces bothersome side effects such as Parkinson-like symptoms. Because of the numerous side effects and problems with these medications, newer atypical antipsychotic medications are frequently used.

Dosing information: Perphenazine (Trilafon) is available in tablets, concentrate, and ampules for injection. The usual therapeutic dose is between 12 and 64 mg. a day. Loxapine (Loxitane) is available in capsules, concentrate, and an injectable form. The usual therapeutic dose is between 20 and 60 mg. a day. Molindone (Moban) is used less frequently than the other two agents and is available only in tablet and concentrate. Its therapeutic range is between 50 and 100 mg. a day, though physicians may prescribe up to 225 mg. a day for severe symptoms.

Common side effects: The intermediate-potency conventional antipsychotic agents are less sedating than the low-potency antipsychotic medications and cause fewer movement abnormalities than the high-potency

antipsychotics. The most common side effects are sedation, sexual dysfunction, orthostatic hypotension, and
mild to moderate anticholinergic effects, including dry
mouth, blurred vision, constipation, difficulty in urinating,
and confusion. Since all conventional anti-psychotics
block dopamine receptors in the hypothalamus, the intermediate-potency agents may increase blood prolactin
levels, leading to breast enlargement and milk secretion in
both women and men. Weight gain is common, except
with molindone (Moban). All may produce rashes and
photosensitivity (an increased susceptibility to sunburn),
and anyone taking these medications should apply sunscreen before going outdoors.

Precautions: All antipsychotic medications may
lower the seizure threshold, although this seems less
likely with molindone (Moban).

Men with enlarged prostates may experience difficulty
in urinating and urinary retention. Individuals with narrow-
angle glaucoma may have dangerous increases in the internal eye pressure, leading to visual disturbances and even
blindness. Because of the effects of antipsychotic medications on the hypothalamus, individuals become very
sensitive to extreme heat and should use caution in high
temperatures.

All antipsychotic medications have the potential to produce neurologic side effects. Although these are more
likely with the high-potency agents, the intermediate-
potency conventional agents may produce dystonia (muscle
spasms in the tongue, jaw, and neck); pseudo-Parkinsonism,
characterized by a pill-rolling tremor, muscle stiffness,
stooped posture, mask-like face, drooling, akinesia (a decrease in voluntary motor movements so the person walks
stiffly); and akathisia (an inner sense of restlessness that
causes people to become agitated, pace constantly, and
wring their hands). Doctors sometimes confuse akathisia
with psychotic depression. If the problem is psychotic de-

pression, an increase in antipsychotic medication may be required.

The intermediate-potency conventional antipsychotic agents may produce excessive weight gain. Since excessive weight is associated with an increased risk of diabetes, hypertension, heart disease, and premature death, people who gain excessive weight should participate in medically supervised programs to reduce this weight gain (diet, exercise, and medication). Also, periodic weight checks are encouraged, while on the medication.

≷⊘≷ **Warnings:** Intermediate-potency antipsychotics can lead to a potentially life-threatening condition, neuroleptic malignant syndrome (NMS), where there is an elevation of body temperature, severe muscle stiffness, rigidity, paralysis of the eye muscles, and a significant increase in heart rate, blood pressure, and sweating. Increases in white-blood-cell counts and blood-chemistry abnormalities also frequently occur. The person may also become delirious, leading to coma. NMS is a medical emergency requiring immediate hospitalization and treatment in an intensive-care unit. NMS can occur with any conventional antipsychotic drug but may be more common with high-potency agents such as haloperidol (Haldol).

People who take antipsychotic medication for a prolonged period of time may develop a condition called tardive dyskinesia, marked by involuntary movements of the tongue, fingers, and upper extremities, jaw movements, facial grimacing, smacking of the lips, twisting of the upper extremities and body, grunting while breathing, and various abnormal movements of the lower extremities. This condition does not affect mental function, but can be so severe that walking, eating, and even breathing become difficult. The risk of developing tardive dyskinesia appears to be related to the cumulative dose and length of treatment with antipsychotic medication. Individuals who are in state mental hospitals have rates in the range of 20 to 40 percent. The incidence rises with age, and women are at greater risk. Unfortunately, there is no known treatment for tardive dyskinesia, and it may be irreversible. Tapering off of the antipsychotic medication is recommended, but the condition may worsen in the short term.

Alcohol: Individuals who are taking antipsychotic medications should not drink alcohol, since alcohol leads to even greater sedation, a significant side effect of these drugs.

Food and beverages: There are no restrictions. Individuals should be discouraged from smoking, since nicotine lowers the blood levels of antipsychotic medications.

Possible drug interactions: Certain antacids may decrease absorption of antipsychotic drugs. Antihypertensive medications such as propranolol (Inderal), clonidine (Catapres), or guanethidine (Ismelin) should be closely monitored when taken with intermediate-potency conventional antipsychotic medications because the antipsychotic drugs also lower blood pressure. Other medications that produce sedation, such as benzodiazepines, antihistamines, and narcotic-type pain medications like meperidine (Demerol), hydrocodone (Vicodin), and others, should be avoided because these drugs may interfere with an individual's breathing when combined with antipsychotics.

Use in pregnancy and breast-feeding: Pregnancy Category C

Women who are contemplating becoming pregnant or who are pregnant should not, whenever possible, take antipsychotic agents. Women who breast-feed should not take an antipsychotic medication because it passes into the breast milk and is absorbed into the baby's bloodstream, leading to potential adverse effects upon the child's developing nervous system.

Use in children: Molindone (Moban), perphenazine (Trilafon), and loxapine (Loxitane) have not been systematically studied in children and are usually not recommended for children under the age of twelve. If a child requires antipsychotic medication, it should be prescribed and monitored by a child psychiatrist.

Use in seniors: Because intermediate-potency antipsychotic drugs produce less orthostatic hypotension and fewer anticholinergic side effects, such as blurred vision, dry mouth, difficulty urinating, constipation, and confusion, they are preferred for seniors over the low-potency, conventional antipsychotic medications.

Overdosage: The most common effects of overdosage are excessive tiredness, decrease in blood pressure, confusion, irregular heartbeats (arrhythmias), seizures, and significant muscle rigidity or spasms. People who take an overdose should always be brought to a hospital emergency room. Bring the bottle of medication to the emergency room with the person, since the date it was prescribed and the number of pills remaining in the bottle can provide helpful information to the treating physician.

Special considerations: As a rule, the newer atypical antipsychotic medications, such as risperidone (Risperdal), olanzapine (Zyprexa), or quetiapine (Seroquel), are preferred over intermediate-potency conventional antipsychotics. While the cost of the newer atypical antipsychotic medications is much higher, they have a much lower risk of tardive dyskinesia, acute dystonic reactions (see page 291), pseudo-Parkinsonian side effects, and allergic reactions.

HIGH-POTENCY CONVENTIONAL ANTIPSYCHOTIC MEDICATIONS

GENERIC NAME	BRAND NAME	DRUG CLASS
fluphenazine	Prolixin	Phenothiazine
haloperidol	Haldol	Butyrophenone
pimozide	Orap	Butyrophenone
thiothixine	Navane	Thioxanthene
trifluoperazine	Stelazine	Phenothiazine

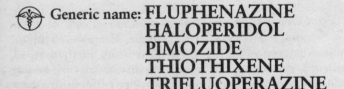 Generic name: **FLUPHENAZINE HALOPERIDOL PIMOZIDE THIOTHIXENE TRIFLUOPERAZINE**

 Available in generic form: Yes

 Brand name: Prolixin, Haldol, Orap, Navane, Stelazine

 Drug class: Phenothiazine, butyrophenone, butyrophenone, thioxanthene, phenothiazine

Prescribed for: Schizophrenia, schizoaffective disorder, acute mania, psychotic depression, severe obsessive-compulsive disorder, agitation in persons with dementia.

🦉 **General information:** The conventional or "typical" antipsychotic medications most in use today are the high-potency agents. Two of them, haloperidol (Haldol) and fluphenazine (Prolixin), have long-acting injectable forms called Haldol Decanoate and Prolixin Decanoate. The person receives Haldol Decanoate injections every four weeks or Prolixin Decanoate every two to three weeks. There is a significant advantage to this "depot" form, the term for decanoate preparations: It assures that an individual "takes" the medication. Compliance with the dosing regimen for typical antipsychotic agents is often a problem because people often do not like the side effects, especially akathisia (a subjective sense of restlessness), weight gain, akinesia (decreased motor activity), and pseudo-Parkinsonian symptoms. Many psychiatrists show a slight preference for Haldol Decanoate over Prolixin Decanoate because it reportedly produces fewer side effects and can be administered monthly, rather than every two to three weeks.

As indicated in the introduction to this chapter, many neuroscientists believe that the psychotic symptoms of schizophrenia result in part from an excess of the neurotransmitter dopamine, increased sensitivity of the dopamine receptors, or altered activity in specific dopamine pathways within the brain. Conventional antipsychotic medications are believed to work by blocking dopamine receptor sites in the hypothalamus. The blocking of dopamine receptors also produces troublesome side effects, such as Parkinson-like symptoms. Because of the numerous side effects and problems with these medications, newer atypical antipsychotic medications are used more frequently.

Pimozide (Orap) is an FDA-approved treatment for Tourette's syndrome and other tic disorders, although it has not been approved to treat schizophrenia and other psychotic disorders. However, psychiatrists have found pimozide to be an effective alternative to other high-potency antipsychotic agents. It is believed to produce tardive dyskinesia less frequently than the other antipsychotic agents, although this has not been conclusively proven.

Dosing information: A usual maintenance dose of haloperidol (Haldol), fluphenazine (Prolixin), or pimozide (Orap) may be 4 to 10 mg.; a dose of thiothixene (Navane) or trifluoperazine (Stelazine) is in the 8- to 20-mg. range. Acutely psychotic persons may require higher doses of all the agents except pimozide (Orap). Pimozide doses above 10 mg. require periodic electrocardiograph monitoring because of its effect on the heart and unexpected deaths in persons taking such doses.

Common side effects: The high-potency agents are much less sedating than the low-potency drugs and are less likely to lower blood pressure or produce orthostatic hypotension. However, they are more likely than intermediate- or low-potency agents to produce extrapyramidal symptoms that mimic those of Parkinson's disease: pill-rolling tremor, shuffling gait, mask-like facial expression, and agitation. To counteract these side effects, psychiatrists frequently prescribe anticholinergic medications such as benztropine (Cogentin) or trihexyphenidyl (Artane).

Other common side effects are sedation and sexual dysfunction. Since antipsychotics block dopamine receptors in the hypothalamus, they may increase blood prolactin levels, leading to breast enlargement and milk secretion in both women and men. Weight gain may be significant. All the conventional antipsychotic medications may produce rashes and photosensitivity (an increased susceptibility to sunburn). Anyone taking these drugs should apply sunscreen before going outdoors.

Precautions: All antipsychotic medications may lower the seizure threshold.

All antipsychotic medications have the potential to produce neurologic side effects, but these are most likely to
occur with the high-potency agents. They include dystonia
(muscle spasms in the tongue, jaw, and neck); pseudo-
Parkinsonism characterized by a pill-rolling tremor, muscle stiffness, stooped posture, mask-like face, drooling;
akinesia (a decrease in voluntary motor movements so the
person walks stiffly); and akathisia (an inner sense of motor restlessness that causes people to become agitated,
pace constantly, and wring their hands). Doctors sometimes confuse akathisia with psychotic depression. A
decrease in antipsychotic medication may improve symptoms in cases of akathisia. If the problem is psychotic depression, an increase in antipsychotic medication may be
required.

Men with enlarged prostates may experience difficulty
in urinating and urinary retention. Individuals with
narrow-angle glaucoma may have dangerous increases in
the internal eye pressure, leading to visual disturbances
and even blindness. Because of the effects of antipsychotic
medications on the hypothalamus, individuals become
very sensitive to extreme heat and should use caution in
high temperatures.

The high-potency conventional antipsychotic agents may
produce excessive weight gain. Since excessive weight is
associated with an increased risk of diabetes, hypertension, heart disease, and premature death, people who gain
excessive weight should participate in medically supervised
programs to reduce this weight gain (diet, exercise, and
medication). Also, periodic weight checks are encouraged,
while on the medication.

§⃠§**Warnings:** High-potency antipsychotics can lead to
a potentially life-threatening condition, neuroleptic
malignant syndrome (NMS), where there is an elevation of
body temperature, severe muscle stiffness, rigidity, paralysis of the eye muscles, and a significant increase in heart

rate, blood pressure, and sweating. Increases in white-blood-cell counts and blood-chemistry abnormalities also frequently occur. The person may also become delirious, leading to coma. NMS is a medical emergency requiring immediate hospitalization and treatment in an intensive-care unit. NMS can occur with any conventional antipsychotic drug but may be more common with high-potency agents such as haloperidol (Haldol).

People who take an antipsychotic medication for a prolonged period of time may develop a condition called tardive dyskinesia, marked by involuntary movements of the tongue, fingers, and upper extremities, jaw movements, facial grimacing, smacking of the lips, twisting of the upper extremities and body, grunting while breathing, and various abnormal movements of the lower extremities. This condition does not affect mental function, but can be so severe that walking, eating, and even breathing become difficult. The risk of developing tardive dyskinesia appears to be related to the cumulative dose and length of treatment with antipsychotic medication. Individuals who are in state mental hospitals have rates in the range of 20 to 40 percent. The incidence rises with age, and women are at greater risk. Unfortunately, there is no known treatment for tardive dyskinesia, and it may be irreversible. Tapering off of the antipsychotic medication is recommended, but the condition may worsen in the short term.

Alcohol: Individuals who are taking antipsychotic medications should not drink alcohol, since alcohol leads to even greater sedation, a significant side effect of these drugs.

Food and beverages: There are no restrictions. Individuals should be discouraged from smoking, since nicotine lowers the blood levels of antipsychotic medications.

Possible drug interactions: Certain antacids may decrease absorption of the drugs. Antihypertensive medications such as propranolol (Inderal), clonidine (Catapres), or guanethidine (Ismelin) should be closely monitored when taken with high-potency conventional antipsychotic medications because the antipsychotic drugs also lower blood pressure. Other medications that produce sedation, such as benzodiazepines, antihistamines, and narcotic-type pain medications like meperidine (Demerol), hydrocodone (Vicodin), and others, should be avoided because these drugs may interfere with an individual's breathing when combined with antipsychotics.

Use in pregnancy and breast-feeding:
Pregnancy Category C

Women who are contemplating becoming pregnant or who are pregnant should not, whenever possible, take antipsychotic agents. Women who breast-feed should not take an antipsychotic medication because it passes into the breast milk and is absorbed into the baby's bloodstream, leading to potential adverse effects on the child's developing nervous system.

Use in children: These medications have been used in children over the age of six months, but they should be prescribed cautiously by a child psychiatrist with special expertise in treating childhood schizophrenia, a relatively rare condition. The newer atypical antipsychotic medications are a recommended alternative.

Use in seniors: Because high-potency antipsychotic drugs have fewer anticholinergic side effects and produce much less orthostatic hypotension, they are often preferred for seniors over the low-potency conventional antipsychotic drugs.

Overdosage: The most common effects of overdosage are excessive tiredness, decreased blood pressure, confusion, irregular heartbeats (arrhythmias), seizures, and significant muscle rigidity or spasms. People who take an overdose should always be brought to a hospital emergency room. Bring the bottle of medication to the emergency room with the person, since the date it was prescribed and the number of pills remaining in the bottle can provide helpful information to the treating physician.

Special considerations: For the most part, haloperidol (Haldol) and other high-potency conventional antipsychotics remain the mainstay of treatment for a first psychotic episode. However, high-potency agents are more likely to produce extrapyramidal side effects and acute dystonia. This is especially true of young men, who do not tolerate these effects very well; consequently, intermediate-acting agents may sometimes be prescribed for them. If individuals need to continue antipsychotic medication for a long period of time, psychiatrists often will prescribe the newer atypical antipsychotics, such as risperidone (Risperdal), olanzapine (Zyprexa), or quetiapine (Seroquel), because they have a much lower risk of tardive dyskinesia and people find them easier to tolerate.

ATYPICAL ANTIPSYCHOTIC MEDICATIONS

 Generic name: CLOZAPINE

 Available in generic form: No

 Brand name: Clozaril

 Drug class: Atypical antipsychotic: dibenzodiazepine

℞ **Prescribed for:** Schizophrenia, schizoaffective disorder, acute mania, psychotic depression, agitation in persons with dementia. Clozapine may be especially beneficial in treating the "negative" symptoms of schizophrenia: lack of motivation, withdrawal, isolation from others, apathy, and inability to experience pleasure.

General information. Clozapine, used in Europe for nearly twenty years, has been available in the United States since 1989. It is used for persons with treatment-resistant schizophrenia or for those unable to tolerate the side effects of the typical antipsychotic medications. Since one-third of individuals taking conventional antipsychotics continue to experience residual symptoms, especially the "negative" symptoms of schizophrenia, clozapine has provided a significant benefit.

This medication is unique in that it is believed to work by blocking specific types of dopamine receptors as well as by affecting serotonin receptors. Clozapine may affect more of the dopamine systems involved in thinking and behaving than those that control motor activity. As a result, it produces fewer extrapyramidal side effects and rarely produces tardive dyskinesia. However, approximately 1 percent of all persons may experience severe agranulocytosis (an absolute decrease in the number of white blood cells), and some deaths have been reported. Consequently, a clozapine Patient Management System was formed by the pharmaceutical company that markets the drug. The prescribing physician enters the patient into this registry when first prescribing clozapine, and a physician and pharmacist review the weekly blood-cell counts. The FDA has reduced the requirement of weekly blood tests to measure white-blood-cell counts to include only the first six months of treatment. After this period, white-blood-cell counts can be monitored every other week.

Dosing information: Clozapine is available in 25- and 100-mg. tablets. The usual starting dose is 25 mg. at bedtime, with 25-to-50-mg. increases every four to five days until a dose of approximately 200 mg. is reached after three weeks. If necessary, the dose of clozapine may be increased thereafter to up to 600 mg. a day. At doses greater than 600 mg., the risk of seizures increases considerably, to nearly 15 percent of individuals. Because some people may require doses in the 600-to-900-mg.-a-day range, psychiatrists often recommend taking anti-seizure medications whenever a dose exceeds 600 mg.

Common side effects: Clozapine produces most of the same side effects as the more traditional low-potency antipsychotic agents. Common side effects include sedation, lowered blood pressure, especially orthostatic hypotension, an increased heart rate, gastrointestinal distress, flulike symptoms, excessive drooling (especially at night), and sexual dysfunction. Significant anticholinergic effects have been reported, including dry mouth, blurred vision, constipation, difficulty in urinating, and confusion. Most people taking clozapine also gain weight. Clozapine may also produce rashes and photosensitivity (an increased susceptibility to sunburn). Anyone taking this medication should apply sunscreen before going outdoors.

Precautions: All antipsychotic medications have the potential to produce neurologic side effects. Although these are more likely to occur with the high-potency agents, clozapine infrequently may produce dystonia (muscle spasms in the tongue, jaw, and neck), pseudo-Parkinsonism characterized by a pill-rolling tremor, muscle stiffness, stooped posture, mask-like face, drooling, akinesia (a decrease in voluntary motor movements so the person walks stiffly); and akathisia (an inner sense of motor restlessness that causes people to become agitated, pace constantly, and wring their hands). Doctors sometimes confuse akathisia with psychotic depression. A decrease in antipsychotic medication may improve symptoms in cases of akathisia. If the problem is psychotic depression, an increase in antipsychotic medication may be required.

Men with enlarged prostates who take low-potency antipsychotics may experience difficulty in urinating and urinary retention. Individuals with narrow-angle glaucoma may have dangerous increases in the internal eye pressure, leading to visual disturbances and even blindness. Because of the effects of antipsychotic medications on the hypothalamus, individuals become very sensitive to extreme heat and should use caution in high temperatures.

Of all the atypical antipsychotic medications, clozapine produces the greatest amount of weight gain. Since excessive weight is associated with an increased risk of diabetes, hypertension, heart disease, and premature death, people who gain excessive weight should participate in medically supervised programs to reduce this weight gain (diet, exercise, and medication). Also, periodic weight checks and blood pressure readings are strongly encouraged, while on the medication.

〰◎〰**Warnings:** The major concern in persons taking clozapine is agranulocytosis. Weekly blood tests during the first six months of treatment and biweekly tests thereafter decrease the likelihood of death or a serious infection since the white-blood-cell count returns to normal levels when the medication is stopped. Another major concern is the increased rate of seizures, especially with doses over 500 mg. a day. An anti-seizure medication may be added by the physician in these higher dose ranges.

Clozapine can lead to a potentially life-threatening condition, neuroleptic malignant syndrome (NMS), where there is an elevation of body temperature, severe muscle stiffness, rigidity, paralysis of the eye muscles, and a significant increase in heart rate, blood pressure, and sweating. Increases in white-blood-cell counts and blood-chemistry abnormalities also frequently occur. The person may also become delirious, leading to coma. NMS is a medical emergency requiring immediate hospitalization and treatment in an intensive-care unit.

People who take an antipsychotic medication for a prolonged period of time may develop a condition called tardive dyskinesia, marked by involuntary movements of the tongue, fingers, and upper extremities, jaw movements, facial grimacing, smacking of the lips, twisting of the upper extremities and body, grunting while breathing, and various abnormal movements of the lower extremities. The risk of tardive dyskinesia for persons on clozapine is much less than with conventional antipsychotics; in fact, it is quite rare. The risk of developing this condition appears to be related to the cumulative dose and length of treatment with antipsychotic medication. Individuals who are in state mental hospitals have rates in the range of 20 to 40 percent. The incidence rises with age, and women are at greater risk. Unfortunately, there is no known treatment for tardive dyskinesia, and it may be irreversible. Tapering off of the antipsychotic medication is recommended, but the condition may worsen in the short term.

Alcohol: Individuals taking clozapine should not drink alcohol, since alcohol may lead to even greater sedation, a significant side effect.

Food and beverages: There are no restrictions. Do not smoke, since nicotine lowers blood levels of clozapine.

Possible drug interactions: Certain antacids may decrease the absorption of clozapine. Because clozapine may reduce the white-blood-cell count, it should not be combined with other medications that are known to decrease the production of white blood cells, such as the anti-seizure medication carbamazepine (Tegretol). Certain antidepressants may increase blood levels of clozapine, but this is not usually a significant problem.

Antihypertensive medications such as propranolol (Inderal), clonidine (Catapres), or guanethidine (Ismelin) should be closely monitored when taken with clozapine because it lowers blood pressure. Other medications that produce sedation, such as benzodiazepines, antihistamines, and narcotic-type pain medications like meperidine (Demerol), hydrocodone (Vicodin), and others, should be avoided because these drugs may interfere with an individual's breathing when combined with clozapine.

Use in pregnancy and breast-feeding: Pregnancy Category B

Women who are contemplating becoming pregnant or who are pregnant should not, whenever possible, take clozapine. Women taking an antipsychotic medication should not breast-feed because it passes into the breast milk and is absorbed into the baby's bloodstream, leading to potential adverse effects on the child's developing nervous system.

Use in children: Clozapine has not been studied in children and is not recommended in children under the age of sixteen.

Use in seniors: Because of the increased rate of seizures and its blood-pressure-lowering effect, clozapine should be prescribed cautiously in seniors. The dose must be increased at a much slower rate than in younger adults; lower doses are usually effective in seniors.

Overdosage: The most common effects of overdosage are excessive tiredness, decreased blood pressure, confusion, hypersalivation (drooling), irregular heartbeats (arrhythmias), seizures, respiratory depression,

coma, and aspiration pneumonia. People who take an overdose should always be brought to a hospital emergency room. Bring the bottle of medication to the emergency room with the person, since the date it was prescribed and the number of pills remaining in the bottle can provide helpful information to the treating physician.

 Special considerations: Clozapine is an outstanding new atypical antipsychotic medication for persons with schizophrenia who have failed to respond to more traditional antipsychotic agents or who have residual symptoms. Individuals with pronounced negative symptoms (apathy, withdrawal, and lack of motivation) are particularly likely to benefit. Because of the frequent blood monitoring required and the potentially life-threatening effect of reduced white-blood-cell counts, clozapine should be reserved for these individuals. Those with treatment-refractory bipolar disorder may also benefit. The cost of the weekly and later biweekly blood counts is quite high; however, most commercial health-insurance companies and federal programs (Medicaid, Medicare) will pay a portion of these costs.

Generic name: OLANZAPINE

 Available in generic form: No

 Brand name: Zyprexa

 Drug class: Atypical antipsychotic: thienobenzodiazepine

 Prescribed for: Schizophrenia, schizoaffective disorder, acute mania, psychotic depression, severe obsessive-compulsive disorder, agitation in persons with dementia. Olanzapine may be especially beneficial in treating the negative symptoms of schizophrenia: lack of motivation, withdrawal, isolation from others, apathy, and inability to experience pleasure.

General information: Olanzapine is an atypical antipsychotic that was approved by the FDA in 1996. Like risperidone (Risperdal) and quetiapine (Seroquel), it has an effect on serotonin receptors as well as dopamine receptors. Individuals generally tolerate this medication well and have a much lower frequency of extrapyramidal and Parkinson-like symptoms (muscle spasms, muscle stiffness, mask-like facial expression, stiff arm movements) and akathisia (an internal sense of physical restlessness) than with the conventional antipsychotic agents. In contrast to clozapine (Clozaril), olanzapine does not produce a decrease in the white-blood-cell count (leukopenia) or cause the bone marrow to stop producing white blood cells (agranulocytosis). There are some reports that olanzapine may improve depressive symptoms in persons suffering from schizophrenia, but this has not been proven. Olanzapine is sometimes added to lithium or divalproex (Depakote) to treat psychotic symptoms in bipolar individuals with mania when other medications have not been successful.

Dosing information: Olanzapine is available in 2.5-, 5-, 7.5-, and 10-mg. tablets. The usual starting dose is 5 mg. a day. After a week or two, the dose may be increased to 10 mg. a day. The usual maximum dose is 15 mg. a day, although some people may require doses as high as 20 mg.

Common side effects: The most common side effects are sedation, a decrease in blood pressure and orthostatic hypotension, dizziness, tiredness, and tremor. In addition, olanzapine produces mild anticholinergic side effects such as dry mouth, blurred vision, constipation, and urinary retention, a particular problem for men who have an enlarged prostate. These symptoms are much less prevalent than with the conventional antipsychotics. Many people complain of weight gain, which is a problem with almost all the antipsychotic medications. Since olanzapine blocks dopamine receptors in the hypothalamus, it may increase blood prolactin levels, leading to breast enlargement and milk secretion in both women and men.

Precautions: Early studies reported that olanzapine increased some liver enzymes, an indication of liver impairment; therefore it should be used cautiously in people with liver disease. Also, because studies conducted prior to its approval showed an increased rate of seizures, as in other conventional and atypical antipsychotic agents, olanzapine should be used with caution in people with a history of seizures and of medical conditions, such as dementia, that may lower the seizure threshold. While all antipsychotic medications have the potential to produce neurologic side effects, olanzapine produces fewer extrapyramidal side effects such as dystonia (muscle spasms in the tongue, jaw, and neck), akinesia (a decrease in voluntary motor movements so the person walks stiffly), and akathisia (an inner sense of motor restlessness that causes people to become agitated, pace constantly, and wring their hands). Doctors sometimes confuse akathisia with psychotic depression. A decrease in antipsychotic medication may improve symptoms in cases of akathisia. If the problem is psychotic depression, an increase in antipsychotic medication may be required. Individuals with narrow-angle glaucoma may have dangerous increases in internal eye pressure, leading to visual disturbances and even blindness. Because of the potential effects of olanzapine on the hypothalamus, individuals become very sensitive to extreme heat and should use caution in high temperatures.

Olanzapine may produce excessive weight gain, although somewhat less than clozapine. Since excessive weight is associated with an increased risk of diabetes, hypertension, heart disease, and premature death, people who gain excessive weight should participate in medically supervised programs to reduce this weight gain (diet, exercise, and medication) or should be switched to an atypical antipsychotic that produces less weight gain, such as risperidone. Also, periodic weight checks and blood-pressure readings are strongly encouraged, while on the medication.

⚠ **Warnings:** Olanzapine has the potential to produce neuroleptic malignant syndrome and tardive dyskinesia, although risks are less than with conventional antipsychotics. Psychiatrists need more experience with the use of olanzapine over longer periods of time in order to identify all its potential dangers. In contrast to clozapine (Clozaril), olanzapine does not cause agranulocytosis.

Atypical antipsychotics can lead to a potentially life-threatening condition, neuroleptic malignant syndrome (NMS), where there is an elevation of body temperature, severe muscle stiffness, rigidity, paralysis of the eye muscles, and a significant increase in heart rate, blood pressure, and sweating. Increases in white-blood-cell counts and blood-chemistry abnormalities also frequently occur. The person may also become delirious, leading to coma. NMS is a medical emergency requiring immediate hospitalization and treatment in an intensive-care unit.

People who take an antipsychotic medication for a prolonged period of time may develop a condition called tardive dyskinesia, marked by involuntary movements of the tongue, fingers, and upper extremities, jaw movements, facial grimacing, smacking of the lips, twisting of the upper extremities and body, grunting while breathing, and various abnormal movements of the lower extremities. The condition does not affect mental function, but can be so severe that walking, eating, and even breathing become difficult. The risk of developing tardive dyskinesia appears to be related to the cumulative dose and length of treatment with antipsychotic medication. Individuals who are in state mental hospitals have rates in the range of 20 to 40 percent. The incidence rises with age, and women are at greater risk. Tapering off of the antipsychotic medication is recommended, but the condition may worsen in the short term.

Alcohol: Individuals who are taking antipsychotic medications should not drink alcohol, since alcohol leads to even greater sedation, a significant side effect.

Food and beverages: There are no restrictions. Individuals should be discouraged from smoking, since nicotine lowers the blood levels of antipsychotic medications.

Possible drug interactions: Certain antacids may decrease the absorption of olanzapine. The concurrent use of carbamazepine (Tegretol) lowers blood levels of olanzapine. Antihypertensive medications such as propranolol (Inderal), clonidine (Catapres), or guanethidine (Ismelin) should be closely monitored when taking olanzapine because they lower blood pressure. Other medications that produce sedation, such as benzodiazepines, antihistamines, and narcotic-type pain medications like meperidine (Demerol), hydrocodone (Vicodin), and others, should be avoided because these drugs may interfere with an individual's breathing when combined with olanzapine.

Use in pregnancy and breast-feeding: Pregnancy Category C
Women who are contemplating becoming pregnant or who are pregnant should not, whenever possible, take

antipsychotic agents. Women who breast-feed should not take an antipsychotic medication because it passes into the breast milk and is absorbed into the baby's bloodstream, leading to potential adverse effects on the child's developing nervous system.

Use in children: Olanzapine has not been studied and is not recommended in children.

Use in seniors: The usual starting dose in seniors is 2.5 mg. a day because this medication produces orthostatic hypotension. Doses should be increased more slowly than in younger adults, to a recommended maximum level of between 5 and 10 mg. a day.

Overdosage: Olanzapine is generally not dangerous in overdose. However, when combined with other medications, especially alcohol and barbiturates, the risk of death may increase considerably. People who take an overdose should always be brought to a hospital emergency room. Bring the bottle of medication to the emergency room with the person, since the date it was prescribed and the number of pills remaining in the bottle can provide helpful information to the treating physician.

Special considerations: Olanzapine represents a significant advantage over conventional antipsychotic agents. It generally has fewer side effects than these drugs and is more effective in treating negative symptoms and persons with schizoaffective disorder. A significant disadvantage is its high cost when compared to risperidone (Risperdal) and especially to traditional antipsychotic medications. However, olanzapine is about half as expensive as clozapine (Clozaril) and may be a suitable alternative for those who fail to respond to risperidone (Risperdal) and who are reluctant to use clozapine (Clozaril). Olanzapine can also be useful for certain individuals who have a bipolar disorder with psychotic symptoms that have not responded to mood stabilizers.

 Generic name: QUETIAPINE

 Available in generic form: No

 Brand name: Seroquel

 Drug class: Atypical antipsychotic: dibenzothiazepine

Prescribed for: Schizophrenia, schizoaffective disorder, acute mania, psychotic depression, severe obsessive-compulsive disorder, agitation in persons with dementia.

General information: Quetiapine, the newest of the atypical antipsychotic agents, was approved by the FDA in 1997. Like risperidone (Risperdal) and olanzapine (Zyprexa), it blocks both serotonin receptors and dopamine receptors and has a low incidence of extrapyramidal side effects: muscle spasms, akinesia (decreased motor movement), akathisia (internal sense of physical restlessness), and dystonia (muscle stiffness).

Dosing information: Quetiapine is available in 25-, 100-, and 200-mg. tablets. The usual starting dose is 25 mg. twice a day with gradual increases up to 300 to 750 mg. a day, taken at least twice a day. Because quetiapine produces significant sedation, the dose of quetiapine is increased slowly and the major portion is usually taken in the evening. Because of its short half-life, quetiapine must be taken at least twice a day.

 Common side effects: The most common side effects are tiredness, sedation, a general slowing of motor activity, dizziness, and orthostatic hypotension. These side effects are most pronounced during the initial weeks of treatment. As with many antipsychotic agents, people who take quetiapine usually gain weight, but this may not occur as frequently as with the traditional antipsychotic medications or olanzapine.

Precautions: Clinical studies prior to the drug's approval noted some increase in liver enzymes but concluded that these changes were temporary and not serious. However, individuals with liver disease should undergo careful monitoring of their liver enzymes. Similar to other conventional and atypical antipsychotic agents, quetiapine increases the risk of seizures and should be used cautiously in those with a history of seizures and of medical conditions, such as dementia, that may lower the seizure threshold. Quetiapine may also increase triglyceride and cholesterol levels; consequently, it should be given carefully to people with elevated lipid levels and cardiovascular disease. Because of potential effects of quetiapine on the hypothalamus, individuals become very sensitive to extreme heat and should use caution in high temperatures. Quetiapine may produce excessive weight gain. Since excessive weight is associated with an increased risk of diabetes, hypertension, heart disease, and premature death, people who gain excessive weight should participate in medically supervised programs to reduce this weight gain (diet, exercise, and medication) or should be switched to an atypical antipsychotic that produces less weight gain, such as risperidone. To decrease the likelihood of weight gain, periodic weight checks are encouraged, while on the medication.

Warnings: Animal studies prior to the drug's approval found that quetiapine produces cataracts in dogs. Consequently, the manufacturer recommends that individuals undergo an ocular examination before taking this medication and every six months during treatment. While many psychiatrists believe this is unnecessary, if the drug is to be taken for a long period of time such testing seems a reasonable precaution until long-term use has demonstrated that this side effect does not occur. Quetiapine may have the potential to produce neuroleptic malignant syndrome and tardive dyskinesia.

Atypical antipsychotics can lead to a potentially life-threatening condition, neuroleptic malignant syndrome (NMS), where there is an elevation of body temperature, severe muscle stiffness, rigidity, paralysis of the eye muscles, and a significant increase in heart rate, blood pressure, and sweating. Increases in white-blood-cell counts and blood-chemistry abnormalities also frequently occur. The person may also become delirious, leading to coma. NMS is a medical emergency requiring immediate hospitalization and treatment in an intensive-care unit.

People who take antipsychotic medication for a prolonged period of time may develop a condition called tardive dyskinesia, marked by involuntary movements of the tongue, fingers, and upper extremities, jaw movements, facial grimacing, smacking of the lips, twisting of the upper extremities and body, grunting while breathing, and various abnormal movements of the lower extremities. The condition does not affect mental function, but can be so severe that walking, eating, and even breathing become difficult. The risk of developing tardive dyskinesia appears to be related to the cumulative dose and length of treatment with antipsychotic medication. Individuals who are in state mental hospitals have rates in the range of 20 to 40 percent. The incidence rises with age, and women are at greater risk. Tapering off of the antipsychotic medication is recommended, but the condition may worsen in the short term.

There are no reports that quetiapine produces agranulocytosis or other blood abnormalities.

Alcohol: Individuals who are taking antipsychotic medications should not drink alcohol, since alcohol leads to even greater sedation, a significant side effect.

Food and beverages: There are no restrictions. Do not smoke, since nicotine may lower blood levels of quetiapine.

Possible drug interactions: Certain antacids may decrease absorption of this medication. The anti-seizure medications carbamazepine (Tegretol) and phenytoin (Dilantin) may decrease quetiapine's blood levels. Consequently, when these agents are used with quetiapine, higher doses of quetiapine may have to be given. Antihypertensive medications such as propranolol (Inderal), clonidine (Catapres), or guanethidine (Ismelin) should be closely monitored when taking quetiapine because it lowers blood pressure. Other medications that produce sedation, such as benzodiazepines, antihistamines, and narcotic-type pain medications like meperidine (Demerol), hydrocodone (Vicodin), oxycodone (Percodan), and others, should be avoided because these drugs may interfere with an individual's breathing when combined with quetiapine.

Use in pregnancy and breast-feeding: Pregnancy Category C
Women who are contemplating becoming pregnant or who are pregnant should not, whenever possible, take antipsychotic agents. Women who breast-feed should not take an antipsychotic medication because it passes into the breast milk and is absorbed into the baby's bloodstream, leading to potential adverse effects on the child's developing nervous system.

Use in children: The safety and effectiveness of quetiapine in children have not been established.

Use in seniors: Because quetiapine produces a much greater likelihood of orthostatic hypotension, seniors taking this medication should be cautioned to be careful to avoid falls.

Overdosage: The most common effects of overdosage are excessive tiredness, decreased blood pressure, confusion, irregular and rapid heartbeats (arrhythmias), seizures, and significant muscle rigidity or spasms. People who take an overdose should always be brought to a hospital emergency room. Bring the bottle of medication to the emergency room with the person, since the date it was prescribed and the number of pills remaining in the bottle can provide helpful information to the treating physician.

Special considerations: For people who cannot tolerate the adverse side effects of the traditional antipsychotic medications, especially extrapyramidal symptoms, quetiapine is a reasonable alternative. Like risperidone (Risperdal), it must be taken at least twice a day. If adherence to a medication schedule is a significant issue, a single daily dose of olanzapine (Zyprexa) may be a better option. If difficulty sleeping or agitation is a problem, quetiapine, which is more likely to produce sedation, may be a good choice.

 Generic name: **RISPERIDONE**

 Available in generic form: No

 Brand name: Risperdal

 Drug class: Atypical antipsychotic: benzisoxazole

℞ Prescribed for: Schizophrenia, schizoaffective disorder, acute mania, psychotic depression, severe obsessive-compulsive disorder, agitation in persons with dementia.

General information: Like quetiapine (Seroquel) and olanzapine (Zyprexa), risperidone, an "atypical" antipsychotic, blocks both serotonin and dopamine receptors. Risperidone has several significant advantages: As long as the dose is kept under 6 mg., it produces far fewer extrapyramidal symptoms (such as tremor, muscle spasms, muscle stiffness, and mask-like face) than conventional antipsychotic agents like haloperidol (Haldol). Consequently, individuals tolerate the medication much better and are more likely to stay on it for a longer period of time. Risperidone is less likely to produce tardive dyskinesia, but it is not as effective as clozapine (Clozaril) in treating negative symptoms.

Dosing information: Risperidone is available in 1-, 2-, 3-, and 4-mg. tablets and in a liquid form. The usual starting dose is 1 mg. twice a day in the first week, with an increase to 2 mg. twice a day in the second week. The dose may be gradually increased to 3 mg. twice a day as needed. The usual therapeutic dose is between 4 and 6 mg. a day. People generally have fewer side effects if they take less than 6 mg. a day. When the medication was first released, the manufacturers advised a rapid increase of the dose to 6 mg. a day within the first week; clinical experience has found that a more gradual increase leads to improved tolerance and compliance. For persons under age sixty-five, the entire dose may be given at bedtime because of the drug's sedative properties.

Common side effects: The most common side effects are sedation, dizziness, orthostatic hypotension, agitation, headache, nausea, constipation, gastrointestinal upset, insomnia, runny nose, rash, and a rapid heart rate. At doses greater than 6 mg., people may experience extrapyramidal side effects, including muscle spasms (dystonia), decrease in normal arm swing (bradykinesia), absence of facial expression, and a restless feeling (akathisia). At doses below 6 mg., extrapyramidal side effects are less common than with traditional antipsychotic medications.

Precautions: All antipsychotic medications lower the seizure threshold, but this side effect may be less frequent with risperidone.

All antipsychotic medications have the potential to produce neurologic side effects. Although these are more likely to occur with the high-potency agents, the atypical antipsychotics may produce dystonia (muscle spasms in the tongue, jaw, and neck); pseudo-Parkinsonism characterized by a pill-rolling tremor, muscle stiffness, stooped posture, mask-like face, drooling, akinesia (a decrease in voluntary motor movements so the person walks stiffly); and akathisia (an inner sense of motor restlessness that causes people to become agitated, pace constantly, and wring their hands). Doctors sometimes confuse akathisia with psychotic depression. A decrease in antipsychotic medication may improve symptoms in cases of akathisia. If the problem is psychotic depression, an increase in antipsychotic medication may be required.

While risperidone may cause excessive weight gain, the risk is less than with clozapine or olanzapine. Since excessive weight is associated with an increased risk of diabetes, hypertension, heart disease, and premature death, people who gain excessive weight should participate in medically supervised programs to reduce this weight gain (diet, exercise, and medication), or should take an atypical antipsychotic that produces less weight gain, such as risperidone. Periodic blood-pressure readings and weight checks are strongly encouraged while on the medication.

Warnings: Atypical antipsychotics, like the traditional antipsychotics, can lead to a potentially life-threatening condition, neuroleptic malignant syndrome (NMS), where there is an elevation of body temperature, severe muscle stiffness, rigidity, paralysis of the eye muscles, and a significant increase in heart rate, blood pressure, and sweating. However, the risk of this medical emergency occurring in risperidone-treated persons is lower than with the conventional antipsychotic agents. NMS is a medical emergency requiring immediate hospitalization and treatment in an intensive care unit.

At higher doses (greater than 6 mg.), risperidone has the potential to produce tardive dyskinesia, marked by involuntary movements of the tongue, fingers, and upper extremities, jaw movements, facial grimacing, and twisting of the upper extremities and body, grunting while breathing, and various abnormal movements of the lower extremities. The risk of developing this condition appears to be related to the cumulative dose and length of treatment with antipsychotic medication. However, this risk is much less than with the conventional antipsychotic medications and probably slightly greater than clozapine (Clozaril) because doses of 6 mg. or less of risperidone have a minimal effect on dopamine.

Alcohol: Individuals taking risperidone should not drink alcohol, since alcohol may lead to even more sedation, which is a significant side effect of this medication.

Food and beverages: There are no restrictions. Do not smoke, since nicotine may lower blood levels of risperidone.

Possible drug interactions: Use of an SSRI (selective serotonin receptor inhibitor) with risperidone may increase the blood levels of risperidone, leading to an increased risk of orthostatic hypotension, sedation, and extrapyramidal side effects. Carbamazepine (Tegretol) may decrease the blood levels of risperidone.

Antihypertensive medications such as propranolol (Inderal), clonidine (Catapres), or guanethidine (Ismelin) should be closely monitored when taken with risperidone (Risperdal) because antipsychotic drugs also lower blood pressure. Other medications that produce sedation, such as benzodiazepines, antihistamines, and narcotic-type pain medications like meperidine (Demerol), hydrocodone (Vicodin), and others, should be avoided because these drugs may interfere with an individual's breathing when combined with risperidone.

Use in pregnancy and breast-feeding: Pregnancy Category C

Risperidone should not be taken by pregnant women because of a possible increase in birth defects, although there are no studies of this drug in humans. Women who are contemplating becoming pregnant should not take this medication. It is not known whether risperidone passes into breast milk, but because it probably does, women who are taking risperidone should not breast-feed.

Use in children: Risperidone has not been systematically studied in children and is not recommended for use in children.

Use in seniors: The usual starting dose in seniors is 0.5 mg. once or twice a day, with a weekly increase of 0.5 mg. to a recommended dose of 2 to 4 mg. a day in two equal doses. The greatest concern for seniors is the risk of falls because of orthostatic hypotension. Consequently, in contrast to younger adults, all the medication should generally not be given in a single dose at bedtime, but should be administered twice a day.

Overdosage: The most common effects of over-dosage are excessive drowsiness, hypotension, confusion, rapid and irregular heartbeats, seizures, and significant muscle rigidity. People who take an overdose should always be brought to a hospital emergency room. Bring the bottle of medication to the emergency room with the person, since the date it was prescribed and the number of pills remaining in the bottle can provide helpful information to the treating physician.

Special considerations: Risperidone represents a significant advance in the available antipsychotic agents to treat schizophrenia and other severe psychotic disorders. It is much better tolerated by people than the conventional antipsychotic agents, especially high-potency agents such as haloperidol (Haldol) or low-potency agents such as chlorpromazine (Thorazine). Other new atypical antipsychotics, such as olanzapine (Zyprexa), may be more effective for those resistant to treatment or with significant residual or negative symptoms. However, risperidone costs less than olanzapine (Zyprexa), and recent studies have proven its efficacy in treating agitation in acutely psychotic patients.

 Generic name: **ZIPRASIDONE**

 Available in generic form: No

 Brand name: Geodon

 Drug class: Atypical antipsychotic

Rx **Prescribed for:** Schizophrenia, schizoaffective disorder, acute mania, psychotic depression, severe
obsessive-compulsive disorder, agitation in persons with
dementia. Ziprasidone may be beneficial in treating negative symptoms of schizophrenia: lack of motivation, withdrawal, isolation from others, apathy, and inability to
experience pleasure.

General Information: Ziprasidone is an atypical
antipsychotic that was approved by the FDA in
February 2001. Like other atypical antipsychotics, the
drug effects its action on serotonin and dopamine receptors. As with other atypical agents, the low frequency
of extrapyramidal and Parkinson-like symptoms (muscle
spasms, muscle stiffness, mask-like facial expression,
stiff arm movements) and akathisia (internal sense of
physical restlessness) contribute to ziprasidone's greater
tolerability than conventional antipsychotic agents. Because ziprasidone inhibits the synaptic reuptake of serotonin and norepinephrine, actions similar to those of
antidepressants, it may improve depressive symptoms in
persons suffering from schizophrenia, but this has not
been proven.

Dosing information: Ziprasidone is available in
20-, 40-, 60- and 80-mg. capsules. The usual starting dose is 20 mg. twice a day, and the dosage may be increased, as needed, up to 80 mg. twice a day. The usual
maximum dose is 200 mg. a day. To ensure the use of the
lowest effective dose, adequate time should be allowed for
clinical response before considering dosage adjustment upward. Ziprasidone should be taken with food to improve
its absorption.

Common side effects: The most frequently reported
side effects of ziprasidone have been sedation, nausea, difficulty in breathing, dizziness, and constipation. In

addition, ziprasidone produces extrapyramidal side effects, a restless feeling (akathisia), rash, and orthostatic hypotension, although these symptoms are much less prevalent than with conventional antipsychotics. Interestingly, ziprasidone seems to induce the least amount of weight gain when compared to other atypical agents, such as olanzapine (Zyprexa) and clozapine (Clozaril). Ziprasidone, like other dopamine (D2) antagonists, may elevate prolactin levels in humans, leading to breast enlargement in men and women, milk secretion, irregular menstruation, and impotence.

Precautions: A small percentage of people taking ziprasidone developed rash and/or hives. The occurrence of rash appeared to be related to higher doses of the drug, as well as to the duration of treatment. Ziprasidone may induce orthostatic hypotension, especially in the elderly, including dizziness, rapid heartbeat, and fainting in some patients. For these individuals, special caution is indicated when ziprasidone is combined with certain antihypertensive drugs.

All antipsychotic drugs may lower the seizure threshold, so ziprasidone should be used cautiously in persons with a history of seizure disorders.

While all antipsychotic medications have the potential to produce neurologic side effects, ziprasidone produces fewer extrapyramidal reactions than with conventional agents like haloperidol (Haldol) and fluphenazine (Prolixin). Akathisia has been reported with ziprasidone. A decrease in antipsychotic medication may improve symptoms in cases of akathisia.

Warnings: Clinical studies have shown that ziprasidone prolongs that segment of a heartbeat (as measured by electrocardiogram) known as the Q-T interval. Q-T prolongation induced by ziprasidone is dose-related (i.e., worsens with higher doses), and may be increased when used with other drugs, such as quinidine, thiorida-zine, and pimozide, that also prolong the Q-T interval. The prolongation of Q-T interval has been associated with the risk of fatal arrhythmias (irregular heartbeat). There-fore, ziprasidone should be used cautiously in people with heart disease or arrhythmia, and should not be used by those who are taking other medication that may prolong the Q-T interval. The manufacturer has warned that ziprasidone is contraindicated in such cases.

Moreover, low levels of serum potassium (hypokalemia) may increase the risk of Q-T prolongation and arrhyth-mia. Low serum potassium may result from diuretic therapy, diarrhea, and other causes. When indicated, serum potassium and other electrolytes should be moni-tored to minimize the risk of Q-T prolongation when tak-ing ziprasidone.

All antipsychotic drugs, including atypical agents like ziprasidone, can lead to potentially life-threatening neu-roleptic malignant syndrome (NMS), where there is an elevation of body temperature, severe muscle stiffness, rigidity, paralysis of the eye muscles, and a significant in-crease in heart rate, blood pressure, and sweating. In-creases in white-blood-cell counts and blood-chemistry abnormalities also frequently occur. The person may be-come delirious, leading to coma. NMS is a medical emer-gency requiring immediate hospitalization and treatment in an intensive-care unit.

The risk of tardive dyskinesia with ziprasidone is un-known. The risk is expected to be similar to that of other atypical antipsychotics: much less than with with conven-tional antipsychotic agents.

Alcohol: Individuals who are taking ziprasidone should not drink alcohol, since alcohol may lead to even more sedation, which is a significant side effect of this medication.

Food and Beverages: Ziprasidone should be taken with food, which can increase its absorption as much as twofold. It is best to take ziprasidone immediately before meals, at the same time each day. Unlike other antipsychotics, smoking does not significantly alter the metabolism, and hence blood levels, of ziprasidone because nicotine and ziprasidone are metabolized by different enzyme systems in the liver.

Possible drug interactions: Ziprasidone should not be used with other medications that prolong the Q-T interval. The manufacturer has issued this warning as a contraindication.

Because ziprasidone can potentially lower blood pressure, it may enhance the effects of certain antihypertensive medications when these drugs are taken together. Blood pressure should be closely monitored when ziprasidone is taken along with antihypertensive medications.

The concurrent use of carbamazepine (Tegretol) may potentially lower blood levels of ziprasidone. Ketoconazole (Nizoral), an antifungal agent, may increase blood levels of ziprasidone. Unlike other atypical antipsychotics, antacids do not effect blood levels of ziprasidone.

Use in pregnancy and breast-feeding: Pregnancy Category C

There are no studies or current data that indicate whether ziprasidone has any harmful effect on the fetus. Whenever possible, women who are contemplating pregnancy or who are pregnant should not take antipsychotic agents.

It is not known whether ziprasidone or its metabolites are excreted in human milk. It is recommended that women who are taking ziprasidone not breast-feed.

Use in children: The effectiveness and safety of ziprasidone have not been studied in children and the drug is not recommended in children.

Use in seniors: In general, clinical studies have showed few differences in tolerability, and no reduced clearance, of ziprasidone in seniors as compared to younger patients. The greatest concern is the risk of falls, because seniors may be more susceptible to the side effects of the medication, such as orthostatic hypotension. Doses should be increased more slowly in this population, although the manufacturer states that dosage adjustments are not required on the basis of age.

Overdosage: There has been limited experience with ziprasidone overdosage. In a patient who had overdosed on the largest confirmed amount of 3,240 mg., the only symptoms reported were sedation, slurring of speech, and transitory elevation of blood pressure; the patient survived without serious consequences. In general, an overdose of ziprasidone alone is not as dangerous as when it is combined with other medications, especially alcohol and barbiturates. In those cases, the risk of death may increase significantly.

People who take an overdose should always be brought to a hospital emergency room. Bring the bottle of medication to the emergency room with the person, since the date it was prescribed and the number of pills remaining in the bottle can provide helpful information to the treating physician.

Special considerations: Ziprasidone is the latest atypical antipsychotic agent introduced in the United States. Like other atypical agents, it offers significant advantages over conventional antipsychotics. In general, it has fewer side effects than the older antipsychotics and is more effective against negative symptoms in treatment of schizophrenia and schizoaffective disorder. Moreover, ziprasidone appears favorable from the standpoint of weight gain; as compared to other atypical agents, it induced the least amount of weight gain. Like other atypical agents, the cost of ziprasidone is relatively high. However, because at present the manufacturer has priced all strengths the same, at higher doses the current daily cost of ziprasidone may be lower than that of other atypical antipsychotics.

CHAPTER 7

Medications Used to Treat Attention-Deficit Hyperactivity Disorder in Adults

To learn more general information about this class of medications, read the first part of the chapter. To read about a specific drug used to treat attention deficit hyperactivity disorder (ADHD), turn to the page indicated in this chapter. See Chapter 10 for information on attention deficit hyperactivity disorder (ADHD) in children.

SLIGHTLY MORE THAN A DECADE AGO, MENTAL-HEALTH professionals assumed that what is now termed attention deficit hyperactivity disorder (ADHD)—the most common psychiatric diagnosis in childhood—was strictly kid stuff. They were wrong. About half of youngsters with this condition do not outgrow their restless, often reckless ways at puberty but continue to have attention problems in adolescence. Half of these individuals— that is, 25 percent of all children who develop attention deficit hyperactivity disorder (ADHD)—continue to have the disorder as adults; more may experience some residual symptoms, even though they do not have the full-blown disorder. (Chapter 10 discusses attention deficit hyperactivity disorder [ADHD] in children.)

Attention deficit hyperactivity disorder (ADHD), a term that has replaced the older terms *minimal brain dysfunction* and *hyperactivity,* refers to a spectrum of difficulties in controlling motion and sustaining attention. Its primary symptoms—hyperactivity, impulsivity, and distractibility— are less obvious in adults than in youngsters. Rather than scooting around a room, grown-ups with attention problems may tap their fingers or jiggle their feet. Some appear calm and organized on the surface but cannot concentrate long enough to finish reading a paragraph or follow a list of directions. Others, on a whim, go on buying sprees or take wild dares. Such behavior does not happen only at some times or in some circumstances; it is chronic and pervasive, meaning that it goes back for as long as the individuals can remember and continues to affect every aspect of their lives.

How Common Are Attention Disorders in Adults?

In all, 1 to 2 percent of adult men and women in the United States, perhaps as many as 5 million individuals, have problems in sustaining attention or controlling their movements and impulses. These problems are even more common in children, affecting 3 to 10 percent of youngsters, about three-quarters of them boys.

In adulthood, men and women seem equally prone to attention problems. It is possible that boys, who usually develop more visible (and vexing) symptoms, are more readily diagnosed at a young age than girls, whose symptoms may be more subtle. It is also possible that attention problems may develop later in females than in males.

What Causes Attention Disorders?

Attention deficit hyperactivity disorder (ADHD) may stem from an abnormality in brain functioning. Using sophisticated brain-imaging techniques, researchers at the National Institute of Mental Health (NIMH) have measured metabolic activity in the brains of adults who have had symptoms of attention deficit hyperactivity disorder (ADHD) since childhood and who have at least one child with the disorder. These images, when compared with those of normal volunteers, show that individuals with attention deficit hyperactivity disorder (ADHD) metabolize glucose, the brain's main energy source, at a slower rate, particularly in regions of the brain that regulate movement and attention.

Vulnerability to this problem may be inherited. ADHD

tends to run in families and is more common among close relatives of people with this disorder than in the general population. Approximately one-third of children diagnosed with ADHD have a parent or sibling with the same problem. In cases that are not familial, something may go amiss during pregnancy, probably during the second trimester, that affects the development of specific areas of the brain.

Despite years of controversy, there is no proof that culprits such as food allergies, additives, sugar, head injury, or fluorescent lights cause ADHD. However, preliminary findings from ongoing studies do suggest that a thyroid disorder may account for a small fraction of cases.

How Attention Disorders Feel in Adults

Individuals with attention disorders live in a confusing and often frustrating world. Their thought processes are different from others', and they can be very easily distracted. On the way from an office building to the post office on the corner, for example, they may forget their objective, wander into a store, and impulsively buy an expensive coat or watch. As long as they are working or talking one to one (as during an interview or while working at a computer), they may perform perfectly well, but when they have to stand in line, do chores, attend meetings, or wait for a delayed flight, they become enormously aggravated.

Men and women who grew up before the late 1960s and early 1970s, when attention problems were first widely recognized in children, may always have sensed that something was wrong but never knew what. Unaware of attention problems, their teachers may have viewed them as underachievers. Their employers may have thought or may still think of them as goof-offs, and their families may remember them as difficult, demanding youngsters who grew up to be irresponsible adults.

While children with ADHD find it hard to filter out

extraneous noises or activities, adults report what some describe as "an internal distractibility." They fail to pay close attention to details; make careless mistakes; and find it hard to focus, sustain attention, keep track of several projects at the same time, or organize their thoughts coherently. Just like youngsters with ADHD, they may act or speak without thinking. Some rush into decisions or business ventures without taking the time to weigh potential disadvantages. Because of this tendency, other people may assume that they are immature or have poor judgment.

Adults with attention disorders can lead successful lives, although they are less likely to do so in more conventional ways. The individuals with undiagnosed ADHD who make their way into therapists' offices with their troubled children are usually the luckier ones. Through determination, talent, or sheer grit, they have found ways to cope, perhaps by going to the gym every night to sweat away their restlessness or by pushing themselves to work harder and longer merely to keep up with everyone else. Some have chosen jobs, such as retail sales or taxi driving, that do not demand sustained concentration. In one study that followed more than 100 boys with ADHD into their twenties, a smaller than expected number completed college or graduate school, while a much higher percentage went into business for themselves.

For some adults, the inability to focus or control impulses is a serious handicap. They drift from job to job and place to place, never really settling down. Their relationships tend to be short and stormy. Their lives often become a jumble of dead ends, wrong turns, frustrations, and failures. They are more prone to abuse alcohol or drugs, to get into accidents or trouble with the law, to develop other mental disorders, and to commit suicide.

There is one major difference between individuals who were diagnosed and treated for attention disorders or hyperactivity as children and those first identified as having ADHD as adults. Those who have been struggling with this problem all their lives but never knew what it was and who may have been ostracized, criticized, or ridiculed as stupid or lazy tend to have much lower self-esteem and to feel more depressed than persons who knew the nature of their problem from childhood.

Risks and Complications

Attention disorders take a toll on mental health. People with these problems have a higher than normal incidence of anxiety disorders, mild depression, and mood swings. They also tend to abuse alcohol or drugs, but not in typical ways. Rather than trying to get high or euphoric, they reach for a drink or a drug to become more calm and focused. Teens and young adults with ADHD experience four times as many car accidents as their non-ADHD counterparts and are more likely to be at fault in an accident.

Treating Attention Disorders

Adults with ADHD benefit from the same therapy as children with this disorder. The most successful approaches involve a combination of medication, psychotherapy, and appropriate academic or vocational education.

Medication

The primary medications—methylphenidate (Ritalin), dextro-amphetamine (Dexedrine), dextro-methamphetamine hydrochloride (Desoxyn), and pemoline (Cylert)—are stimulants that produce a high-intensity rush of euphoria in most people. In those with ADHD, however, they have a paradoxical effect, aiding in concentration and reducing restlessness. Most adults need the same low daily doses as children, do not feel high, do not take more than they need, and do not become tolerant to the therapeutic effects of the medications.

The most common side effects of these stimulants are difficulty in falling asleep and loss of appetite. Adjustments in dosage and timing can ease such reactions. Some people report stomachaches or headaches. Much rarer is the development of tics, which go away once the drug is discontinued. About 60 to 80 percent of adults improve after taking stimulants. When these medications don't work, tricyclic antidepressants, such as desipramine (Norpramin), nortriptyline (Pamelor), and imipramine (Tofranil), or newer antidepressants such as bupropion (Wellbutrin or Zyban) may help. Physicians use the same doses to treat ADHD as they would to treat depression.

The length of time adults must continue to take medication varies. Some need it only until they finish school or learn coping strategies. Others take it for many years but eventually find ways to manage without it. Many report that medication makes them less short-tempered, less distractible, less impulsive, less moody, less vulnerable to stress, and more organized and more responsive to others. For adults who require long-term treatment on a stimulant, abuse and dependence are usually not problems.

 Generic name: **DEXTROAMPHETA-MINE**

 Available in generic form: Yes

 Brand name: Dexedrine

 Drug class: Stimulant

 Prescribed for: Attention deficit hyperactivity disorder (ADHD), narcolepsy (a sleep disorder characterized by an inability to stay awake and episodes of sudden onset of sleep), depression (especially in people who have medical illnesses), fatigue and lethargy from chronic medical illness such as AIDS or cancer.

General information: Dextroamphetamine, one of the first agents that could be classified as a mind/mood drug, was developed to treat what was called minimal brain dysfunction in children, a condition renamed attention deficit hyperactivity disorder (ADHD) in the *DSM-IV*. The d-isomer form of dextroamphetamine, D-amphetamine, is used to treat ADHD and other conditions.

Dosing information: Dextroamphetamine is available in 5- and 10-mg. tablets, spansules of 5, 10, and 15 mg., and an elixir at a dose of 5 mg. per 5 cc. The usual dosage form is the tablet, which is initially prescribed in adults at a dose of 5 mg. twice a day. The usual therapeutic range is between 10 and 40 mg. a day. The spansule capsules provide a slow-release form of the drug that may be taken in a single daily dose, which may be especially beneficial for those who find it difficult to take medication twice a day.

Common side effects: Common side effects of dextroamphetamine are sleep disturbance, racing heart, increased blood pressure, and various gastrointestinal side effects (especially nausea and diarrhea). Weight loss and a decreased appetite also frequently accompany use of the medication.

Precautions: High doses of all amphetamines may produce paranoid psychotic symptoms that are indistinguishable from those of persons with schizophrenia who are experiencing a psychotic episode.

⅗∅⅗ **Warnings:** Another form of amphetamine, methamphetamine, in particular a crystalline form whose street name is "ice," is a dangerous drug of abuse that can be smoked or injected intramuscularly. It is one of the most common causes of emergency-room admissions. Because of the significant risk of abuse and dependence, people with a history of alcohol or substance abuse should not take dextroamphetamine. The current diagnosis of attention deficit hyperactivity disorder (ADHD) is essential before dextroamphetamine is prescribed because many people who believe they have the disorder are actually suffering from another psychiatric disorder, most often bipolar disorder or major depressive disorder; they too should not use dextroamphetamine. This drug should be used with caution in individuals with schizophrenia or other psychotic disorders because high doses of dextroamphetamine may produce psychosis. Dextroamphetamine may worsen a tic disorder or Tourette's syndrome. There may also be an increased risk of seizures in persons taking this medication.

Dextroamphetamine should not be used with an MAO inhibitor; the combination is potentially dangerous. Two weeks should elapse after stopping an MAOI before beginning dextroamphetamine. Also, individuals should wait two weeks after stopping dextroamphetamine before starting an MAOI.

▽ **Alcohol:** People with attention deficit hyperactivity disorder (ADHD) who are taking dextroamphetamine should not drink alcohol, since alcohol may worsen their symptoms.

Food and beverages: There are no restrictions. However, nicotine and caffeine may increase nervousness and anxiety.

Possible drug interactions: People taking MAO inhibitors should never take dextroamphetamine, which can cause dangerous increases in blood pressure. Individuals taking weight-loss medications must be cautious, since these agents increase the probability of agitation, anxiety, and psychosis. Dextroamphetamine may contribute to increases in blood pressure and heart rate; consequently, it should be used cautiously in people with hypertension, especially in those taking antihypertensive medications. Stimulants may also increase cortisol levels.

Use in pregnancy and breast-feeding:
Pregnancy Category C
Dextroamphetamine has been found to produce birth defects in animals, but there have been no systematic studies in pregnant women. Dextroamphetamine should be used in pregnancy only if the benefits to the mother greatly outweigh any potential risks to the fetus. Women on dextroamphetamine should not breast-feed, since the effects on the baby are unknown.

Use in children: As discussed in Chapter 10, children take the same doses as adults. Dextroamphetamine is not approved for use in children under age three.

Use in seniors: Dextroamphetamine has not been studied systematically in seniors. It is sometimes prescribed in older people to increase concentration or alertness. Seniors with serious medical illnesses, such as cancer, who become depressed but are unable to tolerate antidepressants also may benefit from dextroamphetamine.

Overdosage: People who overdose with dextroamphetamine may experience significant agitation, confusion, hallucinations, psychosis, and hypertension. They

356 Methamphetamine Hydrochloride

should be taken to the emergency room. Bring the bottle of medication to the emergency room with the person, since the date it was prescribed and the number of pills remaining in the bottle can provide helpful information to the treating physician.

Special considerations: Dextroamphetamine is an excellent drug for the treatment of attention deficit hyperactivity disorder (ADHD) in children or adults. However, people who have a history of alcohol or substance abuse should not use it because of its addictive potential. Because high doses may produce psychotic symptoms indistinguishable from schizophrenia, individuals with a history of psychosis or schizophrenia should use this medication with caution.

Generic name: METHAMPHETAMINE HYDROCHLORIDE

 Available in generic form: No

 Brand name: Desoxyn

 Drug class: Stimulant

Prescribed for: Attention deficit hyperactivity disorder (ADHD), narcolepsy (a sleep disorder characterized by an inability to stay awake and episodes of sudden onset of sleep), depression (especially in those who have medical illnesses), fatigue and lethargy from chronic medical illness such as AIDS or cancer.

General information: Methamphetamine hydrochloride was developed to treat what was called minimal brain dysfunction in children, a condition renamed attention deficit hyperactivity disorder (ADHD) in the *DSM-IV*.

Dosing information: Methamphetamine hydrochloride is available in 5-mg. tablets and 5-, 10-, and 15-mg. slow-release tablets. The usual dosage form is the standard tablet, which is initially prescribed in adults at a dose of 5 mg. twice a day. The usual therapeutic range is between 10 and 40 mg. a day. The slow-release tablets provide a single daily dose, which is especially beneficial for children because they do not have to take the medication during the day at school.

Common side effects: Common side effects of methamphetamine hydrochloride are sleep disturbance, racing heart, increased blood pressure, and various gastrointestinal side effects (especially nausea and diarrhea). Weight loss and a decreased appetite also frequently accompany use of the medication.

Precautions: High doses of all amphetamines may produce paranoid psychotic symptoms that are indistinguishable from those of persons with schizophrenia who are experiencing a psychotic episode.

Warnings: A crystalline form of methamphetamine, also known by its street name, "ice," is a dangerous drug of abuse that can be smoked or injected intramuscularly. It is one of the most common causes of emergency-room admissions. Because of the significant risk of abuse and dependence, people with a history of alcohol or substance abuse should not take methamphetamine hydrochloride. Diagnosis of attention deficit hyperactivity disorder (ADHD) is essential before methamphetamine hydrochloride is prescribed because many people who believe they have the disorder are actually suffering from another psychiatric disorder, most often bipolar disorder or major depressive disorder; they too should not use methamphetamine hydrochloride. This drug should be used with caution in individuals with schizophrenia or other psychotic disorders, because high doses of methamphetamine hydrochloride may produce psychosis. Methamphetamine hydrochloride may worsen a tic disorder or Tourette's syndrome. There may also be an increased risk of seizures in individuals taking this medication.

Methamphetamine hydrochloride should not be used with an MAO inhibitor; the combination is potentially dangerous. Two weeks should elapse after stopping an MAOI before beginning methamphetamine hydrochloride. Also, individuals should wait two weeks after stopping methamphetamine hydrochloride before starting an MAOI.

Alcohol: People with attention deficit hyperactivity disorder (ADHD) who are taking methamphetamine hydrochloride should not drink alcohol, since alcohol may worsen their symptoms.

Food and beverages: There are no restrictions. However, nicotine and caffeine may increase nervousness and anxiety.

Possible drug interactions: People taking MAO inhibitors should never use methamphetamine hydrochloride, which can cause dangerous increases in blood pressure. Individuals taking weight-loss medications must be cautious, since these agents increase the probability of agitation, anxiety, and psychosis. Methamphetamine hydrochloride may also contribute to increases in blood pressure and heart rate; consequently, it should be used cautiously by people with hypertension and especially those taking antihypertensive medications. Stimulants may also increase cortisol levels.

Use in pregnancy and breast-feeding: Pregnancy Category C

Methamphetamine hydrochloride has been found to produce birth defects in animals, but there have been no systematic studies in pregnant women. Methamphetamine hydrochloride should be used in pregnancy only if the benefits to the mother greatly outweigh any potential risk to the fetus. Women on methamphetamine hydrochloride should not breast-feed, since the effects on the baby are unknown.

Use in children: As discussed in Chapter 10, children take the same doses as adults. Methamphetamine hydrochloride is not approved for use in children under age three.

Use in seniors: Methamphetamine hydrochloride has not been studied systematically in seniors. It is sometimes prescribed in older people to increase concentration or alertness. Seniors with serious medical illnesses, such as cancer, who become depressed but are unable to tolerate antidepressants may also benefit from methamphetamine hydrochloride.

Overdosage: People who overdose with methamphetamine hydrochloride may experience significant agitation, confusion, hallucinations, psychosis, and hypertension. They should be taken to the emergency room. Bring the bottle of medication to the emergency room with the person, since the date it was prescribed and the number of pills remaining in the bottle can provide helpful information to the treating physician.

Special considerations: Methamphetamine hydrochloride is an excellent drug for the treatment of attention deficit hyperactivity disorder (ADHD) in children or adults. However, people who have a history of alcohol or substance abuse should not use it because of its addictive potential. Because high doses may produce psychotic symptoms indistinguishable from schizophrenia, those with a history of psychosis or schizophrenia should use this medication with caution.

 Generic name: **PEMOLINE**

 Available in generic form: No

 Brand name: Cylert

 Drug class: Stimulant

Prescribed for: Attention deficit hyperactivity disorder (ADHD), narcolepsy (a sleep disorder characterized by an inability to stay awake and episodes of sudden onset of sleep), depression (especially in those who have medical illnesses), fatigue and lethargy from chronic medical illness such as AIDS or cancer.

General information: The d-isomer form of pemoline, Cylert, is used to treat attention deficit hyperactivity disorder (ADHD) and other conditions. Some psychiatrists believe there is less potential for abuse with pemoline than with the other stimulants, and animal studies support this observation. However, there is still some potential for abuse and dependence with pemoline.

Dosing information: Pemoline is available in 18.75-, 37.5-, and 75-mg. tablets and a 37.5-mg. chewable tablet. The usual therapeutic dose is between 18.75 and 150 mg. a day. The initial dose is an 18.75-mg. tablet twice a day, with a 37.5-mg. increase in daily dose weekly. The chewable tablet offers a more gradual onset of action.

Common side effects: Common side effects of pemoline are sleep disturbance, racing heart, increased blood pressure, and various gastrointestinal side effects (especially nausea and diarrhea). Weight loss and a decreased appetite also frequently accompany use of the medication.

Precautions: High doses of pemoline may produce paranoid psychotic symptoms that are indistinguishable from those of persons with schizophrenia who are experiencing a psychotic episode.

Warnings: Because of the significant risk of abuse and dependence, people with a history of alcohol or substance abuse should not take pemoline. The diagnosis of attention deficit hyperactivity disorder (ADHD) is essential before pemoline is prescribed because many people who believe they have the disorder are actually suffering from another psychiatric disorder, most often bipolar disorder or major depressive disorder; they too should not use magnesium pemoline. This drug should be used with caution in individuals with schizophrenia or other psychotic disorders because high doses of pemoline may produce psychosis. Pemoline may worsen a tic disorder or Tourette's syndrome. There also may be an increased risk of seizures in persons taking this medication. Pemoline has been reported to increase liver enzymes and, in rare cases, to produce liver failure. For this reason, other stimulants should be tried before pemoline. In addition, your physician may order periodic blood tests of liver enzymes at the beginning of treatment and periodically thereafter.

Pemoline should not be used with an MAO inhibitor; the combination is potentially dangerous. Two weeks should elapse after stopping an MAOI before beginning pemoline. Also, individuals should wait two weeks after stopping pemoline before starting an MAOI.

Y **Alcohol:** People with attention deficit hyperactivity
disorder (ADHD) who are taking pemoline should
not drink alcohol, since alcohol may worsen their symptoms.

Food and beverages: There are no restrictions.
However, nicotine and caffeine may increase nervousness and anxiety.

Possible drug interactions: People taking MAO
inhibitors should never take pemoline, which can
cause dangerous increases in blood pressure. Individuals
taking weight-loss medications must be cautious, since
these agents increase the probability of agitation, anxiety,
and psychosis. Pemoline may also contribute to increases
in blood pressure and heart rate; consequently, it should
be used cautiously in people with hypertension and especially those taking antihypertensive medications. Stimulants may also increase cortisol levels.

Use in pregnancy and breast-feeding:
Pregnancy Category B

Pemoline has not been systematically studied in pregnant
women. Pemoline should be used in pregnancy only if the
benefits to the mother greatly outweigh any potential, unknown risks to the fetus. Women on pemoline should not
breast-feed, since the effects on the baby are unknown.

Use in children: As discussed in Chapter 10, children take the same doses as adults. Pemoline is not
approved for use in children under age six and is recommended in children only if other medications have not
helped. Because of the risk of liver damage, especially in
children, monthly or periodic blood tests of liver function
are usually ordered by the physician.

🏠 **Use in seniors:** Pemoline has not been studied systematically in seniors. It is sometimes prescribed for older people to increase concentration or alertness. Seniors with serious medical illnesses, such as cancer, who become depressed but are unable to tolerate antidepressants also may benefit from pemoline.

☠ **Overdosage:** People who overdose with pemoline may experience significant agitation, confusion, hallucinations, psychosis, and hypertension. They should be taken to the emergency room. Bring the bottle of medication to the emergency room with the person, since the date it was prescribed and the number of pills remaining in the bottle can provide helpful information to the treating physician.

☞ **Special considerations:** Pemoline is an effective drug for the treatment of attention deficit hyperactivity disorder (ADHD) in children or adults. However, people who have a history of alcohol or substance abuse should not use it because of its addictive potential. Because high doses may produce psychotic symptoms indistinguishable from schizophrenia, those with a history of psychosis or schizophrenia should use this medication with caution. Pemoline produces fewer side effects than dextroamphetamine (Dexedrine), methamphetamine hydrochloride (Desoxyn), or methylphenidate (Ritalin). Since its onset of action may be more gradual, it may take several weeks or longer before individuals report improvement. However, because of the risk of liver damage and liver failure, especially in children, it should be reserved for adults or children who have failed to respond to dextroamphetamine (Dexedrine), methamphetamine hydrochloride (Desoxyn), or methylphenidate (Ritalin).

Generic name: **METHYLPHENIDATE**

 Available in generic form: Yes

 Brand name: Ritalin

 Drug class: Stimulant

Prescribed for: Attention deficit hyperactivity disorder (ADHD), narcolepsy (a sleep disorder characterized by an inability to stay awake and episodes of sudden onset of sleep), depression (especially in those who have medical illnesses), fatigue and lethargy from chronic medical illness such as AIDS or cancer.

General information: Methylphenidate, one of the first agents that could be classified as a mind/mood drug, was developed to treat what was called minimal brain dysfunction in children, a condition renamed attention deficit hyperactivity disorder (ADHD) in the *DSM-IV*. Methylphenidate is basically similar to dextroamphetamine (Dexedrine), but it may be slightly shorter-acting. People who cannot tolerate dextroamphetamine because of its gastrointestinal side effects may tolerate methylphenidate better.

Dosing information: Methylphenidate is available in 5-, 10-, and 20-mg. tablets and a 20-mg. slow-release tablet. The usual starting dose is 5 mg. twice a day of the normal-release tablet. The usual therapeutic dose is between 10 and 80 mg. a day.

Common side effects: Common side effects of methylphenidate are sleep disturbance, racing heart, increased blood pressure, and various gastrointestinal side effects (especially nausea and diarrhea). Weight loss and a decreased appetite also frequently accompany use of the medication.

Precautions: High doses of all amphetamines may produce paranoid psychotic symptoms that are indistinguishable from those of persons with schizophrenia who are experiencing a psychotic episode.

Warnings: Because of the significant risk of abuse and dependence, people with a history of alcohol or substance abuse should not take methylphenidate. The diagnosis of attention deficit hyperactivity disorder (ADHD) is essential before methylphenidate is prescribed because many people who believe they have the disorder are actually suffering from another psychiatric disorder, most often bipolar disorder or major depressive disorder; they too should not use methylphenidate. This drug should be used with caution in individuals with schizophrenia or other psychotic disorders, because high doses of methylphenidate may produce psychosis. Methylphenidate may worsen a tic disorder or Tourette's syndrome. There may also be an increased risk of seizures in persons taking this medication.

Methylphenidate should not be used with an MAO inhibitor; the combination is potentially dangerous. Two weeks should elapse after stopping an MAOI before beginning methylphenidate. Also, individuals should wait two weeks after stopping methylphenidate before starting an MAOI.

Alcohol: People with attention deficit hyperactivity disorder (ADHD) who are taking methylphenidate should not drink alcohol, since alcohol may worsen their symptoms.

Food and beverages: There are no restrictions. However, nicotine and caffeine may increase nervousness and anxiety.

Possible drug interactions: People taking MAO inhibitors should never take methylphenidate, which can cause dangerous increases in blood pressure. Individuals taking weight-loss medications must be cautious, since these agents increase the probability of agitation, anxiety, and psychosis. Methylphenidate may also contribute to increases in blood pressure and heart rate; consequently, it should be used cautiously by people with hypertension and especially those taking antihypertensive medications. Stimulants may also increase cortisol levels.

Use in pregnancy and breast-feeding:
Pregnancy Category B
Methylphenidate has not been systemically studied in pregnant women. It should be used in pregnancy only if the benefits to the mother greatly outweigh any potential risk to the fetus. Women on methylphenidate should not breast-feed, since the effects on the baby are unknown.

Use in children: As discussed in Chapter 10, children take the same doses as adults. Methylphenidate is not approved for use in children under age three.

Use in seniors: Methylphenidate has not been studied systematically in seniors. It is sometimes prescribed for older people to increase concentration or alertness. Seniors with serious medical illnesses, such as cancer, who become depressed but are unable to tolerate antidepressants also may benefit from methylphenidate.

Overdosage: People who overdose with methylphenidate may experience significant agitation, confusion, hallucinations, psychosis, and hypertension. They should be taken to the emergency room. Bring the bottle of medication to the emergency room with the person since the date it was prescribed and the number of pills remaining in the bottle can provide helpful information to the treating physician.

Special considerations: Methylphenidate is an excellent drug for the treatment of attention deficit hyperactivity disorder (ADHD) in children or adults. However, people who have a history of alcohol or substance abuse should not use it because of its addiction potential. Because high doses may produce psychotic symptoms indistinguishable from schizophrenia, those with a history of psychosis or schizophrenia should use this medication with caution.

CHAPTER 8

Cognitive-Enhancing Medications

To learn more general information about dementia and this class of medications, read the first part of the chapter. To read about a specific cognitive-enhancing drug, turn to the page indicated below.

THE AGING BRAIN

Although the brain literally becomes smaller as we age, basic mental abilities do not necessarily diminish. Reaction time, intellectual speed and efficiency, nonverbal intelligence, and the maximum speed at which we can work for short periods may decline somewhat by the age of seventy-five. However, understanding, vocabulary, the ability to remember key information, and verbal intelligence remain about the same. A grandfather playing a computer game with his fourteen-year-old grandson will lose every time, because instead of responding in a fifth of a second like the boy, he needs two-fifths of a second. But in tests that involve experience and acquired knowledge, the grandfather has the edge.

Although certain aspects of memory falter with time, most people can compensate by relying on simple coping strategies, such as taking notes, making lists, or—if they arrive in a room but forget what they wanted there—retracing their thoughts and actions before heading there. Some people have better memories in their sixties than others do in their thirties. And at any age, people can improve their recall.

Middle-aged and older individuals may find it more difficult to recall newly learned information than younger ones because they have not learned it well in the first place. Older people often fail to spend as much time organizing the material they want to master as young people do. In preparing for a written driving test, for example, they may not use learning skills, such as highlighting key words or making a list of key points, that could enhance their mastery.

The most common problem for people over sixty is remembering the name of an object or a person. They recognize the individual or know how to use the object, but they cannot produce the right word, especially if it's someone or something they don't refer to often. For example, trying to recall the word for a game played with a small white ball and paddles, they think of tennis rather than Ping-Pong. Running into an old acquaintance, they frantically flip through their mental Rolodex, trying to match the face with a name. The more anxious they get, the more difficult remembering becomes.

Although occasional forgetfulness, memory lapses, and misplacement of everyday objects are common at any age, about 5 to 15 percent of people over the age of seventy develop more serious symptoms of diminished mental capacity, such as errors in judgment and impaired thinking. A general term used to describe such changes in intelligence, attention, concentration, memory, level of consciousness, and other higher brain functioning is *organic brain syndrome*. The term *organic* means that there is a medical or neurological cause for the change in brain functioning. A number of illnesses, including depression, kidney disease, alcoholism, and Alzheimer's disease, can cause organic brain syndrome. Thorough medical and neurological examinations may be able to pinpoint the specific cause.

Dementia and Alzheimer's Disease

One of the most common organic brain syndromes is dementia. Fifty to 60 percent of people who develop dementia—a total of 4 million men and women over the age of sixty-five—suffer from the type called Alzheimer's disease, a progressive deterioration of brain cells and mental capacity. About 20 percent have a form of dementia called vascular dementia, in which the person suffers a series of small strokes that damage or destroy tissue in the affected areas of the brain. In contrast to Alzheimer's disease, in which there is a progressive loss of higher intellectual abilities, people with vascular dementia have a step-wise decline in mental capacity. Parkinson's disease, a disorder characterized by a pill-rolling tremor, lack of facial expression, and a stooped, shuffling walk, can also cause dementia in the elderly. A high percentage of Parkinson's disease patients develop depression and psychosis. As described elsewhere in the book, physicians will frequently prescribe antidepressants (see Chapter 2) to treat the depression and antipsychotic medications (see Chapter 6) to treat psychosis.

There have been major advances in unraveling the keys to Alzheimer's disease, a disorder that robs individuals of their memories, their intellects, their personalities, and eventually their lives. Often the illness progresses slowly, stealing bits of a person's mind and memory a little at a time. Individuals who realize that something is going wrong may make initial efforts to cope by establishing a rigid schedule for daily life and avoiding any changes in that schedule. As the disease progresses, those who have periods of awareness of their condition can become upset and depressed. In time, these lucid periods become less frequent, memory is severely impaired, and they eventually lose the ability to recall words or form sentences.

The personalities of individuals with dementia often change. Its victims may withdraw into a world of their own, become quarrelsome or irritable, and say or do inappropriate things. Some become stubborn or impulsive, others apathetic. Those who develop increasing suspiciousness may accuse others of thefts, betrayal, or plotting against them. As cognitive impairment worsens, demented persons often lose inhibitions and may masturbate or take off their clothes in public. Some become aggressive or violent. Eventually they may forget their closest relatives, their former occupations, even their own names. Because they may wander away from home and get lost, close supervision may become necessary, either at home or in a nursing facility.

The early signs of dementia—insomnia, irritability, increased sensitivity to alcohol and other drugs, and decreased energy and tolerance of frustration—are usually subtle and insidious. Diagnosis requires a comprehensive assessment of an individual's medical history, physical health, and mental status and often involves brain scans and a variety of other tests.

Medications

Nothing can save a brain in the process of being destroyed by an organic brain disease such as Alzheimer's. However, medications can control difficult behavioral symptoms and enhance or partially restore cognitive ability. Low doses of antipsychotic medications (see Chapter 6) ease symptoms such as agitation, wandering, hallucinations, paranoid delusions, and hostility. Tacrine (Cognex) and donepezil (Aricept), the first specific medications for Alzheimer's, produce some cognitive and behavioral improvement in about a third of individuals. Often therapists diagnose other medical or psychiatric problems, such as depression, and treating these conditions can lead to dramatic improvement. Antidepressant drugs (see Chapter 2), for example, may improve sleep, appetite, energy, and involvement with others.

For those with vascular dementia, low-dose aspirin can help prevent blood clots and repeated brain damage. Other medications may also be helpful; as in Alzheimer's, antipsychotic drugs may lessen agitation, wandering, and paranoid delusions. As many as 30 percent of those with dementia not related to Alzheimer's also suffer from depression, but there are few data on whether antidepressants can help them.

Adequate rest, exercise, intellectual stimulation, social contacts, balanced and regular meals, and elimination of nonessential drugs can benefit even those with severe dementia. Most people with dementia do best in consistent, familiar surroundings, with daily routines, prominently displayed clocks and calendars, night-lights, checklists, and diaries to help with orientation.

 Generic name: DONEPEZIL

 Available in generic form: No

 Brand name: Aricept

 Drug class: Reversible cholinesterase inhibitor

 Prescribed for: Treatment of mild to moderate dementia of the Alzheimer's type.

General information: Donepezil was the second cholinesterase inhibitor approved in the mid-1990s by the FDA to treat mild to moderate dementia. It is a reversible, central cholinesterase inhibitor that works by increasing brain acetylcholine levels and activity in cholinergic neurons. This effect is believed to lead to an improvement in memory and other associated cognitive abilities. Although donepezil does not reverse the cognitive decline associated with Alzheimer's disease, it does slow the rate of decline in cognitive functioning associated with this disease. When people begin donepezil, they may report a rapid improvement in memory and overall cognitive ability. However, with time, most individuals, whether treated with donepezil or not, begin to show a further decline in their cognitive functioning.

Donepezil has a number of advantages over tacrine (Cognex), the first approved agent. It is given in a single daily dose and not four times a day like tacrine. It does not require frequent liver-enzyme monitoring. Although there have not been direct comparisons with tacrine, clinical reports from physicians and patients indicate that donepezil is better tolerated.

Dosing information: Donepezil is available in 5- and 10-mg. tablets. The usual initial dose is 5 mg. a day in the morning. The dose is increased to 10 mg. after four to six weeks. If the dose is increased more rapidly than this, such as an increase to 10 mg. after one week on the 5 mg. dose, a much greater frequency of nausea, diarrhea, insomnia, fatigue, vomiting, muscle cramps, and lack of appetite is reported. A slow increase lowers the risk of these side effects. Donepezil should be taken in the evening just prior to going to bed.

Common side effects: The most common side effects reported in clinical trials were nausea, diarrhea, insomnia, fatigue, vomiting, muscle cramps, and lack of appetite. Some people report a slowing of their heart rate, dizziness, and orthostatic hypotension.

Precautions: People who may be undergoing surgery should let their anesthesiologist know they are taking donepezil, since it may affect the action of succinylcholine-type muscle relaxants. In contrast to tacrine, taking donepezil does not require periodic blood tests to measure liver enzymes.

Warnings: Because of its effect on heart rate, individuals who have a low heart rate, who are taking medication or who have a history of dizziness related to this condition must take donepezil with caution. There also may be a slightly increased risk for seizures, although this has not been observed with usual doses of this medication.

Alcohol: People taking donepezil should not drink alcohol. Alcohol increases the rate of metabolism of most drugs, including donepezil (Aricept), and may further interfere with cognitive functioning.

Food and beverages: No restrictions. If taking donepezil on an empty stomach upsets your stomach, try it with food or immediately after eating.

Possible drug interactions: Donepezil has a minimal effect on the metabolism of other drugs, and other medications reportedly have a minimal effect on the metabolism of donepezil. There appear to be no significant drug interactions.

Use in pregnancy and breast-feeding: Pregnancy Category C
There are no adequate or well-controlled studies in pregnant women. Animal studies do not show any evidence of potential risk on the fetus. However, it would be highly unusual for a woman contemplating pregnancy to be taking donepezil, since even the earliest stages of Alzheimer's disease usually do not appear until after the childbearing years. This medication has not been studied in nursing mothers, but again, women who are nursing are not likely to need donepezil.

Use in children: This medication has not been studied in children and is not recommended in children.

Use in seniors: Most of the clinical trials were conducted in seniors, and all the information previously discussed applies principally to this patient population.

Overdosage: Overdosage with donepezil may produce a cholinergic crisis where the person experiences severe nausea and vomiting, sweating, salivation, slowing of the heart rate, a significant drop in blood pressure, seizures, and muscle weakness. Because of the potential seriousness of an overdose with donepezil, individuals should be taken to the emergency room. Bring the bottle of medication to the emergency room with the person, since the date when it was prescribed and the number of pills remaining in the bottle can provide helpful information to the treating physician.

Special considerations: Physicians greatly prefer donepezil over tacrine (Cognex) to decrease the rate of cognitive decline in those suffering from the early to middle stages of Alzheimer's disease.

 Generic name: TACRINE

 Available in generic form: No

 Brand name: Cognex

 Drug class: Reversible cholinesterase inhibitor

 Prescribed for: Mild to moderate dementia of the Alzheimer's type.

General information: Tacrine was the first medication approved by the FDA to treat the cognitive decline associated with Alzheimer's disease. It is a reversible, central cholinesterase inhibitor that works by increasing brain acetylcholine levels and activity in cholinergic neurons. This effect is believed to lead to an improvement in memory and other associated cognitive abilities. Although tacrine does not reverse the cognitive decline associated with Alzheimer's disease, it does slow the rate of decline in cognitive functioning associated with this disease. When people begin taking tacrine, they may report a rapid improvement in memory and overall cognitive ability. However, with time, most patients, whether treated with tacrine or not, begin to show a further decline in their cognitive functioning. The major limitations of tacrine are its side effects, in particular, high rates of nausea and diarrhea and the elevation of certain liver enzymes. This latter effect may make it necessary to stop this medication.

Dosing information: Tacrine is available in 10-, 20-, 30-, and 40-mg. tablets. The usual initial dose is 10 mg. four times a day. After one to two months, the daily dose is then increased to 80 mg. a day; in another four to six weeks, to 120 mg.; and, eventually, if the person is able to tolerate the medication, to 160 mg. a day. The goal in treatment is a daily dose of 120 to 160 mg., which produces a greater improvement in cognitive functioning. However, higher doses also cause increased side effects.

Common side effects: The most common side effects are nausea and vomiting, diarrhea, upset stomach, anorexia, abdominal pain, difficulty with walking (ataxia), dizziness, agitation, lack of appetite, tremor, and elevated liver enzymes, reflecting possible liver damage.

Precautions: Because this medication can increase liver enzymes, it should not be used in people with liver disease. People who may be undergoing surgery should tell their anesthesiologist about this medication, since it may affect the action of succinylcholine-type muscle relaxants. Because it may slow the conduction of electrical impulses through the heart, it should be used cautiously in persons with arrhythmias (irregular heartbeats).

Warnings: Up to 50 percent of people taking tacrine develop an elevation in liver enzymes. In clinical trials, 7 percent of people prescribed tacrine experienced elevations in liver enzymes more than ten times normal. Most people who have increased liver-enzyme levels do not experience any symptoms, and it is not known whether irreversible liver damage or death may result from an elevation of liver enzymes. Because of the frequency of this side effect, physicians obtain blood tests of liver enzymes every other week from week four to week sixteen of treatment, the period when the increase in liver enzymes is most common. After sixteen weeks of treatment with tacrine, liver-enzyme monitoring may be reduced to every three months. If the elevation of the liver enzymes ALT and SGPT is greater than two times the upper limit of normal, the physician usually reduces the dose of the medication. If these liver-enzyme levels become five times greater than normal, tacrine must be stopped. Once liver-enzyme levels fall within acceptable limits, the individual may restart tacrine. In many cases, an increase in liver enzymes does not recur.

Alcohol: People taking tacrine should not drink alcohol. Alcohol increases the rate of metabolism of most drugs and may further interfere with cognitive functioning.

Food and beverages: No restrictions. If taking tacrine on an empty stomach upsets your stomach, take it with food or immediately after eating.

Possible drug interactions: Tacrine inhibits the metabolism of theophylline, a medication frequently found in non-prescription cold or asthma preparations. The anti-ulcer medication cimetidine (Tagamet) may increase serum tacrine levels by over 50 percent. Because tacrine enhances acetylcholine, it inhibits the action of anticholinergic agents and may cause extrapyramidal symptoms (tremor, muscle stiffness, rigidity) in persons who are taking anticholinergic agents to treat Parkinson's disease. Tacrine also increases the effect of succinylcholine- and cholinergic-type agents such as bethanechol (Urecholine) and other cholinesterase inhibitors that are used to improve urination in men who have enlarged prostates.

Use in pregnancy and breast-feeding: Pregnancy Category C

No animal studies have been conducted with tacrine, and it is not known whether tacrine can cause fetal abnormalities. Women who are pregnant, planning a pregnancy, or hoping to breast-feed should not take tacrine, since its effect on the fetus is not known. However, because mild to moderate dementia usually occurs in women past childbearing years, this situation is not likely to arise.

Use in children: This medication is not indicated for use in children and should generally not be used in this population.

Use in seniors: Seniors, of course, are the patient population in which this medication has been studied the most. No special considerations are indicated.

Overdosage: Overdosage with tacrine may produce a cholinergic crisis, in which the person experiences severe nausea and vomiting, sweating, salivation, slowing of the heart rate, a significant drop in blood pressure, seizures, and muscle weakness. Because of the potential seriousness of an overdose with tacrine, individuals should be taken to the emergency room. Bring the bottle of medication

to the emergency room with the person, since the date when the medication was prescribed and the number of pills remaining in the bottle can provide helpful information to the treating physician.

Special considerations: Tacrine is an effective medication that decreases the rate of cognitive decline in individuals suffering from the early or middle stages of Alzheimer's disease. It is not believed to be effective in the later stages of this illness. Because of tacrine's potential for producing significant nausea, vomiting, and other gastrointestinal side effects, the medication must be increased slowly over a long period of time. Because tacrine may increase liver enzymes, blood tests are necessary during the first four to sixteen weeks of treatment. Because of these limitations, donepezil, a newer medication, has generally replaced tacrine as the treatment of choice for cognitive decline associated with dementia.

CHAPTER 9

Herbal Medications and "Natural" Mind/Mood Substances

To learn general information about this class of medications and the conditions for which they are used, read the first part of the chapter. To learn more about a specific medication, turn to the page indicated below.

THE LAST DECADE HAS SEEN AN ENORMOUS INCREASE in interest in and use of a broad range of therapies sometimes called "alternative," "unconventional," or "holistic." According to national surveys, 40 to 45 percent of Americans have tried at least one nontraditional treatment, including herbs or "natural" enzymes. In 1991, just 3 percent of Americans reported using herbal medicine; by 1998, 37 percent had tried an herbal remedy at least once. By 1999, the herbal-medicine and natural-products market had grown to an estimated $12 billion in annual sales, approaching the $17 billion that Americans spend each year on over-the-counter drugs.

Many people assume that because products are "natural," they also are safe—or at least "safer" than synthetic drugs. This is not the case. Heroin and cocaine are among many natural substances that have potentially deadly effects. Consumers of products that bear the ubiquitous label "natural" have to be especially wary because these preparations, which almost always undergo some processing before being marketed, have been largely unregulated. Like synthetic drugs—drugs that have been created, or synthesized, by pharmaceutical companies—they too can cause adverse side effects and possible drug interactions; however, these are largely unknown. Some alternative therapies are expensive and overly hyped by unqualified "experts." Furthermore, individuals with serious disorders who turn to unproven herbal remedies first may delay getting proven effective treatments.

The FDA categorizes herbs as "dietary supplements," which are not subject to the same rigorous efficacy and safety trials that all prescription and nonprescription drugs must undergo. The companies that manufacture herbal preparations can market them without submitting proof of purity, standardization of ingredients, or medicinal efficacy to the FDA. Herbal products cannot be marketed for the diagnosis, treatment, cure, or prevention of diseases. However, under the provisions of the 1994 Dietary Supplement Health and Education Act, herbal-medicine manufacturers can advertise the supposed benefits of their wares as long as they do not claim that the products affect a specific illness. As a result, consumers are bombarded with high-pressure advertising featuring general health claims (such as enhanced mood or improved memory) that may be untested, unproven, or simply untrue.

There are other problems with herbal medicines. The potency of herbal preparations varies greatly, depending on the form in which they are used. Because of the lack of regulation, potency also can vary from brand to brand and batch to batch. The U.S. Pharmacopoeia, a nonprofit organization that sets strength and purity standards for prescription and over-the-counter drugs, has published standards for some popular botanicals. Those that meet these standards have "NF" (national formulary) on the package.

The FDA also now requires a "supplement facts" panel on the label, similar to the nutritional facts panel on most foods. It contains information on which part of the plant was used to make the product and how much is an appropriate amount to use. Throughout this chapter, we provide dosage information based on the active ingredient of the preparation. As detailed on the supplements facts label, this translates into different recommended amounts, depending on whether the product comes in the form of dried herbs, tinctures, capsules, pills, or tea bags.

Despite ongoing attempts to improve the quality of herbal preparations, these products are often contaminated with other compounds that may produce adverse side effects. Purity is a significant issue, and some natural products have been withdrawn from the market after consumers suffered serious side effects from preparations that may not have been produced under hygienic conditions.

Consumers increase the likelihood of an adverse reaction when they combine natural remedies with prescription medications and do not inform their doctors that they are using an herbal medicine. While little is known about potential drug interactions, there are increasing reports of hazards, such as bleeding problems among individuals taking ginkgo biloba extract, advertised as a memory aid, along with anti-coagulant and anti-platelet drugs.

Many people have reported benefits from various herbal medications. Unfortunately, few systematic studies have been conducted to prove or disprove actual benefits and potential risks. The National Center for Complementary and Alternative Medicine (NCCAM), created in 1998 as part of the National Institutes of Health, is conducting and supporting studies on nontraditional treatments using the same rigorous standards applied to conventional medicine. The National Institute of Mental Health has launched a $4 million study of the efficacy and safety of St. John's wort as a treatment for mild to moderate depression. It will take several years to obtain conclusive results.

Because of the lack of information on both the efficacy and toxicity of herbal preparations, it is difficult for physicians to provide informed guidance to individuals who may wish to try such products. As a general guideline, based on the wide range of potency and unknown effects of herbal preparations, we recommend that children and women who are pregnant or nursing avoid their use. Seniors should use them with caution and should check with their physicians about possible interactions with other medications they are using and about the need for lower doses.

We urge all consumers, before trying any alternative mind/mood treatment, to gather the latest and most authoritative information available. Talk with your physician, and ask about potential benefits, possible interactions with medications you are taking, and other risks. In addition, several on-line databases cover clinical and scientific research on alternative medicine, including the NCCAM's Citation Index, which provides approximately 180,000 bibliographic records on complementary and alternative medicine (CAM) research. The Web site address is: http://altmed.od.nih.gov/nccam/resources/cam-ci/.Botanical Medicine Information Resources, a Web site from Columbia University, provides a comprehensive listing of links to Web sites related to herbal medicine; its address is: http://cpmc net.columbia.edu/dept/rosenthal/Botanicals.html.

This chapter includes summaries of the most commonly used herbal preparations for mind/mood problems in the United States today as well as information on two "natural" products: SAM-e, which is often taken to boost mood and fight depression, and melatonin, which is frequently used for insomnia and especially jet lag.

Name: GINKGO BILOBA

Source: *Ginkgo biloba* tree. The *Ginkgo biloba* is found in China, Japan, and Korea. The dry extract from the leaf is made up of several active compounds, including flavonoids, bioflavonoids, and terpenoids.

Indications: Ginkgo has been used to treat mild dementia, or memory impairment.

General information: Ginkgo biloba extract is promoted for use in improving cognitive function and blood flow. It is believed to work by inhibiting the aggregation, or clumping, of platelets. There have been several controlled trials of ginkgo to treat persons with mild dementia. The major benefits—seen most often in those with the greatest degree of memory impairment—were slightly improved memory and concentration, increased energy, reduced anxiety, and improved mood. Ginkgo may be less effective in individuals with milder memory impairment. In other research studies those suffering from dementia of the Alzheimer's type and cardiovascular dementia (resulting from many small strokes) reported some improvement with ginkgo. However, there have not been enough long-term research trials to provide conclusive evidence of ginkgo's benefits, and the FDA has not approved its use as a medical treatment for dementia or any other medical condition. It also is not clear whether ginkgo can help age-related memory impairment; there is no evidence of benefits in normal, healthy men and women.

Dosing information: Gingko biloba extract is available in both liquid and pill forms. The usual dose is 60 to 120 mg. taken two times a day. Read the supplements information label for the equivalent amount.

Common side effects: Common side effects are headache and mild gastrointestinal symptoms, such as nausea and abdominal cramps. Ginkgo may also produce allergic skin reactions.

Warnings: Ginkgo may increase bleeding time or, if a person is taking anticoagulants, produce bleeding problems. There have been several reports of spontaneous bleeding. Individuals who are taking anticoagulants such as warfarin (Coumadin), or medications such as aspirin, should avoid ginkgo.

Alcohol: Avoid alcohol.

Food and beverages: No restrictions.

Possible drug interactions: Ginkgo may interact with anticoagulants such as warfarin (Coumadin) and aspirin and may increase bleeding time, resulting in bleeding complications.

Use in pregnancy and breast-feeding: Not recommended.

Use in children: Not recommended.

Use in seniors: It is not known whether ginkgo can improve memory in healthy seniors with memory problems.

Overdosage: The major risks from an overdose are bleeding problems.

Special considerations: Ginkgo has been used extensively in Europe and also in China. Although there are no conclusive data, it may be beneficial for individuals who are experiencing memory disturbance related to dementia, whether the Alzheimer's type or caused by a stroke. Do not use if you are taking anticoagulants. Report any unusual bleeding or bruising, new-onset headaches, or vision changes to your physician immediately.

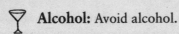
Name: ST. JOHN'S WORT

Source: *Hypericum perforatum.* The *Hypericum perforatum* is a perennial plant found throughout Europe, Western Asia, and Northern Africa, and it is culti-

vated in Australia, New Zealand, and Eastern Asia.
St. John's wort is comprised of the above-ground parts of
the plant, which are dried quickly after the plant is cut at
the start of the flowering season.

℞ **Indications:** Anxiety and depression.

General information: Most commercial St. John's
wort products consist of an 0.3 percent extract of
hypericin, the active ingredient. More than twenty controlled studies, mostly in Germany, have been conducted
on St. John's wort and suggest that it has antidepressant
effects, although it seems less useful for severe major depression than for mild depression. There have been no
controlled data comparing St. John's wort's efficacy with
that of the SSRIs; however, NIMH has launched a study
that should provide this information within several years.

Dosing information: St. John's wort is available in
various forms, including extracts, teas, and crude
plant material. The recommended dose is 300 mg. of the
standard hypericin extract taken three times a day. Read
the supplements information label for the equivalent
amount.

Common side effects: Side effects include gastrointestinal symptoms (nausea, diarrhea, constipation,
or cramping), dizziness, sedation, dry mouth, restlessness,
and photosensitivity.

Warnings: German research has identified hypericin, the active ingredient in St. John's wort, as a
monoamine oxidase (MAO) inhibitor. However, this has
been challenged by at least one American study. Nonetheless, anyone taking an MAO inhibitor should avoid
St. John's wort because of the risk of a dangerous increase

in blood pressure. There have been no reported instances of an interaction between St. John's wort and tyramine-containing foods, which anyone taking an MAO inhibitor must avoid, as discussed in Chapter 2.

There is some laboratory evidence that St. John's wort may affect the neurotransmitters serotonin, dopamine, and norepinephrine. Because the combined effects of St. John's wort with prescription antidepressants may not be safe, consumers taking any antidepressant should not use St. John's wort. They also should be cautious about starting a prescription antidepressant after recent use of St. John's wort. Hypericin has a half-life of twenty-four to forty-eight hours, and as a precaution, it is advisable to wait two weeks before starting treatment with antidepressant medication.

St. John's wort may increase photosensitivity, and individuals regularly exposed to bright sunlight should avoid its use or use sunscreen before going outdoors.

Alcohol: Unknown.

Food and beverages: No restrictions.

Possible drug interactions: Individuals taking MAO inhibitors or other prescription antidepressants should not use St. John's wort.

Use in pregnancy and breast-feeding: Women who are pregnant or who are breast-feeding should not take St. John's wort.

Use in children: Not recommended.

Use in seniors: Lower doses may be recommended for seniors.

Overdosage: Unknown.

Special considerations: Anyone who is sufficiently depressed or anxious who is considering taking St. John's wort would benefit from an examination by a physician. Clinically significant anxiety or depression may require professional treatment, including use of an anti-anxiety agent or antidepressant. Do not combine these medications with St. John's wort.

Name: VALERIAN

Source: *Valeriana officinalis*. This plant is found in Europe and in the warmer climates of Asia. The root and other underground parts of the plant provide the active agent.

Indications: Anxiety and insomnia.

General information: Valerian has been used throughout the world for a variety of purposes, but primarily to treat anxiety and mild insomnia. It is believed to work by stimulating gamma-aminobutyric acid (GABA) receptors, which may reduce anxiety—the same mechanism of action thought to characterize the benzodiazepines. Although valerian has not been systematically studied in controlled trials, health professionals have reported that it has anxiety-relieving effects.

Dosing information: Dosage for valerian ranges from 2 to 3 g. of the dried root, often taken in a tea-like preparation three times a day for anxiety or at bedtime for insomnia. Read the nutrition supplements information label for the equivalent amount.

Common side effects: Gastrointestinal symptoms are rare. Individuals may experience headaches, restlessness, or sleep problems. Valerian has also been used externally as an addition to bathwater. The efficacy of this use is unproven. When taken orally, there are few adverse side effects.

Warnings: The sedative effects of valerian may be increased if taken with other anti-anxiety agents such as benzodiazepines. Anyone taking a benzodiazepine should not take valerian.

Alcohol: Avoid alcohol because its sedating properties can compound the sedative actions of valerian.

Food and beverages: No restrictions.

Possible drug interactions: Because this herbal preparation may produce increased sedation, avoid the use of other sedating medications, such as benzodiazepines, antihistamines, and pain medications.

Use in pregnancy and breast-feeding: Women who are pregnant or who are breast-feeding should not take valerian.

Use in children: Not recommended.

Use in seniors: Lower doses may be recommended for seniors.

Overdosage: Unknown; but profound sedation can be expected.

Special considerations: People who are sufficiently anxious or who are experiencing sleeping problems to such an extent that they are considering taking valerian would benefit from an examination by a physician. Clinically significant anxiety or insomnia may require professional treatment, including use of an anti-anxiety agent, antidepressant, or sleep medication.

Name: KAVA, KAVA-KAVA

Source: *Piper methysticum.* The plant is found in the South Sea Islands. The medicinal part of the plant is the rhizome, which has been separated from the roots.

Indications: Anxiety and insomnia.

General information: Kava has been used in the South Pacific for its sedative and anxiety-relieving properties. It is believed that the herb acts on gamma-aminobutyric acid (GABA) receptors, which may produce its anti-anxiety effects. The active compound of kava is the lactone preparation. In comparison to benzodiazepines, kava may have an advantage; it does not produce coordination or cognitive problems.

Dosing information: Kava is usually prescribed in a dose of 100 mg. of the kava extract twice a day (for anxiety) or at bedtime (for insomnia).

Common side effects: There have been reports of gastrointestinal symptoms, such as nausea, vomiting, diarrhea, and constipation. Other side effects include dilation of the pupils, decreased responsiveness of the eyes to changes in light, and a decrease in visual acuity. Higher doses have been reported to produce a scaling of the skin on the extremities, possibly related to vitamin B deficiency.

Warnings: Because kava may interact with benzodiazepines, individuals taking benzodiazepines should not take kava; the combination could produce significant sedation. Some individuals who take this preparation for sleep report daytime drowsiness upon wakening. Because of its sedative properties, depressed individuals who are taking antidepressants should not use kava.

Alcohol: Avoid alcohol.

Food and beverages: No restrictions.

Possible drug interactions: Avoid benzodiazepines, sedative antidepressants, or other medications that cause sedation as a side effect.

Use in pregnancy and breast-feeding: Women who are pregnant or breast-feeding should not take kava.

Use in children: Not recommended.

Use in seniors: Unknown.

Overdosage: Not reported.

Special considerations: People who are sufficiently anxious or who are experiencing insomnia to such an extent that they are considering taking kava would benefit from an examination by a physician. Clinically significant anxiety or insomnia may require professional treatment, including use of an anti-anxiety agent, antidepressant, or sleep medication.

Name: GINSENG or KOREAN GINSENG

Source: *Panax ginseng.* The medicinal part is the dried root of this plant. *Panax ginseng* is found in China, Korea, Japan, and Russia. This form of ginseng is different from Siberian ginseng, which has a different active ingredient and for which less information has been published in the U.S. medical literature.

Indications: Decreased energy and fatigue.

General information: Ginseng is used for a wide variety of conditions, including fatigue, to improve endurance, to relieve stress, and to enhance concentration.

Dosing information: Ginseng is available in many forms, including pills, capsules, and extracts. The average daily dose is 1 to 2 g. of the root. Read the supplements information label for the equivalent amount.

Common side effects: Common side effects are insomnia, restlessness, and anxiety. Some individuals have reported euphoria, gastrointestinal side effects such as diarrhea, and hypertension.

Warnings: Individuals using MAO inhibitors should not take ginseng because of the risk of dangerous increases in blood pressure. Individuals who take stimulants, especially caffeine, may become agitated. Individuals with hypertension or diabetes also should not use ginseng.

Alcohol: Avoid drinking alcohol, because alcohol increases fatigue and obscures any positive benefits of ginseng.

Food and beverages: Avoid large amounts of caffeine-containing beverages.

Possible drug interactions: Individuals taking prescribed stimulants, such as methylphenidate (Ritalin) or amphetamines, and those who drink large quantities of coffee or cola preparations that contain caffeine should not use ginseng. Individuals who are hypertensive and suffer from diabetes should be cautious about its use. People with sleep problems should avoid ginseng, since it frequently worsens sleep.

Use in pregnancy and breast-feeding: Women who are pregnant or breast-feeding should not take ginseng.

Use in children: Not recommended.

Use in seniors: Older individuals may experience sleeplessness, agitation, confusion, increase in blood pressure, and edema (fluid retention). Use with caution, and discuss the dosage with your physician.

Overdosage: Unknown.

Special considerations: People who are sufficiently tired or fatigued that they are considering taking ginseng would benefit from an examination by a physician. Clinically significant fatigue may be a symptom of an underlying medical illness or psychotic disorder, especially depression.

 Brand and Generic Name: MELATONIN

 Drug class: Hormone

Indications: Jet lag and insomnia resulting from shift work.

 General information: Melatonin is a hormone produced by the pineal gland in the brain during the early stages of sleep. Taking a low dose of melatonin in the early evening may cause the pineal gland to produce melatonin before it would normally be produced, causing individuals to fall asleep earlier and more quickly. Melatonin preparations are promoted as ways to assist the body in adjusting to different time zones (jet lag) or to new sleep patterns required by rotating work shifts. Melatonin is available in a synthetic form and as an extract obtained from a cow's pineal gland (a part of the brain). The synthetic form is preferable because it avoids possible impurities in the animal preparation.

Despite its popularity and the much-hyped claims for its usefulness, melatonin has not proven to be better than a placebo for alleviating jet-lag symptoms. In a comparison of three different dosage regimens of melatonin with a placebo in a group of 257 Norwegian doctors who were flying to Oslo from New York, researchers measured jet-lag severity by questioning the subjects daily about nine common symptoms: fatigue, daytime sleepiness, impaired concentration, decreased alertness, trouble with memory, clumsiness, weakness, lethargy, and light-headedness. Ratings were done on the day of travel and for the next six days. There was a marked increase in symptoms on the first day after arrival, with 63 percent of the doctors reporting at least moderate jet lag. Thereafter, symptoms improved steadily in all participants, with no significant difference among the four treatment groups. The apparent effectiveness of melatonin in previous studies may have represented a placebo effect.

Dosing information: The correct dose to take for treating jet lag or insomnia caused by shift work is unknown. The most common over-the-counter preparations are 3-mg. tablets that should be taken in the early evening. While smaller doses of 0.1 or 0.3 mg. are adequate, these may not be found in health-food stores.

Common side effects: The only side effect is mild sedation, which is desirable.

Warnings: None.

Alcohol: Individuals who are experiencing sleep problems should not drink alcohol because alcohol will further interfere with their sleep.

Food and beverages: Anyone with insomnia should restrict caffeine-containing beverages.

Possible drug interactions: Unknown.

Use in pregnancy and breast-feeding: Women who are pregnant or breast-feeding should not use melatonin.

Use in children: This has not been studied.

Use in seniors: Seniors, who often experience sleep problems, should discuss the best options for sleep improvement with their physicians.

Overdosage: Unknown.

Special considerations: If jet lag or insomnia resulting from shift work is a problem, consult your physician, who may prescribe medication known to be effective in treating these conditions, such as a benzodiazepine or non-benzodiazepine sleeping pill (see Chapter 5).

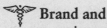

Brand and generic name: S-ADENOSYLME-THIONINE, or SAM-e (pronounced "sammy")

Source: SAM-e is a natural substance made from the amino acid methionine and the energy-producing compound adenosine triphosphate.

Indications: Mild depression.

General information: SAM-e is believed to work in the brain by enhancing the impact of serotonin and dopamine, although it is not known if it slows their breakdown, speeds up the production of receptors for these neurotransmitters, or makes the receptors more responsive.

SAM-e's impact on mood has been studied since the 1970s; it became available as a dietary supplement in the United States in March 1999. There have been about forty clinical studies, most of them small, and SAM-e has not won FDA approval as a treatment for any disorder. None of the research has shown SAM-e to be more effective than prescription antidepressants, although it may produce fewer side effects. There also is some evidence that SAM-e enhances the action of conventional antidepressants. One small study showed faster improvement in persons taking the tricyclic antidepressant imipramine who also were given 400 mg. of SAM-e daily. SAM-e can be expensive (costs range from $2.50 to $18 a pill), and pharmaceutical-grade (full-strength) SAM-e can be hard to obtain.

Dosing information: It is generally suggested that SAM-e be started at a dosage of 200 mg. taken twice a day, with a gradual increase to 400 mg. twice a day. The recommended maximum dose for mood improvement is generally 800 mg. twice a day.

Common side effects: Nausea and stomach upset.

Warnings: Individuals with bipolar disorder (manic depression) should not take SAM-e because of the risk of mood swings and worsened symptoms.

Alcohol: Unknown.

Food and beverages: Taking SAM-e on an empty stomach is believed to increase absorption. Enteric-coated capsules, which dissolve only in the intestine, also improve absorption and decrease gastrointestinal side effects.

Possible drug interactions: Because of its effects on liver function, SAM-e may speed the clearance of some drugs, but no information is available on specific drugs.

Use in pregnancy and breast-feeding: Women who are pregnant or who are breast-feeding should not take SAM-e.

Use in children: Not recommended.

 Use in seniors: SAM-e is also promoted for relieving arthritis pain and inflammation, common problems among seniors. Some see this as an additional potential benefit for older individuals with mild depression.

Overdosage: Unknown.

Special considerations: People who are sufficiently depressed to be considering taking SAM-e would benefit from an examination by a physician. Clinically significant depression may require professional treatment, including the use of antidepressant medication.

CHAPTER 10

Special Considerations for Women, Children, and Seniors

THE PREVIOUS CHAPTERS DISCUSSED THE USE OF MIND/ mood medications to treat psychiatric disorders in adults. This chapter focuses on three groups—women, children, and seniors—and special considerations involving their use of medications to treat mental disorders. Although the drug profiles in the previous chapters include specific information about drugs for these groups, this chapter discusses broader aspects of mind/mood treatments for them.

WOMEN

Women around the world are twice as likely to suffer depression than men; they are also more vulnerable to many anxiety disorders, including panic disorder and generalized anxiety disorder. Yet even though women are more likely to use mind/mood medications, most of these agents have been tested only in men. Although we need far more gender-specific research, we already know that mind/mood pills have different effects in women. In general, when taking the same doses as men, women have higher blood levels of these medications, especially if they are also using oral contraceptives or hormone-replacement therapy. Birth-control pills can raise blood levels of some agents so high that a woman may require only a fraction of the standard dose. Some medications also have stronger or weaker effects at different times in the menstrual cycle and may require adjustments in dose. Women have reported a worsening of certain conditions premenstrually, including depression and anxiety disorders, yet we know very little about the need to change dosage strengths during this time.

In the past, when tricyclics were the treatment of choice for depression, men generally reported greater benefits while women experienced more side effects. The advent of serotonin-boosting drugs—the SSRIs and other agents like nefazodone (Serzone) and fluvoxamine (Luvox)—has revolutionized treatment for women. These medications cause far fewer side effects in both sexes and have proven safer and easier to use, but they are especially beneficial to women, not only for depression, but also for phobias, panic disorder, obsessive-compulsive disorder, premenstrual mood disorders, bulimia, and mood disorders.

In general, antipsychotic medications are more effective in women than in men. However, women are more likely to suffer adverse reactions such as hypothyroidism and abnormal movements. Moreover, we do not yet fully understand how these drugs affect and are affected by oral contraceptives and hormone-replacement therapy.

Of all the special concerns regarding women and mind/mood pills, the one that has received the greatest attention over the years is pregnancy. The following section discusses what we know about the risks and benefits of drug treatment during pregnancy and after giving birth.

Pregnancy

Women who are contemplating pregnancy or who are pregnant should discuss the use of mind/mood medications with their primary-care physician and/or obstetrician-gynecologist. Whenever possible, women taking these drugs should discontinue them prior to conception or as soon as they realize they are pregnant. Since the blood flow from the mother through the placenta into the baby does not fully develop until two to three weeks after conception, the fetus is usually not exposed to medication between the time of conception and the first missed menstrual cycle. As noted in the previous chapters, the use of certain drugs is of most concern in the first trimester, when major organs are developing. Approximately 90 percent of women take one or more medications during pregnancy; as many as 35 percent take a psychoactive drug. The major risk of mind/mood pills is organ malformations, which are most likely to occur in the first twelve weeks of gestation.

Table 10-1 summarizes the major effects of mind/mood medications on the developing fetus and the FDA's pregnancy classifications for these drugs. As you will note, there is a wide range of effects upon the fetus. While we might wish not to use drug treatment during pregnancy, certain psychiatric disorders may worsen or first become evident during pregnancy, so it is not always possible or advisable to avoid mind/mood medications.

For women who are being treated for depression with antidepressants, newer medications—SSRIs, nefazodone (Serzone), venlafaxine (Effexor), and mirtazapine (Remeron)—are generally believed to be safe and not cause adverse effects on the baby's development, mind, mood, or temperament. In themselves, MAO inhibitors do not have adverse effects on the fetus, though they may produce a dangerous rise in blood pressure—a hypertensive crisis—in the mother. Researchers generally feel that tricyclic antidepressants, the most widely studied mind/mood drugs, do not cause congenital abnormalities, although babies may experience withdrawal symptoms at the time of birth because of the anticholinergic properties of such agents as amitriptyline (Elavil), desipramine (Norpramin), and nortriptyline (Pamelor). These include jitteriness, irritability,

Table 10-1: Potential Effects of Psychiatric Medications upon the Fetus

MEDICATION CLASS	DRUG	FDA RISK CATEGORY	POTENTIAL EFFECTS ON THE FETUS
Antidepressants	Tricyclic antidepressants (Elavil, Norpramin, etc.)	C/D	Increased heart rate and abnormal beats, withdrawal symptoms (jitteriness, irritability, lethargy, decreased muscle tone), anticholinergic effects (constipation, bowel obstruction, inability to urinate)
	MAO inhibitors	C	Rare effects on the fetus, hypertensive crisis in mother
	SSRIs (Prozac, Zoloft, Luvox, Paxil, Celexa)	C	Unknown
	Serzone	C	Unknown
	Effexor	C	Unknown
	Remeron	C	Unknown
Anti-anxiety and hypnotic agents	Benzodiazepines	D/X	Cleft palate, withdrawal symptoms, "floppy baby," decreased growth
	BuSpar	B	Unknown

Table 10-1: Potential Effects of Psychiatric Medications upon the Fetus (continued)

MEDICATION CLASS	DRUG	FDA RISK CATEGORY	POTENTIAL EFFECTS ON THE FETUS
Antipsychotic agents	Low-potency agents (Thorazine, Serentil, Mellaril)	C	Nonspecific abnormalities, jaundice, anticholinergic effects (constipation, inability or decreased ability to urinate)
	Intermediate- and high-potency agents (Haldol, Navane, others)	C	Unknown
	Atypical agents (Risperdal, Seroquel, Zyprexa)	C	Unknown
	Clozaril	B	Unknown
Mood stabilizers	Lithium	D	Heart abnormalities, decreased muscle tone, poor suck reflex, decreased blood sugar, goiter, cyanosis (blue baby with decreased oxygen)

Table 10-1: Potential Effects of Psychiatric Medications upon the Fetus (continued)

MEDICATION CLASS	DRUG	FDA RISK CATEGORY	POTENTIAL EFFECTS ON THE FETUS
Mood stabilizers (continued)	Depakote	D	Neural-tube defects (spina bifida), craniofacial defects, decreased development of fingernails, heart abnormalities
	Tegretol	C	Neural-tube defects (spina bifida), craniofacial defects, decreased development of fingernails, heart abnormalities
	Neurontin	C	Unknown
	Lamictal	C	Unknown

FDA Pregnancy Risk Categories

A=Controlled studies show no risk to humans.

B=No evidence of risk in humans but adequate human studies have not been performed.

C=Risk cannot be ruled out.

D=Positive evidence of risk to humans; risk may be outweighed by potential benefit.

X=Potential risks to the fetus outweigh benefits of the drug. The drug should not be used during pregnancy.

lethargy, decreased muscle tone, constipation (and even bowel obstruction), and decreased ability to urinate.

Some investigators have noted a significant increase in cleft palate and other facial abnormalities in babies whose mothers used benzodiazepines during pregnancy. Infants also may experience decreased growth in the womb, withdrawal symptoms, have problems feeding, and have "floppy baby" syndrome (decreased muscle tone). The risk of cleft palate may be greater with alprazolam (Xanax) and diazepam (Valium) than other benzodiazepines, but the data are still unclear. For women who have generalized anxiety disorder, buspirone (BuSpar) is a reasonable alternative to these drugs, since it has not been found to produce fetal abnormalities.

As a rule, women suffering from schizophrenia must continue use of their antipsychotic medication. Traditional high-potency agents such as haloperidol (Haldol) are believed to be safe. Low-potency agents such as chlorpromazine (Thorazine) or thioridazine (Mellaril) may produce anticholinergic effects in the baby, such as constipation and decreased ability to urinate. In addition, these drugs are associated with a higher incidence of newborn jaundice and other nonspecific abnormalities. The atypical agents, such as risperidone (Risperdal) and clozapine (Clozaril), have not been reported to produce any adverse effects in babies. However, because they are relatively new, we need more experience with these medications before we can draw definite conclusions about their safety for the fetus.

Mood stabilizers, such as lithium, divalproex (Depakote), and carbamazepine (Tegretol), pose a greater potential risk to the fetus than other mind/mood medications. Sometimes it is possible for women with bipolar disorder who want to get pregnant to taper off their medications gradually and, if no relapse occurs, to discontinue them prior to conception. However, there are times when the risk of a relapse is too great to try this approach, and medication must be continued because the danger of a manic episode is greater than the risk associated with mood stabilizers.

In such instances, lithium is often the preferred mood stabilizer during pregnancy; it carries a lower risk of producing abnormalities in a developing baby than does divalproex or carbamazepine. This does not mean it is entirely safe, however. The use of lithium in the first trimester has been associated with a rare cardiac defect called Ebstein's anomaly, in which one of the heart valves is displaced into the right ventricle. The estimated likelihood of this happening is about 1 in 1,000 cases. Lithium's use in the third trimester has been linked with floppy baby syndrome, which is characterized by decreased muscle tone. A study has found no adverse outcomes of any type in five-year-old children exposed to lithium in pregnancy.

First-trimester use of carbamazepine has been associated with a 1 percent rate of neural-tube defects, as well as developmental delays and head and facial anomalies. With divalproex, there is a 1 to 2 percent risk of spina bifida (incomplete development of the spinal cord) with exposure in the first trimester. Folate supplements before and after conception, which are recommended for all women planning a pregnancy, may reduce the risk of neural-tube defects in women using these mood stabilizers. It is not yet known whether newer medications, such as Neurontin (gabapentin) and Lamictal (lamotrigine), produce defects in the developing fetus. A reasonable alternative to medication for a pregnant woman with mania is electroconvulsive therapy (ECT), which produces fewer adverse effects.

Breast-feeding

The general recommendation is that mothers taking mind/mood medications not nurse their babies. Most psychiatric medications are absorbed into the breast milk, and so would also be absorbed into the baby's bloodstream. Since the level of medication that eventually reaches the baby's developing central nervous system is small, the seriousness of this problem may be relatively mild. However, there are no controlled studies that have examined the effects of various mind/mood medications on babies, so women taking these drugs should avoid breast-feeding.

Postpartum

Approximately 85 percent of women may experience some degree of postpartum "blues," a condition characterized by tearfulness, sadness, rapidly shifting moods, anxiety, and depression that usually begins a few days after birth and ends within a week or two. Women with a history of premenstrual depressive symptoms or a family history of depression are probably at greater risk of this condition.

Approximately 10 percent of all women experience a full-blown major depression following delivery. In women with a prior history of major depression, the risk of postpartum depression increases to 24 percent; in those who have previously experienced such a depression, it rises to 50 percent. Women with a family and a personal history of bipolar disorder are at even greater risk. The treatment of postpartum depression is similar to that used for other major depressive disorders. The same cautions discussed above concerning breast-feeding apply to women taking antidepressants.

In approximately 1 of every 1,000 births, the mother may develop postpartum psychosis. This risk is greater in women who have a history of bipolar disorder, and is estimated to be 35 percent. For women who have had a previous postpartum psychosis, the risk of another episode ranges from 20 to 30 percent.

CHILDREN AND ADOLESCENTS

Many of the mind/mood problems that occur in adults also develop in children: depression, anxiety, attention disorders, eating disorders, sleep problems, substance abuse disorders, and psychotic disorders. Certain other disorders are unique to childhood and adolescence or require special consideration in young people. These include disruptive behaviors—problems of attention, conduct, or opposition—that can be difficult for parents to assess. Some youngsters may simply be testing the limits to find out what is acceptable and accepted behavior and what isn't. In other cases, there may be an underlying problem that is responsible for a child's extreme physical activity, defiance, or aggression.

Choosing a mind/mood medication for a child or young adolescent who requires drug treatment is an important decision that requires expert consultation with a skilled physician, preferably a psychiatrist who is knowledgeable about the use of medications in the young. There are no clinical trials that have examined the long-term effects of psychiatric medications upon a child or adolescent's developing brain, maturation, social development, and overall well-being. As with pregnancy and breast-feeding, the decision to use such medications in children or adolescents should carefully weigh benefits against any potential or unknown dangers.

Unfortunately, in the past, children were excluded from clinical trials, and the FDA had few data to evaluate the effects of psychiatric medications upon children. We do know that children or adolescents metabolize these drugs quite rapidly. Their livers work very efficiently and their kidneys also readily excrete medications. Because of this, children, especially before puberty, are able to tolerate adult doses. However, doses should be started low and gradually increased. By puberty, adolescents begin to metabolize and excrete medications in a manner similar to adults.

The correct dosage of medication in children is determined by either their body weight or surface area, and is usually prescribed in a milligram-per-kilogram ratio. Because children are normally quite active, the milligram-per-kilogram dose is generally greater than it would be in adults. For children who require psychiatric medications, the physician always attempts to avoid the use of multiple agents or keeps them to a minimum. In addition, parents need to understand the reason for the use of the medication, a child or adolescent's normal response to the drug, and how the medication may be adjusted to minimize side effects. Whenever possible, medications are not prescribed to prepubertal children more than twice a day, to avoid the need to take them during school. Some medications, such as certain antidepressants, may be taken in a single dose at bedtime. Others come in an extended-release formulation that enables the child to take the medication prior to going to school.

Attention Deficit Hyperactivity Disorder

The term *hyperactive* has been used so loosely over the years that parents may hear it applied to any child who seems particularly energetic or rambunctious. Although all children become restless and fidgety at times, relatively few—an estimated 3 to 5 percent of school-age children— suffer from an actual disorder. These youngsters are not merely squirmy or distractible. Some consistently cannot focus their attention; others are unable to resist an impulse to blurt out what's on their mind or to grab what they want. At home and at school, the behavior of these youngsters isn't simply more active than that of others their age, but more chaotic, reckless, and disorganized.

Psychiatrists themselves have used different terms to refer to attention and activity problems in children: minimal brain damage, minimal brain dysfunction, hyperactivity, and hyperkinetic syndrome. The current diagnostic term, attention deficit hyperactivity disorder (ADHD), refers to a spectrum of problems, from impulsivity to distractibility, that may or may not include hyperactivity per se (excessive running, jumping, climbing, etc.).

Boys, who usually have more visible symptoms, such as persistent, extremely active behavior, are diagnosed as having ADHD far more often than girls, who tend to develop more subtle signs, such as an inability to concentrate. Many youngsters have symptoms, such as being impulsive or inattentive, that may suggest possible ADHD but do not meet the diagnostic criteria.

For years scientists have debated possible causes of childhood attention problems, including food additives, excessive sugar intake, lead poisoning, head trauma, and dysfunctional families. Carefully controlled studies have failed to show any significant link between sugar consumption, once theorized to be a culprit, and ADHD, nor have any of the other alleged culprits proved to be responsible.

ADHD probably has multiple causes. Genetics plays a role in about 40 percent of cases; these youngsters often have several close biological relatives with the same problem. In some cases, a viral infection may contribute to the condition. The incidence of ADHD increases, for instance, after an outbreak of encephalitis. Other cases may stem from an occurrence in pregnancy—possibly exposure to infection, alcohol, nicotine, cocaine, toxins, or environmental factors—that affected the prenatal development of key areas in the brain that regulate movement and attentiveness. Researchers at the National Institute of Mental Health, using positron emission tomography (PET) scans, have found that children and adults with attention disorders are slower to metabolize glucose, the brain's main energy source.

Seeking Help

Often parents aren't sure whether their pint-sized perpetual-motion machine is hyperactive or simply energetic. It is very difficult to diagnose attention deficit hyperactivity disorder (ADHD) prior to age four or five because preschoolers are typically active and impulsive and may not be able to focus their attention for a sustained period of time. If you are trying to get a handle on your child's behavior, ask yourself whether your child:

- Fidgets or squirms constantly
- Has a hard time sitting still
- Is easily distracted
- Can't wait for a turn in games or groups
- Blurts out answers to questions before they've been completed
- Is unable to follow through on instructions from others
- Finds it hard to concentrate on tasks or play
- Shifts from one uncompleted activity to another
- Has difficulty playing quietly
- Talks excessively
- Interrupts or intrudes on others
- Often doesn't seem to be listening or paying attention
- Constantly loses toys, pencils, books

- Does dangerous things, like running into the
  street, without considering the consequences

If you answer yes to several of these questions, the
problem could be attention deficit hyperactivity disorder
(ADHD). However, the range of symptoms in this disorder
is broad, and even mental-health professionals may find it
hard to distinguish between normal and abnormal behaviors. In making an evaluation, they rely on a comprehensive interview with the child, as well as evaluations from
teachers and parents and standardized assessment scales.
For a diagnosis of ADHD, the behaviors must persist for
at least six months and be so severe that they cause great
distress or impair a child's functioning at home or school
or in social situations. In making the diagnosis, therapists
distinguish between various types of ADHD, depending on
whether symptoms of inattention, hyperactivity-impulsivity,
or a combination predominate.

Treating Attention Deficit Hyperactivity Disorder (ADHD)

A combination of medication, remedial education, behavior modification, individual counseling, and family therapy
is most effective in treating this disorder. Parents can help
by learning as much as possible about the disorder, avoiding stressful situations that may cause fatigue, frustration,
or overstimulation for the child, and establishing regular
routines and consistent limits. Many find classes in parent-
ing skills or programs for parents of hyperactive children
useful.

The primary drugs used in treating attention deficit hyperactivity disorder (ADHD) are stimulants—methylphenidate
(Ritalin), dextroamphetamine (Dexedrine), dextrometham-
phetamine hydrochloride (Desoxyn), and magnesium
pemoline (Cylert)—which have a paradoxical effect on individuals with this condition, reducing rather than height-

ening their activity level. Rather than being stimulating, as they are in those without the disorder, these medications improve performance of various tasks, possibly by enhancing concentration.

Youngsters who do not respond to a particular stimulant may improve with another one or with the antidepressants Norpramin (desipramine), Tofranil (imipramine), or Pamelor (nortriptyline). Short-term side effects, which occur in less than 5 percent of youngsters, include insomnia, loss of appetite and weight, headaches, and stomachaches. Clonidine (Catapres), a drug used to treat hypertension, is sometimes used, usually along with a stimulant, for youngsters with ADHD who are extremely agitated, hyperactive, impulsive, or defiant. It often helps them fall asleep, overcomes their refusal to go to bed, and counteracts the effects of stimulants. However, it can make children drowsy, at least during the initial weeks of treatment.

In follow-up studies, parents, teachers, physicians, or therapists rate 75 percent of hyperactive children given stimulants as improved, compared to 40 percent of those taking a placebo. Nevertheless, although medication helps, particularly in decreasing excessive physical activity, these children typically continue to have some problems. A therapist can teach parents behavioral techniques, such as sending children to a quiet spot for a time-out if they become disruptive, that improve behavior. Supportive psychotherapy helps to deal with low self-esteem and other problems related to ADHD. Family therapy can also be beneficial.

About one-third of children with ADHD continue to show some signs of this disorder in adolescence and adulthood. (Chapter 7 discusses adult attention disorders.) Teens and young adults with the condition are much more likely to cause or be involved in auto accidents than other young drivers. A national support and educational organization, Children with Attention Deficit Disorders (CHADD), can provide helpful information and referrals.

Depressive Disorders

Like adults, children can have mood swings and feel down in the dumps or blue. While symptoms of being depressed, such as feeling sad, are common among youngsters of all ages, major depression is more intense, more enduring, more disabling, and more serious. Clinical depression takes different forms in children of different ages. A preschooler may become listless, lose interest in playing, and cry easily and often. A grade-schooler may pull away from family and friends, have problems with schoolwork, and seem sad and discouraged. A teenager may argue with parents and teachers, refuse to do chores or homework, and drop out of sports or other favorite activities. At any age, depressed youngsters may be irritable and extremely self-critical. Parents may not be able to tell whether their child is "going through a phase" or struggling with depression; mental-health professionals experienced in evaluating and treating children and teenagers can.

By conservative estimates, about 2 percent of children and 4.7 percent of adolescents develop major depression. An additional 3.3 percent of teenagers suffer from chronic mild depression, or dysthymia. Some investigators believe that the incidence of depressive disorders in the young is much higher than these figures suggest. In a study of 508 boys and girls in elementary school who were followed for five years beginning in the third or fourth grade, researchers from Stanford University and the University of Pennsylvania found that 10 to 15 percent were moderately to severely depressed. In a 1988 study of almost 1,500 boys and girls, the percentage of depressed girls zoomed up from about 8 percent in the preteen years—about the same as for boys in childhood and adolescence—to 16 percent among those between the ages of fourteen and sixteen.

As in adults, the causes of depression in children are complex. Some may inherit a biological predisposition, and depressed children often live with a depressed parent, usually their mother. Depression also may develop after extreme stress or a traumatic loss, experiences that can lead to deep feelings of helplessness and hopelessness.

Different factors may have more of an impact at different ages. Among younger children, negative life events, such as divorce, a close relative's death, or a major financial setback for the family, have the greatest impact. As youngsters get older, their way of interpreting an event becomes equally important. Children who blame themselves (for example, concluding that they got a poor report card because they're "stupid" rather than because they didn't study hard), or who take the pessimistic view that more bad things will happen in the future, are most likely to develop depression. In a study of third-, fourth-, and fifth-graders rejected by their classmates, those who blamed the rejection on something wrong with them were likely to become depressed, whereas those who felt they might be able to turn things around were not.

Depression in children can interfere with their personal development and their acquisition of basic social skills. Moreover, once youngsters become moderately depressed, they often don't "get over it"; they may stay that way for a very long time and may be more vulnerable to depression throughout life.

Seeking Help

If you suspect that depression may be a problem, ask yourself whether your child:

- Seems sad, discouraged, bored, or irritable

- Has lost interest in favorite activities

- Has stopped taking part in after-school sports or hobbies

- Is not gaining weight at the expected rate

- Is sluggish and lethargic or becomes agitated and restless
- Feels tired all the time
- Has withdrawn from family and friends
- Pretends to be sick to stay away from school, sports, or play
- Seems to cover up sadness with lots of activity or aggression
- Argues over everything
- Cries easily and often
- Has poor self-esteem and negative feelings about him- or herself and others
- Has no interest in food
- Sleeps much more or less than usual
- Has nightmares or is extremely restless while sleeping
- Gets poor grades
- Argues with teachers
- Cannot get schoolwork done
- Refuses to do chores
- Expresses feelings of hopelessness

If the answer is yes to several of these questions and the symptoms have persisted for two weeks or more, the problem could be a depressive disorder. Mental-health professionals base their diagnosis on a careful interview with the child. They ask questions about his or her mood in age-appropriate terms, such as using the word "cranky" rather than "irritable" with a younger child. In making the diagnosis, they consider all aspects of a child's functioning and physical and mental state. Depression in children may be marked by an irritable mood rather than sadness, and by a failure to gain weight as expected, rather than actually losing weight.

Depression can be a fatal disease. More than half of all teens who attempt suicide are depressed. Because of the risk of suicide, therapists ask depressed children or adolescents whether they have thought about dying or killing themselves, whether they wish to die, and whether a friend or relative has recently committed suicide. Discussing such feelings openly can become an important part of the therapeutic process.

Dysthymia (chronic mild depression) in children and teens can impair schoolwork and relationships with peers and adults. The symptoms of this disorder in youngsters are similar to those in adults, except that their mood may be irritable rather than depressed and they are likely to feel this way for one year, rather than two. In addition to being depressed or irritable, children with dysthymia tend to react to almost everything, including praise or an invitation to participate in a fun activity, in a negative way. They may also eat and sleep much more or less than usual, have little energy, show poor self-esteem, have problems concentrating, and feel hopeless.

Treating Depressive Disorders

The primary treatment for depression in children and teens is psychotherapy—individual, family, or both. Family therapy is especially helpful if other family members also suffer from depression. Interpersonal therapy, which has proved effective in adults, also holds promise for children; it helps them express feelings and communicate better with others, particularly their parents.

Mental-health professionals who work with children usually modify the same approaches they use for adults.

Rather than talking, they may use children's drawings, storytelling, and play, for example, to help youngsters express difficulties. A child's comments about a figure in a drawing or a doll may indicate low self-esteem or feelings of loneliness. Through such interactions, the therapist can point out the many good things about the child or teach new ways of reaching out to others. With older children, therapists may use cognitive-behavioral techniques in the same way they would with adults. If a teenager believes that no one likes her because one group of girls has snubbed her, for instance, the therapist might point out that she is generalizing and encourage her to focus on the much larger number of her peers who are friendly.

For youngsters who do not improve within four to six weeks, child psychiatrists may prescribe antidepressant medications. It is difficult to predict which children will respond to medications—and even more difficult to do so in adolescents, who have a high placebo response. Psychotherapy continues to remain an important part of therapy, not only to help youngsters deal with psychological issues that may have contributed to the depression, but also to deal with what it means to a child to have a "condition," take a pill, and need to work through problems in therapy.

Before prescribing medication, a child psychiatrist may check pulse and blood pressure and order various tests, including a baseline electrocardiogram (EKG), complete blood count, and blood chemistry. Usually an antidepressant is prescribed for eight to twelve weeks to see if it helps. If it proves useful, drug treatment usually continues for nine to twelve months; then the medication is gradually reduced to determine whether the child can do without it. If not, the youngster goes back on medication for another six to twelve months. Maintenance therapy over a period of months or even years, which has proved very helpful in preventing recurrences in adults, has not been studied in children.

Children are at risk for the same medication side effects

as adults (see Chapter 2). Parents should closely supervise administration of medication and keep the pills in a secure place. Youngsters taking certain drugs, such as tricyclic antidepressants, will need monitoring of their blood and heart rates. Children tolerate the newer antidepressants very well and do not require special monitoring.

Anxiety Disorders

Although adults may like to think of children as carefree, worry is common at every age. However, the nature of youngsters' worries and fears varies as they grow. A two-year-old may be terrified of the vacuum cleaner, and a four-year-old be afraid of the dark. In elementary school, children may come to worry most about tests and school performance. In high school, teenagers may worry about being liked by their peers.

Whatever the source of apprehensiveness or fear, there is a difference between feeling anxious and having an anxiety disorder, which is a more serious, longer-lasting problem. The anxiety disorders—the most common mental disorders among children as well as adults—include phobias, such as intense fear of insects or dogs, extreme anxiety when separated from loved ones (usually parents), excessive shrinking from contact with unfamiliar people, and persistent and unrealistic overanxiousness.

Two to 8 percent of children and adolescents develop anxiety disorders, which often overlap with depression. After puberty these are more common in girls than in boys. Many more children suffer from undue anxiety, even though they may not have a true anxiety disorder.

Children with anxiety symptoms or an anxiety disorder benefit greatly from treatments that help them to relax, bring their fears out into the open, and teach them practical coping skills. They often respond well to behavioral techniques such as relaxation training, systematic desensitization, and assertiveness training. Cognitive therapy, for children old enough to grasp the basic concepts, may reduce anxiety by changing self-defeating thoughts. Family therapy can also be useful in dealing with issues that affect not only the youngster but parents and siblings as well. In some cases, mind/mood medication may be part of the treatment.

Obsessive-Compulsive Disorder

Various studies have shown that 0.4 to 1 percent of youngsters develop obsessive-compulsive disorder (OCD), a malfunction of information-relaying mechanisms within the brain that causes repetitive thoughts or ritualistic behaviors to spin out of control. However, many therapists believe that this problem is far more common than the percentages indicate.

OCD can run in families. About 20 percent of affected children have a family member with the disorder. In a study of seventy children with OCD conducted by the Child Psychiatry Branch of the National Institute of Mental Health, the mean age at onset was 10.2 years, with boys outnumbering girls by more than 2 to 1. Most children develop a single obsession or compulsion and then shift to another after a period of months or years. At least three-quarters wash their hands excessively. Teenagers may develop obsessive sexual thoughts, such as fear of AIDS, that trigger the washing. As in adults, obsessions and compulsions can become so severe that they interfere with normal living and make children miserable. OCD tends to be chronic, although symptoms may come and go over the years, often flaring up during times of change or crisis.

Treatment with clomipramine (Anafranil) or an SSRI such as fluoxetine (Prozac), combined with behavioral therapy and psychotherapy, leads to improvement in 75 percent of youngsters with OCD. In severe cases, medications are used for children under ten as well as for older ones. Although symptoms are rarely eliminated entirely, the medication can reduce the force of obsessions and compulsions and greatly improve the quality of a child's life.

SPECIAL MEDICATION ISSUES IN CHILDREN

Medications can play a useful role in relieving symptoms of certain problems, such as attention deficit hyperactivity disorder (ADHD), depression, and certain anxiety disorders, and may enable children to benefit from psycho therapy and other behavioral approaches. Because many medications have not been tested in children, often little is known about possible side effects or optimal doses.

The use of medication in children can be very complicated. Every drug has more than one effect. Because children metabolize and respond to drugs differently from adults, they may have rapid and unpredictable swings in blood levels of a medication, from too much to too little. In addition, youngsters are growing physically, mentally, and emotionally, and medication must not interfere with their development.

Child psychiatrists are best qualified to prescribe and supervise the use of medications in children. They are most experienced in weighing the risks of a disorder with what is known about the relative efficacy and the side effects of medication. Frequent follow-ups are an important part of treatment.

Parents and, to whatever extent is possible, children themselves should learn about how a specific medication works and about its side effects. Parents need to be informed about the complete range of possible effects, including those involving thinking and behavior as well as physical reactions, and they must know when they should call the psychiatrist. It is critical that parents be aware of any dangers of abuse or overdose. Except for certain anti-anxiety agents, psychiatric medications are not addictive.

There is no evidence that children who take medications for a mental or emotional disorder are more likely to develop drug abuse problems later in life.

Medication schedules must be followed conscientiously, with parents supervising their children's drug-taking. Taking medications as directed often requires the cooperation of teachers and child-care providers. If a child refuses medication, if parents don't believe that their child really needs a drug, or if school personnel cannot follow a schedule for giving medication, many of the potential benefits of drug therapy may be lost.

SENIORS

We are getting older, not just as individuals but as a society. Men and women over the age of fifty-five make up more than a fifth of our population. By the year 2010, 1 in 4 Americans—some 74.1 million people—will be over fifty-five; 1 in 7 will be sixty-nine or older. Just as the number of senior citizens is growing every day, so is their life expectancy. Today's sixty-five-year-olds, far healthier than were their parents and grandparents who survived that long, can expect to live nearly two more decades.

Older people face a variety of medical, economic, social, and psychological challenges. They may not get adequate nutrition. They may become increasingly isolated. Impaired mobility or vision may interfere with their ability to function from day to day. Hearing loss can be particularly devastating because it is so isolating. They may think that others are talking about them in deliberately low tones so as not to be overheard; unable to discern what others are saying, they may withdraw and become depressed or suspicious. With the passage of time, many older people develop serious diseases such as arthritis, arteriosclerosis, cancer, and osteoporosis. The death of contemporaries, hospitalization, the loss of a home in a fire or flood, or other unexpected catastrophes can have a much greater impact than they would at earlier stages of life. The cumulative impact of stressful events, one often following another before the individual has had time to adjust, can take a toll on physical and emotional well-being.

The American Psychiatric Association estimates that 15 to 25 percent of the elderly have significant symptoms of mental illness. As many as half of all older people hospitalized for medical or surgical reasons develop psychiatric difficulties, such as delirium. Some of these symptoms are caused by malnutrition, abnormal thyroid activity, drug side effects, or depression, and can be reversed. Severe mental illnesses, including delusions and paranoia, affect nearly 1 million elderly Americans. Many more suffer milder forms of mental disorders or develop age-related problems such as Alzheimer's and other forms of dementia.

Seniors have a decreased ability to excrete medications because of reduced kidney function. Consequently, medications like lithium, which are excreted unchanged in the urine, may rise to dangerous levels. In contrast to children and adults, seniors usually metabolize medications less well, because their livers do not function as efficiently as they did earlier in life. In addition, there is usually less protein in the bloodstream of older individuals. This is important because the active agent in mind/mood medications is believed to be that of the drug that does not bind to proteins. In seniors, more of this unbound active agent is available to be absorbed into the central nervous system to produce desired effects, such as decreased anxiety or depression. As a result, lower doses of medications produce the same effects that higher ones do in younger adults.

Seniors are more sensitive to side effects of drugs, such as the anticholinergic effects caused by certain tricyclics and the older low-potency antipsychotic agents. These effects include a drop in blood pressure when going from a sitting to standing position (orthostatic hypotension), constipation, blurred vision, decreased ability to urinate, dry mouth, and increased risk of dental cavities. In addition, antidepressants and antipsychotic agents are more likely to cause confusion, tremor, and abnormal movements in older individuals.

One of the greatest risks older persons face is the increased potential for falls, especially with benzodiazepines, certain antipsychotic agents, and certain antidepressants such as tricyclic antidepressants and MAO inhibitors. Seniors who do fall and fracture a hip are at much greater risk for complications. Some do not leave the hospital alive; others require nursing-home care; many may suffer another fall. For all these reasons, the standard practice is to prescribe low doses of these medications for seniors and to increase the dose gradually over a longer period of time than in younger adults. A medication that might be increased every three to four days in a younger person may be delayed for seven to ten days in older individuals to decrease the risk of falls as well as other adverse side effects.

Loss and Grief

Life's final years, once described as "the season of loss," may mean the gradual loss or end of many things: a partner, gratifying work, cherished friendships, financial and physical independence. Retiring after a successful career can seem like the end of purposeful existence. As friends and family die or move away, social networks can disintegrate. Diminished physical abilities can change the way individuals view themselves and their future. Those who can no longer see, hear, or get around as well as they once did may mourn the loss of the sense of safety and freedom they once had. Even senior citizens without physical limitations may be fearful—and often justifiably so—of venturing out after dark or walking through certain parks or neighborhoods. Regardless of their current health, many worry about what the future might bring, such as the loss of financial, social, domestic, or physical independence.

Developing effective coping strategies and reaching out for support from family and friends can be crucial in dealing with these difficult issues.

Regardless of age, the loss of a loved one is always the most stressful of life's traumas. This remains true later in life, when grieving survivors drink more alcohol, take more anti-anxiety drugs, and require more frequent hospitalization than others their age. The phases of grief are common to all ages. Initially, individuals feel shock, disbelief, emptiness, confusion, numbness, and free-floating anxiety. They have problems sleeping, lose their appetites, and experience muscle aches and pains. It takes about four to six weeks for the finality of the loss to hit. A widow or widower may yearn to be reunited with a spouse, yet feel anger at being abandoned and left behind. Hallucinations, such as seeing the dead person seated in a favorite chair, are common. About 15 to 25 percent of bereaved individuals still show signs of significant distress, particularly major depression, a year or two after a loss.

In general, widows are more susceptible to mental-health problems, such as depression and anxiety disorders, whereas widowers tend to develop more physical illnesses, particularly heart disease, and face increased risk of dying within a year of their wife's death. Two years after a loss, older men and women seem to fare about the same in terms of depression, life satisfaction, and resolution of their grief.

Depression

Most older people do not become clinically depressed, although symptoms of depression frequently occur. Nonetheless, according to a 1992 report by the National Institutes of Health consensus development panel on depression in late life, about 15 percent of men and women over sixty-five living in the community experience clinically significant depression. In nursing homes the rate ranges from 15 to 25 percent. Recurrences are common, with 40 percent suffering repeated episodes. Older men and women who become depressed are more likely to develop psychotic symptoms, such as hallucinations and delusions, than younger ones.

In late life, as at other times, the causes of depression are complex. Some older individuals have a biological predisposition or a history of depression that makes them vulnerable. Others often have lost a spouse or have few social supports. Health problems and restrictions or a sense of not having fulfilled life expectations may contribute to depression. Some medications, including drugs widely taken for high blood pressure, can also play a role.

Late-life depression can be particularly hard to identify. Some of its classic signs—appetite changes, weight loss, insomnia, and fatigue—may be mistakenly attributed to medical problems, medications, or old age itself. Psychiatrists experienced in geriatric care can sort out the underlying causes of telltale symptoms; other physicians may not be able to do so. In one study of 150 older individuals admitted to a hospital for medical reasons, the examining physician did not detect a single case of depression, yet a psychiatrist who interviewed the same individuals found that 15 percent were severely depressed. In older men and women, psychological symptoms such as tearfulness or sadness may be absent or denied, whereas symptoms such as lack of pleasure and physical complaints are more frequent or intense.

The consequences of not recognizing and treating depression that occurs late in life can be tragic. Depression that develops after an illness or injury, if not identified, can hinder recovery; depression following a heart attack or stroke can increase mortality. Older Americans have the highest suicide rate in our society, with some 8,500 elderly persons killing themselves every year. The suicide rate at age sixty-five is five times higher than that of younger individuals. It continues to increase with age, especially among white men. Mental-health professionals who are working with a depressed elderly person often meet with family members and enlist their aid in getting their older relatives involved in activities and monitoring them for any signs of suicidal thoughts or behavior.

More than 70 percent of the depressed elderly improve dramatically with treatment, which usually consists of a combination of psychotherapy and medication, often along with family counseling. (Similar improvement occurs when cognitive impairment is treated.) Various methods of psychotherapy, including cognitive and behavioral therapies, have proved effective with older men and women. Common issues addressed in treatment include rapid and cumulative losses and a sense of defenselessness and hopelessness.

Antidepressant drugs can help (see Chapter 2), but psychiatrists pay special attention to the increased risk of side effects, such as dizziness on sitting or standing abruptly, in selecting a medication for older individuals. Often lower doses are adequate. Another strategy for decreasing side effects is dividing the dose by taking half the usual amount twice a day rather than the full dose at once.

Because of physiological differences caused by age, older individuals usually respond more slowly to antidepressants than younger persons, and it can take from eight to twelve weeks for benefits to be apparent.

Anxiety Disorders

Anxiety disorders can occur at any age, but in general their incidence decreases with age. According to the National Institute of Mental Health's epidemiological data, the older individuals are, the less the likelihood of their developing a serious anxiety disorder. However, anxiety itself is a common symptom among older persons, with about 20 percent reporting some physical or psychological signs of anxiety. In late life, anxiety symptoms often occur along with depression.

Sometimes particular circumstances, such as increased difficulty in driving, cause episodic anxiety that abates under different circumstances. Caffeine is a common culprit, particularly when individuals combine their usual coffee intake with over-the-counter medications, such as analgesics that contain caffeine or cold remedies with ephedrine. In cases of more intense and persistent anxiety, health problems such as hyperthyroidism or cardiac arrhythmias may be responsible. Withdrawal after long use of certain substances, among them alcohol and the benzodiazepines, can also cause significant anxiety in the elderly.

Counseling that emphasizes behavioral and relaxation techniques can be very helpful in easing anxiety. Medication also has proved effective. Because many drugs remain active in the elderly for much longer periods than in younger people, psychiatrists usually prescribe short-acting benzodiazepines for treatment of anxiety. These drugs must be reduced or discontinued after a few weeks because long-term use can produce cumulative harmful effects, including confusion and psychosis. To avoid withdrawal symptoms, psychiatrists taper off the dose gradually over a week or so. The non-benzodiazepine anti-anxiety agent buspirone (BuSpar) is not sedating, does not interact with alcohol, has no potential for abuse, and does not interfere with a person's ability to perform motor tasks or drive a car. However, it may take somewhat longer than the benzodiazepines—about two to four weeks—for individuals to experience its full benefits.

Sleep Disorders

Sleep changes drastically in both quality and quantity over the course of a lifetime. A twenty-year-old falls asleep in about eight minutes and spends half an hour or longer in the deepest, most restful sleep stages. An eighty-year-old takes eighteen minutes to fall asleep and spends only a few minutes, if any, in deep sleep. The young person spends 95 percent of the night asleep, racking up an average of seven and a half to eight hours. The older person spends only 80 percent of the night asleep, with a total sleep time of about six hours.

In epidemiological surveys, about one-third of older men and women report sleep problems. The most common are insomnia (difficulty falling or staying asleep), breathing-related disorders (such as sleep apnea), periodic leg movements that disturb sleep (nocturnal myoclonus), and a mismatch between sleep-wake patterns and the environment, which in the elderly most often involves falling asleep in the early evening and waking before dawn. Medical and mental disorders, including depression and anxiety, and medications can also contribute to sleep disturbances.

Treatment often depends on identifying and correcting an underlying problem, such as depression or alcohol dependence, that may be causing the insomnia. Improved sleep habits, sometimes combined with relaxation techniques, are the best long-term option for insomnia. For older men and women, the most helpful guidelines are:

- Establishing regular hours for waking, meals, and bedtime

- Not spending too much time in bed during the day

- Not going to bed too early

- Not drinking alcohol to get to sleep

- Getting some exercise every day

- Cutting down or eliminating stimulants, including caffeine

Although sleeping pills are effective as short-term therapy, they have many drawbacks, especially for the elderly (see Chapter 5). They interfere with the brain's signals to the body to resume breathing, which can be critical in sleep apnea, a breathing disorder that is more common in older persons. They can also cause complications in those who have high blood pressure, heart disease, and other chronic medical conditions. Troubling side effects include impaired memory and daytime drowsiness. Older men and women who take sleeping pills are in danger of falls if they wake up in the night confused and disoriented. When medications are necessary, psychiatrists may prescribe low-dose tricyclic antidepressants rather than conventional sleep medications or may choose sleeping pills that have short half-lives.

Problems with Alcohol and Medications

Alcohol dependence and abuse are less common among older men and women than among younger individuals. Less than 5 percent of men and less than 1 percent of women over the age of sixty-five abuse alcohol. Nevertheless, sleeping difficulties and increased stress caused by retirement, illness, isolation, or bereavement may lead to drinking problems.

Alcohol abuse can be particularly harmful for older people because it increases the likelihood of malnutrition, liver disease, heart damage, digestive problems, cognitive impairment, dementia, and falls. Even a small amount of alcohol can make mental confusion and memory problems worse. When severe alcohol dependence or abuse develops, older individuals may require close supervision in a hospital during withdrawal. Possible complications include agitation, delirium, and hallucinations.

Older people, who are more likely to have physical ailments requiring treatment, use one-quarter of all drugs prescribed in the United States and often inadvertently misuse them. Some take ten or more prescription and over-the-counter agents each day. The more medications any person takes, the greater the chance of error. It is wise for seniors to keep a medication chart, organized by days of the week, on which they check off each dose and drug when taken; and to keep their primary physician or their pharmacist aware of all the drugs they consume, both prescription and over-the-counter, so that these professionals can watch out for possible harmful interactions.

Cognitive problems are the number one psychiatric side effect of drugs in the elderly. When older people become confused, forgetful, or paranoid, family members should find out what medications they are taking and check their alcohol intake. Another not-uncommon problem that can cause these symptoms is dependence on sleeping pills or pain medications. Withdrawal from some of these drugs, primarily those in the benzodiazepine family, can be potentially life-threatening and may require careful monitoring in a hospital.

Special Medication Issues in Seniors

As we have noted, the capacity to metabolize or break down drugs within the body declines with age, so medications may remain active in the elderly for a longer period than in younger adults. As a result, older men and women are more sensitive to certain side effects, such as drowsiness or a drop in blood pressure that can cause dizziness and light-headedness on sitting or standing (orthostatic hypotension). Usually psychiatrists prescribe lower doses for older individuals, often about half the amount they would give a younger person, or choose particular agents considered safer for seniors. They also monitor blood levels of psychiatric medications more frequently in older men and women.

Physical problems can complicate drug treatment of psychiatric symptoms. A heart condition may make the use of certain antidepressants risky. Older men with enlarged prostates may develop serious complications from tricyclic antidepressants and many antipsychotic drugs. Every older person should undergo a careful medical assessment before any medications are prescribed.

GLOSSARY OF TERMS

Acetylcholine: A neurotransmitter in the brain that helps to regulate memory. (See also *anticholinergic; cholinergic.*) Medications to treat Alzheimer's disease, such as tacrine (Cognex) and donepezil (Aricept), improve memory by increasing the amount of acetylcholine in the brain.

Addiction: A behavioral pattern characterized by compulsion, loss of control, and continued repetition of a behavior or activity in spite of adverse consequences.

Adrenaline: See *epinephrine.*

Adrenergic: Pertaining to the neurotransmitter epinephrine (adrenaline).

Affect: External expression of emotion, feeling, or mood that accompanies a thought.

Aggression: Forceful behavior with intent to dominate; physical or verbal force directed toward the environment, another person, or oneself.

Agitation: Excessive physical activity, usually associated with tension, such as an inability to sit still, fidgeting, pacing, or wringing of hands.

Agoraphobia: Fear of open spaces, leaving a familiar place (e.g., one's home), or being in places or situations where escape may be difficult or embarrassing or where help may not be available.

Akathisia: A subjective state of uncontrollable motor restlessness and movement, commonly a side effect of certain medications, especially older antipsychotic agents such as haloperidol (Haldol).

Akinesia: A state of reduced movement. This is a common side effect of the older antipsychotic medications, such as thiothixene (Navane), haloperidol (Haldol), and others.

Alcohol dependence: Alcohol use characterized by tolerance or development of withdrawal symptoms when alcohol intake is reduced or eliminated. (Also called alcoholism.)

Alcoholic: An individual who loses control over use of alcohol and develops the characteristic symptoms of alcoholism.

Alcoholism: A chronic, progressive, potentially fatal disease characterized by physical dependence on alcohol, tolerance to its effects, and withdrawal symptoms when consumption is reduced or stopped.

Alzheimer's disease: A form of dementia characterized by progressive deterioration of mental function caused by age-related physiological changes within the brain; symptoms include memory impairment and loss, diminished ability to concentrate, disorientation, depression, apathy, amnesia, and paranoia.

Amnesia: Permanent or temporary loss of memory.

Amphetamines: A group of stimulant medications used to treat attention deficit hyperactivity disorder (ADHD) and often misused in order to overcome fatigue, induce euphoria, reduce appetite, or increase energy.

Analgesics: Medications that relieve pain without inducing a loss of consciousness.

Anhedonia: Lack of pleasure in normally enjoyable activities; a symptom often found in depression.

Anorexia nervosa: An eating disorder in which refusal or inability to maintain normal food intake leads to malnutrition, severe weight loss, medical complications, and possibly death.

Antagonists: Agents that limit or prevent the action of another substance or that block receptors located on neurons in the brain. For instance, nefazodone (Serzone) blocks specific serotonin receptors in the brain.

Anticholinergic: Impeding the action of the neurotransmitter acetylcholine. Anticholinergic side effects of certain antipsychotic, tricyclic antidepressant, and anti-Parkinson drugs include dry mouth, constipation, and blurred vision, problems in urinating, confusion (especially in older people), and a rapid and sometimes irregular heartbeat.

Antidepressants: Drugs developed primarily to treat and relieve symptoms of depression.

Antihistamines: Drugs used to treat allergic reactions and some cold symptoms; sometimes used as sleep aids because they may cause drowsiness. They work by inactivating histamine, a substance found in body tissues that plays a role in allergic reactions.

Antipsychotics: Drugs used to treat the severe distortions in thought, perception, and emotion that characterize psychosis. These medications are also called neuroleptics.

Anxiety: Apprehension or uneasiness about an anticipated danger. Anxiety may be a normal reaction to danger or threat, or occur when no such danger exists and cause troubling symptoms.

Anxiety disorders: A group of conditions characterized by anxiety, affecting an individual's personal or work life, relationships, or emotional well-being. According to the *DSM-IV*, these disorders include agoraphobia, specific (simple) phobia, social anxiety disorder, obsessive-compulsive disorder, posttraumatic stress disorder, acute stress disorder, generalized anxiety disorder, mixed anxiety-depressive disorder, secondary anxiety disorder due to a general medical condition, and substance-induced anxiety disorder.

Anxiolytics: Drugs that reduce anxiety. Prescription medications include the benzodiazepines (lorazepam [Ativan] and others) and the serotonergic agent bupropion (Wellbutrin or Zyban).

Apathy: Indifference, or lack of feeling, emotion, or interest.

Attention deficit hyperactivity disorder (ADHD): A mental disorder that usually develops before the age of seven and is characterized by limited attention span, overactivity, restlessness, distractibility, and impulsiveness. This disorder may last into adulthood.

Atypical depression: A form of major depression characterized by symptoms other than those usually associated with depression (e.g., increased appetite, weight gain, and sleeping more than usual).

Autistic disorder: A developmental disorder that manifests itself in infancy or early childhood and consists of severe impairment of social interaction and communication, behavior, and normal activity; thought to be neurophysiologic in origin.

Barbiturates: An older class of anxiolytic and sedating drugs that depress the central nervous system. Because of their lethality, especially in overdose, they are not generally prescribed by physicians anymore except to treat seizure disorders.

Benzodiazepines: A group of drugs used as anti-anxiety agents or sedatives.

Beta-blocker: An antihypertensive medication that halts or inhibits the action of the beta-adrenergic receptors in the nervous system, which affect the blood vessels, heart, and lungs; in psychiatry, used most often in the treatment of performance anxiety.

Bipolar disorder: According to the *DSM-IV*, a mood disorder characterized by recurrent, alternating episodes of depression and either mania or hypomania (less than full-blown mania). (Formerly called manic depression; see also *cyclothymic disorder*.)

Brain imaging: Techniques used to visualize the structures and/or the functioning of the brain, including computed tomography (CT), positron emission tomography (PET), magnetic resonance imaging (MRI), and functional magnetic resonance imaging (fMRI).

Bulimia nervosa: An eating disorder characterized by recurrent episodes of binge eating followed by vomiting, purging with diuretics and laxatives, or other methods to control weight such as fasting or extreme exercise regimens.

Cataplexy: Sudden loss of muscular strength without loss of consciousness, typically triggered by an emotion such as anger or excitement. This condition occurs in people with the sleep disorder narcolepsy.

Catatonia: A motionless state, characterized by muscle rigidity or inflexibility, seen in states of extreme fear and in some types of psychosis.

Cholinergic: Pertaining to the neurotransmitter acetylcholine. Medications that act by increasing acetylcholine such as atropine are called cholinergic agents.

Cognitive: Pertaining to the mental processes of thinking, understanding, perceiving, judging, remembering, and reasoning, in contrast to emotional processes.

Compulsion: A repetitive behavior (e.g., handwashing) or repetitive mental process (e.g., counting) that serves no rational purpose.

Cross-addiction: A state of physical dependence in which the physiologic need for one psychoactive substance leads to dependence on similar substances.

Cross-tolerance: The capacity to tolerate the effects of a psychoactive substance similar to another substance for which tolerance has already developed.

Cyclothymic disorder: As described in the *DSM-IV*, a bipolar disorder characterized by hypomanic episodes and frequent periods of depressed mood or loss of interest or pleasure. The "ups" and "downs" are not as pronounced or severe as in bipolar disorder.

Delirium: A cognitive disorder characterized by impaired consciousness and attention, and by changes in thinking or other mental processes.

Delusion: A false belief regarding the self or the world that a person persistently holds despite clear evidence to the contrary. This symptom is usually found in people suffering from paranoid schizophrenia.

Dementia: A cognitive disorder characterized by impaired memory, language, thinking, and perception.

Depression: A term that describes feelings of sadness, discouragement, and despair. It can be a normal and transitory reaction to events in a person's life, a symptom occurring in various physical and mental conditions, or a mental disorder in itself. The mental disorder involves slowed thinking, decreased pleasure, feelings of guilt, hopelessness, despair, and helplessness, and problems with eating and sleeping.

Depressive disorders: A group of mood disorders that includes major depressive disorder, dysthymic disorder, and others.

Detoxification: A process that eliminates dependence-producing substances such as alcohol or addictive drugs from the body, usually combined with medication and supportive care.

Diagnostic and Statistical Manual of Mental Disorders: The book that lists diagnostic criteria for all formally recognized mental disorders; used by mental-health professionals in diagnosing mental disorders. It is regularly revised and updated, and is currently in its fourth edition (also called *DSM-IV*), which was published in 1994.

Distractibility: The inability to sustain attention or the tendency to shift focus from one activity or topic to another.

Epinephrine: A substance produced by the adrenal gland; it is responsible for many of the physical manifestations of fear and anxiety. (Also called adrenaline; see also *adrenergic*.)

Estrogen: The sex hormone that plays a major role in the development and maintenance of female secondary sex characteristics. In menopause, the amount of estrogen women's bodies produce is substantially reduced; consequently, they may be prescribed estrogen by their physician (estrogen replacement therapy).

Ethyl alcohol: The intoxicating agent in alcoholic beverages. (Also called ethanol.)

Etiology: Cause, particularly of a disease.

Extrapyramidal syndrome: Involuntary signs and symptoms resulting from malfunction in the part of the central nervous system responsible for coordinating body movements, which include muscle rigidity, tremors, drooling, shuffling gait (Parkinsonism); restlessness (akathisia); peculiar involuntary postures (dystonia); and inertia (akinesia). May be a side effect of antipsychotic or neuroleptic drugs.

Generalized anxiety disorder (GAD): An anxiety disorder characterized by unrealistic or excessive apprehensiveness and worry about life circumstances, which persists for a period of at least six months and interferes with normal functioning.

Geriatric psychiatry (geropsychiatry): A subspecialty of psychiatry concerned with the psychological aspects of aging and mental disorders of the elderly.

Half-life: The length of time a drug remains in the bloodstream. This length, or half-life, determines how frequently the medication needs to be taken in a 24-hour period. The half-life of many psychiatric medications is 24 hours; consequently, these medications need to be taken only once a day. Medications with shorter half-lives, say 8 to 12 hours, need to be taken twice a day.

Hallucinations: A perception of sound (called auditory hallucinations), vision (visual hallucinations), physical sensations, or smells that do not exist.

Hallucinogen: A chemical substance that produces hallucinations in the user.

Hormones: Substances secreted by the endocrine system that are released into the bloodstream and regulate a wide variety of crucial bodily functions such as growth, development, blood pressure, metabolism, and many more.

Hyperactivity: Excessive physical activity that may be purposeful or aimless.

Hypersomnia: A type of sleep disorder called a dyssomnia that is characterized by prolonged sleep or excessive daytime drowsiness.

Hypertension: High blood pressure.

Hypomania: A state of abnormal mood that falls between euphoria (mild mood elevation) and mania (an elevation of mood so pronounced that the person frequently requires hospitalization). Hypomania is characterized by unrealistic optimism, rapid speech and activity, and a decreased need for sleep.

Hypotension: A decrease in blood pressure.

Impulse: A sudden desire to act in a certain way to ease tension or feel pleasure.

Impulse-control disorders: Disorders marked by the inability to resist an impulse or the temptation to perform an act that is harmful to oneself or to others. Problems of impulse control may occur as aspects of other mental disorders or as distinct conditions; among the latter are kleptomania, pyromania, pathological gambling, trichotillomania, and intermittent explosive disorder.

Inhalants: Substances that produce vapors having psychoactive effects when inhaled. Inhalants may produce severe and permanent brain damage and lead to death.

Intoxication: The acute physiological effects of overdosage with a chemical substance.

Labile: Rapidly changing, as applied to emotions; unstable.

Lithium carbonate: A naturally occurring mineral salt used to treat and prevent both mania and depression in bipolar illness.

Major depressive disorder: A depressive disorder characterized by depressed mood, loss of interest in pleasurable activities (anhedonia), changes in sleep or appetite patterns, fatigue, difficulty in concentrating, feelings of worthlessness, and thoughts of death or suicide. People suffering from major depressive disorder frequently will benefit from antidepressant medications.

Mania: A mood disturbance characterized by excessive elation, inflated self-esteem, hyperactivity, agitation, and rapid and often confused thinking and speaking; may occur in bipolar disorder.

Monoamine oxidase (MAO): An enzyme that breaks down certain neurotransmitters called biogenic amines and deactivates them.

Monoamine oxidase inhibitors (MAOIs): A group of chemically related antidepressant drugs that act by inhibiting monoamine oxidase (MAO) in the brain, thereby raising the level of certain neurotransmitters.

Mood disorders: A group of disorders characterized by disturbances in mood; they include depressive disorders, bipolar disorder, and certain disorders caused by a general medical condition or substance use.

Narcolepsy: A sleep disorder consisting of irresistible attacks of sleep during the day, cataplexy (loss of muscle tone) typically associated with intense emotion, and recurrent intrusions of REM sleep into the transitional period between sleep and wakefulness.

Narcotic: Any drug, natural or synthetic, that is derived from, or has a chemical structure related to, that of an opiate; relieves pain and alters mood; addictive.

Negative symptoms: In people suffering from schizophrenia, these symptoms include flattened or inappropriate emotions, lack of will, loss of spontaneous verbal expression, or lack of logic.

Neuroleptics: See *antipsychotics*.

Neuron: Nerve cell; the basic unit of the nervous system.

Neuroscience: The study of brain and nervous-system function and behavior.

Neurotransmitters: Chemicals found in the nervous system that function as messenger molecules by facilitating the transmission of impulses across the synapses between neurons.

Nicotine: The addictive substance in tobacco.

Norepinephrine: A neurotransmitter that is chemically related to epinephrine; when in excess, may play a part in manic states, and when deficient, in certain depressive states. (Also called noradrenaline.) In depression, certain antidepressants, such as bupropion (Wellbutrin), are believed to work by increasing the amount of norepinephrine in the brain.

Opiate: Any chemical derived from opium; relieves pain and produces a sense of well-being; addictive.

Opioids: Synthetic narcotics that are similar to opiates in their chemical structure and their effects; addictive.

Organic disease: An illness that impairs function in an organ or tissue.

Orthostatic hypotension: A drop in blood pressure when moving from a lying to sitting position or from sitting to standing.

Over-the-counter (OTC) drugs: Medications that can be legally obtained without a prescription.

Pain disorder: A somatoform disorder characterized by persistent pain that causes marked distress or impairs a person's normal functioning.

Panic attacks: Sudden, unprovoked, emotionally intense experiences of impending doom, fear of dying, "going crazy," or losing control, and marked by physical symptoms such as palpitations, dizziness, trembling, nausea, or shortness of breath.

Panic disorder: Recurrent panic attacks, at least one of which is followed by a month or more of persisting concern about having further attacks.

Paranoia: A tendency to view the actions of others as deliberately threatening or demeaning; suspicious thinking based on misinterpretation of an actual event.

Paranoid ideation: Suspiciousness about being harassed, persecuted, or treated unfairly.

Pharmacokinetics: The study of how drugs are metabolized.

Physical dependence: The physiological attachment to, and need for, a drug, characterized by tolerance and withdrawal symptoms if the drug is stopped. (See also *addiction; substance dependence; substance use disorders.*)

Posttraumatic stress disorder (PTSD): An anxiety disorder occurring after exposure to an extreme mental or physical stress—usually involving actual or threatened death or serious injury to self or others—and characterized by symptoms that persist for one month or more and include reexperiencing of the event, avoidance of stimuli associated with it, numbing of general responsiveness, and signs of increased arousal (e.g., sleeplessness, irritability, hypervigilance).

Premenstrual dysphoric disorder (PMDD): Depressive disorder—more severe than premenstrual syndrome (PMS)—that occurs prior to the onset of menstruation and abates soon thereafter. It is estimated to occur in 5 to 9 percent of menstruating women. Symptoms are both psychological (e.g., emotional volatility, anxiety, depressed mood) and physical (e.g., sleep problems, breast tenderness or swelling, headaches, overeating or food cravings).

Premenstrual syndrome (PMS): A common condition characterized by physical discomfort and psychological distress that occurs prior to the onset of a woman's menstrual period and abates soon thereafter.

Psychiatrist: A licensed medical doctor (M.D.) who has had specialized training in the diagnosis, treatment, and prevention of mental and emotional disorders; the only mental-health professional licensed to prescribe medication. Board-certified psychiatrists have passed national oral and written examinations ("boards") after completing medical school and a four-year residency program in psychiatry.

Psychiatry: The medical science that deals with the etiology (origin), diagnosis, treatment, and prevention of mental disorders.

Psychoactive: Mood-altering; often used to describe both prescribed medications and illicit drugs that act on the brain to change feelings or emotions.

Psychologist: A licensed professional who has completed a graduate program in psychology that includes clinical training and internships, and who provides care for individuals with mental and emotional problems. An increasing number of psychologists have a doctorate and have undergone postdoctoral training; however, they are not physicians and cannot prescribe medication.

Psychomotor: A term referring to combined physical and mental activity.

Psychomotor agitation: Excessive motor activity associated with a feeling of inner tension.

Psychomotor retardation: Slowing of physical and emotional reactions.

Psychopharmacology: The study of the actions and effects of psychoactive drugs on behavior in both animals and people.

Psychosis: A major mental disorder characterized by gross impairment of a person's perception of reality and ability to communicate and relate to others. A psychosis can be biological or emotional in origin.

Psychotic: See *psychosis*.

Psychotropic: A term used to describe drugs that act in a particular way on the brain and affect the mind.

Rapid cycling: In bipolar disorder, the occurrence of four or more episodes of mood disturbance (mania, depression, or both) within one year.

Rapid eye movement (REM) sleep: A regularly occurring phase of the sleep cycle during which the most active dreaming takes place; comprises about 25 percent of a night's sleep.

Receptors: Specialized molecules on the surface of neurons to which particular neurotransmitters bind after their release from another neuron; receptors receive the chemical "message" to activate or inhibit a nerve, blood vessel, or muscle.

REM latency: The time lag between sleep onset and the first rapid eye movement (REM) sleep.

Schizoaffective disorder: A psychotic disorder where either a major depressive episode or a manic episode develops concurrently with the symptoms of schizophrenia.

Schizophrenia: A major mental disorder with characteristic psychotic or positive symptoms (such as delusions, hallucinations, disorganized behavior, and disordered thought patterns) and often negative symptoms (such as lack of logic or will, apathy, withdrawal). The onset is generally between late adolescence and the mid-thirties. The prognosis varies, although complete remission is uncommon.

Seasonal affective disorder (SAD): A recurrent mood disorder characterized by depressive episodes and related symptoms that develop at particular times of the year, most often in fall or winter, and remit when the season ends.

Selective serotonin reuptake inhibitor (SSRI): A medication that inhibits recapture of the neurotransmitter serotonin by the nerve cells (fluoxetine [Prozac], sertraline [Zoloft], paroxetine [Paxil], and others).

Serotonin: A neurotransmitter found both in the brain and elsewhere in the body that may play a role in several mental disorders, including depression. A number of the newer antidepressants, such as the SSRIs, are believed to work by increasing the amount of serotonin in the body.

Sexual dysfunctions: A group of disorders characterized by disturbances in sexual desire and by psychophysiological changes in the sexual response cycle, which cause marked distress and interpersonal difficulty.

Short-term memory: Technically, the recognition, recall, and reproduction of perceived material ten seconds or longer after initial presentation. The term is popularly used to refer to memory for recent events, as contrasted with events in the past.

Side effect: A person's adverse response to a medication. It accompanies the principal therapeutic response that is the purpose of a medication and, if severe, frequently causes people to stop medication.

Sleep apnea: A breathing-related sleep disorder marked by repeated episodes in which a sleeping individual stops breathing for a short period of time.

Sleep disorders: A group of conditions involving sleep that include primary sleep disorders (dyssomnias and parasomnias), sleep disorders related to another mental disorder (including insomnia), secondary sleep disorder due to a general medical condition, and substance-induced sleep disorder resulting from intoxication or withdrawal.

Sleep terror disorder: A parasomnia characterized by a pattern of abrupt awakening from sleep that is accompanied by a sense of panic and confusion.

Social anxiety disorder: A persistent fear of finding oneself in situations that might lead to scrutiny by others and humiliation or embarrassment.

Social work: A profession whose primary concern is how human needs, both of individuals and of groups, can be met within society.

Somatic therapy: In psychiatry, the biological treatment of mental disorders; examples are psychopharmacological treatment (the use of medications and electroconvulsive therapy [ECT]).

SSRI: See *selective serotonin reuptake inhibitor*.

Stress disorder, acute: An anxiety disorder that develops when or immediately after a person experiences a highly traumatic stressor that includes feelings of intense fear, helplessness, or horror.

Stress disorder/reaction, posttraumatic: See *posttraumatic stress disorder*.

Substance: A chemical agent that is used to alter mood or behavior. (See also *psychoactive*.)

Substance abuse: The compulsive use of a substance, such as alcohol or a drug, despite evidence that it is impairing an individual's social and occupational functioning.

Substance dependence: Chemical dependence, usually defined in terms of tolerance (the need for the person to take higher doses of the substance to achieve the desired effect) or withdrawal (bothersome and often severe physical and psychological symptoms that people experience when they stop taking the substance).

Substance use disorders: Dependence, abuse, intoxication, and withdrawal syndromes associated with episodic or regular use of chemical substances. Use disorders are recognized for amphetamines, caffeine, cannabis, cocaine, hallucinogens, inhalants, nicotine, opioids, phencyclidine (PCP), alcohol and sedative/hypnotic/anxiolytic drugs, and combinations of drugs (polysubstance use).

Suicide: Taking of one's own life.

Synapse: The gap or space between the surface of one nerve cell (neuron) and another.

Syndrome: A group of signs and symptoms that often appear together and which sometimes may suggest a particular cause.

Tardive dyskinesia. A medication-induced neurological disorder consisting of involuntary movements of the tongue, jaw, or extremities that develops with long-term use (usually a period of months or more) of antipsychotic (neuroleptic) medications; sometimes irreversible.

Tic: An involuntary, abrupt, rapid, and recurrent motor movement or vocalization.

Tolerance: A characteristic of substance dependence marked by the need for increasing amounts of the substance to achieve the desired effect.

Tranquilizer: A drug that decreases anxiety and agitation.

Tremor: A trembling or shaking of the body or any of its parts.

Trichotillomania: An impulse-control disorder characterized by pathological hair pulling that results in noticeable hair loss.

Tyramine: A chemical found in many foods and beverages that ordinarily has no effect on normal body functioning but that can cause a dangerous rise in blood pressure when a monoamine oxidase inhibitor (MAOI) drug is taken. Persons using MAOIs must not consume foods and drinks containing tyramine.

Withdrawal: The symptoms and signs that develop within a short period of time (usually hours) after cessation or reduced use of an addictive substance; may include sweating, rapid pulse, hand tremor, nausea or vomiting, agitation, anxiety, or temporary hallucinations or illusions.

MIND/MOOD RESOURCES

GENERAL MEDICAL INFORMATION RESOURCES

American Medical Association
AMA Publications
515 N. State Street
Chicago, IL 60610
(312) 464-5000
http://www.ama-assn.org/

National Institutes of Health (NIH)
9000 Rockville Pike
Bethesda, MD 20892
(301) 496-4000
http://www.nih.gov/

Public Health Service
200 Independence Ave., S.W.
Washington, DC 20201
(202) 619-0257
(202) 690-6867
http://phs.os.dhhs.gov/phs/phs.html
Tel-Med Health Information Service provides taped messages on health concerns.

ALCOHOL, DRUG, AND SUBSTANCE ABUSE

Al-Anon, Alateen, and Adult Children of Alcoholics Al-Anon Family Group Headquarters, Inc.
1600 Corporate Landing Parkway
Virginia Beach, VA 23454-5617
For Free Introductory Literature Packet:
Call Toll Free 24 Hours
(888) 425-2666 USA
(800) 714-7498 Canada
http://www.al-anon-alateen.org/ *A fellowship of relatives and friends of alcoholics.*

Alcohol Hotline
Adcare Hospital
107 Lincoln Street
Worcester, MA 01605
(800) ALCOHOL
(800) 345-3552

Alcoholics Anonymous, Inc.
A.A. General Service Office
475 Riverside Drive
New York, NY 10015
(212) 870-3400
(212) 870-3003
http://www.alcoholics-
anonymous.org/
*Voluntary, nonprofessional,
twelve-step organization of
recovering alcoholics.*

American Council for Drug
Education
204 Monroe Street
Rockville, MD 20850
(301) 294-0600
(800) DRUGHELP
http://www.acde.org/
*Hotline for troubled
students.*

Children of Alcoholics
Foundation
164 West 74th Street
New York, NY 10023
(212) 595-5810 Ext. 7760
http://www.coaf.org/

Cocaine Anonymous World
Services
P.O. Box 2000
Los Angeles, CA 90049-
8000
(800) 347-8998
(310) 559-5833
http://www.ca.org/index.html

*Self-help, nonprofessional,
twelve-step fellowship
program for men and
women in recovery from
cocaine addiction.*

Co-Dependents
Anonymous (CoDA)
P.O. Box 33577
Phoenix, AZ 85067-3577
(602) 277-7991
http://www.codependents.
org/

800-COCAINE
P.O. Box 100
Summit, NJ 07901
*Referrals to local hot lines
only.*

Families Anonymous
World Service Office
P.O. Box 528
Van Nuys, CA 91408
(818) 780-3951
http://www.families
anonymous. org/
*Support group for
recovering narcotics
addicts.*

National Clearinghouse for
Alcohol and Drug
Information
P.O. Box 2345
Rockville, MD 20847-
2345

(800) 729-6686
(301) 468-2600 (Maryland and Washington, DC)

National Drug Abuse Information and Treatment Referral Hotline and National Institute on Drug Abuse Helpline
12280 Wilkins Avenue
Rockville, MD 20852
(800) 662-HELP
(800) 66-AYUDA
(Spanish-speaking callers)

National Drug Information Center of Families in Action
Century Plaza II
2957 Clairmont Road, Suite 150
Atlanta, GA 30329
(404) 248-9676
http://www.emory.edu/NFIA/

National Federation of Parents for a Drug Free Youth
1423 N. Jefferson
Springfield, MO 65082
(417) 836-3709

National Institute on Alcohol Abuse and Alcoholism
6000 Executive Boulevard

Willco Building
Bethesda, MD 20892-7003
(301) 402-1466
http://www.niaaa.nih.gov/

Office for Substance Abuse Prevention
Alcohol, Drug Abuse and Mental Health Association (ADAMHA)
5600 Fishers Lane
Rockwall II Building
Rockville, MD 20852
(301) 443-0365

PRIDE (Parents' Resource Institute for Drug Education)
3610 Dekalb Technology Parkway, Suite 105
Atlanta, GA 30340
(770) 458-9900
http://www.prideusa.org/

Women for Sobriety, Inc.
109 W. Broad Street
P.O. Box 618
Quakertown, PA 18951
(215) 536-8026
(800) 333-1606
http://www.womenfor sobriety.org/
Support group for women with drinking problems. A self-help program "whose purpose is to help all women recover from problem drinking."

ALZHEIMER'S DISEASE

The Alzheimer's
Association National
Headquarters
919 N. Michigan Avenue,
Suite 1000
Chicago, IL 60611-1676
(312) 335-8700
(800) 272-3900
(800) 572-6037 (in Illinois)
http://www.alz.org/

ANXIETY DISORDERS AND PHOBIAS

Anxiety Disorders
Association of America (an
expansion of the Phobia
Society of America)
11900 Parklawn Drive,
Suite 100
Rockville, MD 20852
(301) 231-9350
http://www.adaa.org/

PASS Group, Inc.
6 Mahogany Drive
Williamsville, NY 14221
(716) 689-4399
*Support group to help treat
agoraphobia.*

TERRAP (Territorial
Apprehensiveness)
648 Menlo Avenue, Suite 5

Menlo Park, CA 94025
(415) 327-1312
http://www.terrap.com/
*Headquarters for national
network of treatment
clinics for agoraphobia.*

ATTENTION DEFICIT DISORDERS

National Attention Deficit
Disorder Association
(ADDA)
P.O. Box 1303
Northbrook, IL 60065-
1303
http://www.add.org/
*Information on support
groups.*

Children and Adults with
Attention Deficit
Hyperactivity Disorder
(CHADD)
8181 Professional Place
Suite 201
Landover, MD 20785
(800) 233-4050
(301) 306-7070
http://www.chadd.org/index.
htm

Learning Disabilities
Association of America
(LDA)
4156 Library Road
Pittsburgh, PA 15234

(412) 341-1515
http://www.ldanatl.org/

MOOD DISORDERS

Depression After Delivery, Inc.
P.O. Box 278
Belle Mead, NJ 08502
(908) 575-9121
(800) 944-4PPD
Information Request Line
(215) 295-3994
Professional Inquiries
Support for women suffering from postpartum depression and psychosis.

Depression Awareness, Recognition and Treatment Program (D/ART) National Institute of Mental Health
5600 Fishers Lane
Rockville, MD 20857
(800) 421-4211
http://www.nimh.nih.gov/depression/

Depressives Anonymous
329 E. 62nd Street, Suite 50
New York, NY 10021
(212) 689-2600
Self-help organization for people suffering from depression.

Lithium Information Center
c/o Department of Psychiatry
University of Wisconsin
7617 Mineral Point Road, Suite 300
Madison, WI 53717
(608) 827-2470
www.healthtechsys.com/mimlithium.html

National Alliance for the Mentally Ill
200 N. Glebe Road, Suite 1015
Arlington, VA 22203-3754
(800) 950-NAMI
http://www.nami.org/
Self-help and advocacy organization for persons with schizophrenia and depressive disorders and their families.

National Alliance for Research on Schizophrenia and Depression (NARSAD)
60 Cutter Mill Road, Suite 404
Great Neck, NY 11021
(516) 829-0091
(800) 829-8289
http://www.narsad.org/

National Depressive and Manic-Depressive Association (National

DMDA)
730 N. Franklin Street,
Suite 501
Chicago, IL 60610-3526
(312) 642-0049
(800) 826-3632
http://www.ndmda.org/

National Foundation for
Depressive Illness Inc.
P.O. Box 2257
New York, NY 10116
(800) 248-4344
http://www.depression.org/
*Assists in finding
professional help.*

EATING DISORDERS

American
Anorexia/Bulimia
Association, Inc.
165 W. 46th Street,
Suite 1108
New York, NY 10036
(212) 575-6200
http://www.aabainc.org/
*Self-help group that
provides information and
referrals to physicians and
therapists.*

Anorexia Nervosa and
Related Eating Disorders,
Inc.
P.O. Box 5102

Eugene, OR 97405
(503) 344-1144
http://www.anred.com/
*Provides information and
referrals for people with
eating disorders.*

Bulimia, Anorexia & Self-
Help, Inc.
522 N. New Ballas Road,
Suite 206
St. Louis, MO 63141
(314) 567-4080
(800) 762-3334

Eating Disorders
Awareness and Prevention,
Inc.
603 Stewart Street,
Suite 803
Seattle, WA 98101
(206) 382-3587
(800) 931-2237
Referral hot line
http://www.edap.org/

National Association of
Anorexia Nervosa and
Associated Disorders
P.O. Box 7
Highland Park, IL 60035
(708) 831-3438
(847) 831-3438 HOTLINE
http://www.anad.org/
*Counseling and
information for anorexics,*

bulimics, their families, and professionals.

Overeaters Anonymous
6075 Zenith Court, N.E.
Rio Rancho, NM 87124
(505) 891-2664
http://www.overeaters
anonymous.org/
Self-help fellowship of men and women who wish to stop eating compulsively.

MENTAL HEALTH RESOURCES

American Mental Health Fund
2735 Harland Road Falls Church, VA 22043
(703) 573-2200

American Psychiatric Press, Inc.
1400 K Street, N.W.
Washington, DC 20005
(202) 682-6262
(800) 368-5777
http://www.appi.org/index.html

National Alliance for the Mentally Ill
200 N. Glebe Road, Suite 1015
Arlington, VA 22203-3754

(703) 524-7600
(800) 950-NAMI
http://www.nami.org/
Self-help and advocacy organization for persons with mental disorders and their families.

National Alliance for Research on Schizophrenia and Depression (NARSAD)
60 Cutter Mill Road, Suite 200
Great Neck, NY 11021
(516) 829-0091
(800) 829-8289
http://www.mhsource.com/narsad.html

National Association of Social Workers
750 First Street, N.E., Suite 700
Washington, DC 20002-4241
(202) 408-8600
(800) 638-8799
http://www.naswdc.org/

National Mental Health Association
1021 Prince Street
Alexandria, VA 22314-2971
(703) 684-7722
(800) 969-NMHA
http://www.nmha.org/

National Mental Health Consumers' Self-Help Clearinghouse
1211 Chestnut Street, Suite 1207
Philadelphia, PA 19107
(800) 553-4KEY
(215) 751-1810
http://www.mhselfhelp.org/

Recovery, Inc.
Association of Nervous and Former Mental Patients
802 N. Dearborn Street
Chicago, IL 60610
(312) 337-5661
http://www.recovery-inc.com/ *Self-help group for former mental patients.*

NEUROLOGICAL DISORDERS

National Institute of Neurological Disorders and Stroke
National Institutes of Health
P.O. Box 5801
Bethesda, MD 20824
(301) 496-4000
http://www.ninds.nih.gov/

Tardive Dyskinesia/Tardive Dystonia National Association
4244 University Way, N.E.

P.O. Box 45732
Seattle, WA 98145-0732
(206) 522-3166

OBSESSIVE-COMPULSIVE DISORDERS

Obsessive-Compulsive Foundation, Inc.
337 Notch Hill Road
North Branford, CT 06471
(203) 315-2190
http://www.ocfoundation.org/
A voluntary organization "dedicated to early intervention in controlling and finding cures for OCD, and for improving the welfare of people with this disorder."

PROFESSIONAL ORGANIZATIONS

American Academy of Child and Adolescent Psychiatry
3615 Wisconsin Avenue, N.W.
Washington, DC 20016-3007
(202) 966-7300
http://www.aacap.org/

American Group Psychotherapy Association
25 E. 21st Street, Sixth Floor

New York, NY 10010
(212) 477-2677
http://www.groupsinc.org/

American Mental Health
Counselors Association (a
division of the American
Association for Counseling
and Development)
801 N. Fairfax Street,
Suite 304
Alexandria, VA 22314
(703) 548-6002
(800) 326-2642
http://www.amhca.org/
home.html

American Psychiatric
Association
1400 K Street, N.W.
Washington, DC 20005
(202) 682-6000
http://www.psych.org/

American Psychological
Association
750 First Street, N.E.
Washington, DC 20002-
4242
(202) 336-5500
http://www.apa.org/

Association for the
Advancement of Behavioral
Therapy
15 W. 36th Street

New York, NY 10018
(212) 279-7970

Center for Cognitive
Therapy
University of Pennsylvania
133 S. Thirty-sixth Street,
Room 602
Philadelphia, PA 19104
(215) 898-4100

National Association of
Private Psychiatric
Hospitals
1319 F Street, N.W., #1000
Washington, DC 20004
(202) 393-6700

National Association of
Social Workers
750 First Street, N.E.,
Suite 700
Washington, DC 20002
(202) 408-8600

National Council of
Community Mental Health
Centers
12300 Twinbrook
Parkway,
Suite 320
Rockville, MD 20852
(301) 984-6200

National Institute of
Mental Health
Information Resources and

Inquiries Branch
5600 Fishers Lane, Room
15-C-105
Rockville, MD 20857
(301) 443-4515

National Association for
the Advancement of
Psychoanalysis
80 8th Avenue,
Suite 1501
New York, NY 10011
(212) 741-0515
http://www.naap.org/

SCHIZOPHRENIA

National Alliance for the
Mentally Ill
200 N. Glebe Road,
Suite 1015
Arlington, VA 22203-3754
(800) 950-NAMI
(703) 524-7600
http://www.nami.org/
*Self-help and advocacy
organization for persons
with mental disorders and
their families.*

National Alliance for
Research on Schizophrenia
and Depression (NARSAD)

60 Cutter Mill Road,
Suite 200
Great Neck, NY 11021
(516) 829-0091
(800) 829-8289
http://www.mhsource.com/
narsad.html

·

SLEEP AND SLEEP
DISORDERS

American Narcolepsy
Association
P.O. Box 26230
San Francisco, CA 94126-
6230
(800) 222-6085

American Academy of
Sleep Medicine
6301 Bandel Road,
Suite 101
Rochester, MN 55901
(507) 287-6006
http://www.asda.org/

Better Sleep Council (of the
International Sleep
Products Association)
333 Commerce Street
Alexandria, VA 22314
(703) 683-8371
http://www.bettersleep.org/

INDEX

Note: Drugs in this index are listed by both generic and brand names, with brand names in **boldface**.

ABOUT THE AUTHORS

Robert F. Hales, M.D., is professor and chair of the Department of Psychiatry at the University of California, Davis. He has been named one of the Best Doctors in America annually since 1995, and in an *American Health* survey of all medical specialties in the United States, one of the top ten psychiatrists. Dr. Hales is a past president of the Association for Academic Psychiatry, and a former vice president of the American Association of General Hospital Psychiatrists. He is also a clinical professor of psychiatry at Georgetown University and the Uniformed Services University of the Health Sciences. He has co-authored or co-edited twenty-five major books in mental health, including the American Psychiatric Press *Textbook of Psychiatry* and the immensely popular *Concise Guides Series* of more than thirty paperbacks in the field, as well as many professional articles and book chapters.

Dianne Hales, one of the most widely published and honored freelance writers on health subjects in the country, is most recently the author of *Just Like a Woman: How Gender Science is Redefining What Makes Us Female.* Among her many other books are the award-winning compendium of mental health information, *Caring for the Mind: The Comprehensive Guide to Mental Health,* co-authored with Dr. Robert E. Hales. The recipient of numerous writing awards, she is one of the few journalists to be honored for excellence in magazine writing by both the American Psychiatric Association and the American Psychological Association. She is a contributing editor for *Parade* and *Ladies Home Journal,* and has published more than 1,100 articles in national publications. Her textbook, *Invitation to Health,* now in its ninth edition, is the leading text for college health courses.